## The Springer Series
## on Death and Suicide

ROBERT KASTENBAUM, Ph.D., Series Editor

**Charles A. Corr, Ph.D.,** is Professor in the School of Humanities, Southern Illinois University at Edwardsville, President of the Board of Hospice of Madison County (Granite City, Illinois), and Treasurer of the Illinois State Hospice Organization. His previous publications as co-author or co-editor in the field of death and dying include: *Death Education: An Annotated Resource Guide* (1980), *New Directions in Death Education and Counseling: Enhancing the Quality of Life in the Nuclear Age* (1981), and *Helping Children Cope with Death: Guidelines and Resources* (1982).

**Donna M. Corr, R.N., B.S.N.,** is Instructor in the Nursing Faculty, St. Louis Community College at Forest Park, St. Louis, Missouri. In addition to numerous workshops and presentations on hospice and improving care for dying persons and their families, she is co-author of an extensive, annotated bibliography, "Selected Resources for Hospice Training," which will be published in Volume 2 of *Death Education: An Annotated Resource Guide.*

# HOSPICE CARE

## Principles and Practice

Charles A. Corr, Ph.D.
Donna M. Corr, R.N., B.S.N.
*Editors*

## Springer Publishing Company
### New York

Springer Publishing Company, Inc.
200 Park Avenue South
New York, New York 10003

83 84 85 86 87 88 / 10 9 8 7 6 5 4 3 2 1

*Library of Congress Cataloging in Publication Data*

Main entry under title:

Hospice care, principles and practice.

(Springer series on death and suicide ; 5)
Includes bibliographies and index.
1. Terminal care.  2. Terminal care facilities.  I. Corr, Charles A.
II. Corr, Donna M.  III. Series.  [DNLM: 1. Hospices.  2. Palliative
treatment.  3. Terminal care.  4. Death.  W1 SP685P v.5 / WX 28.61
H8275]
R726.8.H658  1983      362.1′75      82-16736
ISBN 0-8261-3540-4

Printed in the United States of America

To the memory of our fathers who gave us life and taught us love:

Anton Charles Skach (1906–1960)

and

John Joseph Corr (1903–1975)

And to our mothers, Sadie and Betty, whose suffering at the deaths of their husbands might have been lessened, even in a small way, if they had been able to call upon the resources of the hospice philosophy.

# Contents

# Preface

The hospice approach is a distinct and cohesive outlook for assisting human beings at a stressful time in life. This approach primarily reflects lessons that have been learned in caring for dying persons and their families both before and after death. For example, it recognizes that dying and mourning are normal parts of life; that they are not psychiatric illnesses, although they may involve multidimensional stressors; and that it is possible to develop a caregiving program that responds to such stressors by combining professional expertise and humane concern. Despite the publicity that hospice has received, this point of view has not always been well understood. In particular, by focusing on its institutionalization, many have missed the central lesson: *Hospice is a philosophy, not a facility*. It is an approach to the giving of care, rather than a place in which services are offered.

For a number of reasons, the modern hospice movement has given most of its attention to those who are dying, and within that group to persons suffering from cancer. But neither the scope nor the implications of hospice care are rightly confined within these limits. New movements in caregiving display a natural tendency in their early stages to emphasize a particular subset of the overall population. This is often exaggerated by such external considerations as the availability and appropriateness of other modes of care or funding restrictions. But hospice principles are not limited to cancer or to dying. They represent an effort to recover guidelines for caring whenever cure is no longer a likely prospect. In the first place, this constitutes a program to *maximize present quality of living* as long as life continues. Thus, hospice care is continuous with a broad historical and contemporary tradition of palliative care, or care addressed to the amelioration of distressing symptoms even where the underlying pathology cannot be reversed. From another point of view, hospice principles apply equally well to the care of those with chronic illnesses. Most of these people are not dying in any immediate sense, although they may be characterized as what Patricia Downie (see Chapter 12, p. 149) calls "[individuals] with a vulnerable future." Apart from vulnerability to death, such individuals may simply be suffering from long-term, interconnected stressors that call for a program of total care in the hospice mode.

Moreover, hospice care recognizes that a patient is more than a malfunctioning organ or an isolated individual. In a phrase, *dying patients are living human beings*. That may seem to be an elementary truism, but it is full with significance. It means that we must respond to the needs of the whole person. It also means that we must meet such persons where they are in relationship to their needs *as they perceive them*. Dying persons must be permitted to identify their own needs and to maintain autonomy in decision making as much as that is possible. And because persons are always at the center of a web of psychosocial relationships, adequate caregiving must take into account families and friends, both as within the unit receiving care and as included among those who can give care in important ways. Since the problems of these latter people continue and in some respects may worsen after the death, a comprehensive program of care must continue to show its concern and provide care in appropriate ways during the period of bereavement. Finally, carrying through the principle that those who give care also have needs of their own that deserve care, hospice programs have also spoken to the requirements of their own staff members —whether professional or lay, paid or volunteer—for suitable kinds of support.

This book attempts to represent the present state of development in hospice care. Our aim has been to get beyond popular representations and narrow, single-unit reports that have thus far dominated the field. Instead, we have sought to create a comprehensive resource for caregivers and students of the sort that is simply not available at present. To that end, we began by reaching out to contributors from across Great Britain and North America. Many of these authors are well known and need no introduction to readers. Others have not yet gained such wide recognition for their work. We believe that the presence of less well-known contributors and their intermingling with widely recognized counterparts is a necessary and constructive step in the further development of this field. All are authoritative in their respective areas; each draws upon first-hand experience, personal insights, an awareness of the relevant literature, and an ability to articulate lessons in an effective manner.

We have emphasized contributions originating from within the hospice movement, but we have not hesitated to draw on those outside that particular context where it has seemed appropriate. In that way, this book speaks *from* hospice to a much broader audience about well-established hospice principles for improving care. It also speaks *to* hospice workers in order to further their own education and development of services. Hence, the presence here of selections from many sources—chosen solely for their intrinsic quality and for their value to the book as a whole—is essential.

Some 60% of the selections that appear here have been written specifically for this book. These pieces are designed to fill the gaps that are so readily apparent in many areas and topics, and to complement those that are already available in the existing literature. Many experts in particular areas have joined with us to write these new pieces and to shape them to fit both the demands of their subjects and the needs of our book as a whole. We are most grateful to these contributors for their generous cooperation in this difficult and time-consuming task.

Beyond that, we have also drawn upon a number of items that have appeared elsewhere, mostly in professional journals. Although available in principle, pieces of this sort are often neither obvious nor easily locatable for most readers. In fact, our sources are scattered across several countries and a wide range of specialized interests. After an exhaustive review of the existing literature, we chose the best items that are relevant to our subject in order to bring them together in a single convenient source.

We undertook this comprehensive examination of hospice principles and practice in order to learn about a kind of care that is relevant to the real needs of dying persons, their families, and others coping with death or significant limitations in living. Our immediate goal was to make possible better education for students of hospice care and to encourage better caregiving by those who work in hospice settings. As we proceeded, we realized that hospice principles can also be applied in settings that do not bear the title "hospice." The hospice movement that grew out of existing health care systems and particular social contexts is now seeking to return to its origins and to share what it has learned. Thus, our larger ambition is to assist caregivers and society at large to reassess human and professional resources that are already at hand. Even when death is close at hand and cure is no longer within our reach, there is much we can do to meet the needs, alleviate the distress, and improve the lives of our fellow human beings in any setting. Further, serving the dying more effectively is not just a way of benefiting that special group of patients. Ultimately, it illuminates, enriches, and ennobles us all. Our final lesson is that hospice is an effective approach to death and dying because it gives practical application to fundamental values in life and living.

To assist our readers who may not be familiar with some of the proprietary brand names for drugs that are used by our contributors, we provide a table of selected equivalents on page 356.

CHARLES A. CORR, PH.D.
DONNA M. CORR, R.N., B.S.N.

# Contributors

**Mary Baines, M.B., B.Ch.,** is Consultant Physician, St. Christopher's Hospice, London, England

**John Clancy, M.D., FRCP(C),** is Professor of Psychiatry, University of Iowa College of Medicine, Iowa City, Iowa

**Marjory Cockburn, S.R.N., S.C.M., H.V., O.N.C.,** is Matron, St. Luke's Nursing Home, Sheffield, England

**Inge B. Corless, R.N., Ph.D.,** is Program Director, St. Peter's Hospice, Albany, New York

**Anthony G. O. Crowther, M.A., M.B., B.Chir., D.Obst.R.C.O.G.,** is General Practitioner, Sheffield, England; Honorary Lecturer, Department of Community Medicine, University of Sheffield Medical School; and Associate Medical Director, St. Luke's Nursing Home, Sheffield, England

**Patricia A. Downie, FCSP,** is Medical and Nursing Editor, Faber & Faber Ltd. (Publishers), London, England; formerly she was Rehabilitation Officer for the Marie Curie Memorial Foundation, London, England

**Cyril W. K. H. Greaves, B.M., B.Ch.,** is General Practitioner, Sheffield, England; and Teacher of General Practice, St. Luke's Nursing Home, Sheffield, England

**Susan Grinslade, R.N., B.S.N., M.S.Ed.,** formerly was Nursing Supervisor, Continuing Care Unit, Lutheran Medical Center, St. Louis, Missouri; presently she is Level II Coordinator: Medical-Surgical Nursing, School of Nursing, Jewish Hospital, St. Louis, Missouri

**Daniel C. Hadlock, M.D., M.S., FACP,** is Medical Director, Hospice, Inc., Miami, Florida; and Past President, The National Hospice Organization, Washington, D.C.

**Enid Henke,** at the time when she wrote this essay, was a patient at St. Christopher's Hospice, London, England

**E. Richard Hillier, M.D.,** is Consultant Physician, Countess Mountbatten House, Moorgreen Hospital, Southampton, England

**Trevor Hoy, M.Div.,** formerly was Chaplain and Training Coordinator, Hospice of Marin, San Rafael, California; presently he is a consultant to hospices and churches

**Mwalimu Imara, D.Min.,** is Director of Hospice, Methodist Hospital of Indiana, Indianapolis, Indiana

**Eve Kavanagh, R.N., R.C.S.J.,** formerly was Director of Education, Hospice of Central Iowa, Des Moines, Iowa; presently she is Staff Nurse, St. Peter's Hospice, St. Peter's Hospital, Albany, New York

**Sylvia A. Lack, M.B., B.S.,** is consultant in hospice care to St. Mary's Hospital, Waterbury, Connecticut, while on leave for additional study from her position as Medical Director of The Connecticut Hospice (formerly Hospice, Inc.), Branford, Connecticut

**Marcia E. Lattanzi, R. N., M.A.,** is Director of Education and Bereavement, Boulder County Hospice, Boulder, Colorado

**Lawrence LeShan, Ph.D.,** is Research Psychologist, Psychophysical Research Laboratories, Princeton, New Jersey

**Bonnie Lindstrom, R. N., M.Ed.,** is Bereavement Coordinator, St. Mary's Hospice (formerly Hillhaven Hospice), Tucson, Arizona

**Arthur G. Lipman, Pharm.D.,** is Professor and Chairman, Department of Pharmacy Practice, College of Pharmacy, The University of Utah, Salt Lake City, Utah; and President (1982–1983), Hospice of Salt Lake, Inc.

**Nina Millett, R.N., M.S.W.,** is Program Director, Hospice of Madison County, Granite City, Illinois

**Russell Noyes, Jr., M.D.,** is Professor of Psychiatry, University of Iowa College of Medicine, Iowa City, Iowa

**Colin Murray Parkes, M.D., FRCPsych, D.P.M.,** is Consultant Social Psychiatrist, The London Hospital Medical College; and St. Christopher's Hospice, London, England

**Ruth Reko, M.S.W.,** formerly was Program Coordinator, Continuing Care Unit, Lutheran Medical Center, St. Louis, Missouri; presently she is Regional Director, Midwest Division, National Health Screening Council for Volunteer Organizations, Inc.

**Dame Cicely M. Saunders, D.B.E., M.A., M.D., FRCP,** is Medical Director, St. Christopher's Hospice, London, England

**Averil Stedeford, M.B., B.S., MRCPsych,** is Senior Registrar, Department of Psychotherapy, the Warneford Hospital; and Sir Michael Sobell House, The Churchill Hospital, Oxford, England

**Claire B. Tehan, M.A.,** is Hospice Program Director, Hospital Home Health Care Agency, Torrence, California; and Member, Board of Directors, The National Hospice Organization, Washington, D.C.

**Kent Nelson Tigges, M.S., O.T.R.,** is Associate Professor, Department of Occupational Therapy, School of Health Related Professions, State University of New York, Buffalo, New York; and Resident Consultant, Hospice Buffalo, Inc.

**Robert G. Twycross, M.D., D.M., FRCP,** is Consultant Physician, Sir Michael Sobell House, The Churchill Hospital, Oxford, England

**Mary L. S. Vachon, R.N., Ph.D.,** is Research Scientist, The Clarke Institute of Psychiatry; and Associate Professor, Psychiatry and Behavioral Science, University of Toronto, Toronto, Ontario, Canada

**Eric Wilkes, O.B.E., M.A., FRCP, FRCGP, FRCPsych,** is Professor of Community Care and General Practice, University of Sheffield Medical School; and Medical Director, St. Luke's Nursing Home, Sheffield, England

# Acknowledgments

We owe a great deal—surely more than can adequately be acknowledged here—to many people who have contributed to our education in the hospice philosophy and to those who have supported our work in the preparation of this book. We cannot mention all of the individuals—dying persons (many now dead), family members and friends, caregivers, and colleagues —who sustained us over a period of several years, but they will know who they are and that they have our gratitude.

The community of love and care that is St. Luke's Nursing Home in Sheffield, England, received us warmly (along with our three children) during the summer of 1978 and allowed us to work within and explore every aspect of their program without hindrance. We are most grateful to Eric Wilkes, Marjory Cockburn, and the people of this fine unit. During that summer, we were also welcomed for day-long visits at six other British hospice units.

Earlier, one of us had had an opportunity to visit briefly the Palliative Care Service at the Royal Victoria Hospital in Montreal, and to work as a part-time volunteer for 3 months at the (then new) Continuing Care Unit of Lutheran Medical Center in St. Louis. Since then, we have been privileged to share in the home care program of Hospice of Madison County in Granite City, Illinois. Over a period of several years, our interdisciplinary research in this area has received generous encouragement and assistance from the School of Humanities and the Office of Research and Projects in the Graduate School of Southern Illinois University at Edwardsville. More recently, we wish to acknowledge the nursing faculty of St. Louis Community College at Forest Park.

# I

# Needs and Responses— The Hospice Approach

Recently, a participant in one of our day-long workshops on improving care for dying persons and their families asked, "Where have all these dying people suddenly come from?" As soon as the question was asked, she realized what she had said and added, "Of course, the dying have always been with us. But why is there so much interest in them lately?" The issues posed by this nurse are important ones. An adequate response requires some understanding of changes in society in general and in our health care systems in particular.

Caring for dying persons has always been a responsibility of the human community. Originally, it fell mainly upon families and local groups and had strong overtones of religious values. Care was offered, even though curative abilities might have been quite limited. Average life expectancy was relatively short; dying was usually a quick process; and death was accepted as a part of life. With better food, clothing, shelter, sanitary conditions, and transportation systems, things began to change. As scientific medicine became more and more effective, particularly in the 20th century, many communicable diseases were all but eradicated. Mortality rates during pregnancy, at childbirth, in infancy and childhood, and at other vulnerable times were greatly improved. People lived longer, on the average, and dying became more and more an experience of the elderly and a result of degenerative diseases such as cancer.

At the same time, extended families were replaced by the smaller nuclear family, and these were scattered across a mobile society. With more elderly people in the population, many outlived or became isolated from relatives who might formerly have cared for them. Long-term care facilities sprang up to offer nursing and convalescent care. Hospitals increasingly became secular health centers devoted to acute treat-

1

ment and cure. Death and dying gradually became phenomena of institutions set aside from the mainstream of everyday living. They were not matters of vital concern or high priority. And the process compounded itself: Distancing created unfamiliarity and discomfort, which fostered further withdrawal. Dying persons found that their changing needs were less and less effectively met at home by family and over-burdened community resources, while their position became less and less secure in both acute care hospitals and custodial facilities.

We have now begun to realize that we cannot go on in this way. An increasingly aging society will face more—not less—of these problems in the near future. Chronic illnesses and degenerative diseases resist quick cures and will always be with us. In the meantime, it is never true that there is "nothing more that we can do" for other human beings who are troubled by distressful symptoms. If we cannot cure or control the underlying causes of illness and death, we can at least ameliorate their symptomatic manifestations.* Palliative care is an ancient and legitimate tradition both in our social customs and in medical practice. It applies as much to the common cold as to advanced muscular dystrophy or disseminated malignancy. The hospice movement represents a grassroots effort to provide skilled and humane services to those for whom cure may no longer be a feasible option.

In Part I, Dame Cicely M. Saunders introduces these themes in an article based on her work in the early and mid-1960s at St. Joseph's Hospice—that is, her work prior to the founding of St. Christopher's. (Note: This is the only article not reprinted here in full; with Dame Cicely's permission, we have deleted several pages on drug therapies, because principles and practices have since altered and are now more accurately reflected in Part II of this volume.) Dame Cicely reminds us that, while death is always an end to life, for many it can also be a conclusion or, in her word, a "fulfillment." Thus, she speaks of the "privilege" of keeping watch with dying persons and their families, and of assisting them to obtain this outcome as they may choose in their own ways. To a skilled professional who is also a fellow human being, such care is a positive challenge with its own proper achievements and rewards. For those who view dying as a battle and themselves as narrow specialists, death can only be a defeat and a failure. But that depends primarily on what we as caregivers bring to the situation. If we view things differently we can afford to keep company with the dying, not in a passive or negative way, but in an active and positive effort to create the safety of a caring and therapeutic community.

Those who are sympathetic to the hospice approach have the obligation of bringing into clearer focus the real situation of dying persons *in our society. Who are the dying among us? What are their real needs? What do they have in common with the rest of us and with other ill people? And what are the special problems faced by individuals approaching death? Our next three selections speak to these questions by illustrating distinctive difficulties that afflict many dying people and the common concerns that may come to bother them in a special way. First of all, Russell Noyes and John Clancy follow the lead of a famous American sociologist, Talcott Parsons, to recall that, however confused are its boundaries, dying is a very special situation in life. If we cannot allow ourselves to abandon the dying and treat them as if they were already dead, it is equally wrong mindlessly to attack every reversible process and to continue to do investigations or to run tests without regard for their relevance or for the suffering the tests themselves may be causing. Too much of this results from the subtle but forceful expectations that we impose on those around us—from our own ideals, which we assume as a basis for action and transfer to vulnerable people who may not always share them. All too many studies remind us of our failures in this regard. Instead, we must let dying persons and their families be our teachers, so that we may achieve a new appreciation of their actual needs. We must look again with as little bias or professional distortion as possible to see those whom we profess to serve as integral wholes.*

*When we do this, perhaps the first thing that springs to light is an enormous amount of unrelieved pain. Neither dying nor pain—nor, for that matter, cancer—are coextensive. One may be in pain and not be dying, or be dying and not be in pain. But all too many dying persons do experience an unnecessary share of severe or significant pain. One reason for this is that severe chronic pain of long duration that is often associated with dying is quite different from short-term acute pain of the sort that we all know and tend to use as a standard for judgment. Lawrence LeShan's brilliant analysis of the world of the person experiencing severe chronic pain explains its all-consuming and inward-turning nature. We need to acquire a whole new understanding of this sort of pain if we are ever to treat it adequately. This is a prime example in which active listening to real needs is the only antidote for our own inadequate conceptual apparatus.*

*A popular slogan in recent medical and nursing education is "the patient as person." Perhaps more honored in the breach than in practice, it means that care should be addressed not just to a defective organ or biochemical system, but to the whole human being. This is never more true than when the person is chronically ill or dying. The dimensions of severe chronic pain include not merely the physical, but also the psychological, the social, and the spiritual. The whole individual is involved, as are the networks of other people with whom he or she is inevitably enmeshed. Colin Murray Parkes illustrates this well in his account of the emotional impact of progressive, degenerative disease. Notice that the discussion applies to everyone who becomes involved in coping with the disease—patient, family, staff, and society as a whole —and that it is not limited to any particular sort of disfiguring illness. As a general rule, cancer seems to have an emotional impact in our society that is disproportionate to that of other diseases, but all terminal and chronic illnesses can generate these dimensions of stress.*

*In the final selection of Part I, Sylvia A. Lack carries these guidelines from individual behavior to a full-fledged system by describing 10 characteristics of a comprehensive program of hospice care. This schema has been widely accepted as a useful plan to guide the implementation of hospice programs. It serves as an ideal for emerging hospice units and as a rudimentary way to measure their adequacy. For our purposes, Lack's schema is a kind of précis for the detailed expositions that follow in the next five parts of this book.*

# 1

# The Last Stages of Life

*Dame Cicely M. Saunders*

"I thought it so strange. Nobody wants to look at me."

"Will you turn me out if I can't get better?"

These two remarks, made to me by patients on their admission to St. Joseph's Hospice, illustrate the feelings of guilt, failure, and rejection that so often beset the dying.

Although these feelings are indeed those of patients with any long chronic illness, they are all too often a reflection of our own attitudes. Death is feared, all thoughts of it are avoided, and the dying themselves are often left in loneliness. Both in their homes and in hospital, they are emotionally isolated even when surrounded by their families or involved in much therapeutic activity. When we do come near them, we tend to look at them with that pity which is not so far removed from contempt. Concentrating on our own reactions to death, we often fail to learn the respect for the dying that can help us find the real meaning we both need.

This should not be so. The last stages of life should not be seen as defeat, but rather as life's fulfillment. It is not merely a time of negation, but rather an opportunity for positive achievement. One of the ways we can help our patients most is to learn to believe and to expect this.

During the past six years, I have had the privilege of knowing many hundreds of patients during the last days and weeks of their lives, and of helping a community of nuns and nurses look after them.

It seems to me that the way to find a philosophy that gives confidence and permits a positive approach to death and dying is to look continually at the patients, not at their need but at their courage, not at their dependence but at their dignity. Doctors and nurses who have fought hard to save life or to relieve dying rightly comfort themselves with the knowledge that they have done all they could. But those who also realize how well the patient himself played his part can find consolation for loss and courage to face the future.

St. Joseph's is a specialized unit. Often in just such a setting it is easier to see one problem clearly and thus to find general principles that have wide relevance. St. Joseph's does not have the challenge of diagnosis nor the difficult decisions concerning treatment. Others have wrestled with these problems for our patients; those stages of their illness are now over.

We do not have the hope of cure, but it is easier for us to look at our patients as persons in distress and to concentrate on giving them relief. We have the endless fascination of watching each individual come to terms with his illness in his own way and come along his own path to life's ending. Almost invariably it is a quiet ending that leaves behind a sense of real fulfillment. When each patient first comes to us, we do not know what this path will be nor how we can help him. Certainly we have no preconceived ideas about what his death should be like.

We must appreciate, but not judge, each patient's achievements. We may admire some more than others, perhaps, but who is to say who did best—old Mr. Hanson, who somehow managed to stop grumbling for his last two weeks, or young Mrs. Arthur, who filled the ward with gaiety for five months, made all that happened into a sort of party, and never showed us how much it cost her? None of us will forget Mr. Martin, to whom all the nuns brought their special intentions for his prayers, for whom the slowest of the nurses always moved quickly, and whose shaving water was always really hot. But how should we compare him with Mr. Clark, cheerful, untidy, and alcoholic, who always justified Sister's act of faith in letting him spend much time out in the local public house by getting back to the ward just on time, and who was the only person who managed to bring some comfort to the lonely refugee in the next bed?

The time for active treatment is over when patients are admitted to our wards. The decision that all that can now be given is comfort and care, and that too much activity would merely be a useless disturbance of peace, has been made elsewhere. There is the occasional, unexpected remission and discharge and, although these are rare, the possibility is never forgotten. Of course we are delighted when this happens, but we do not look upon these as our only triumphs. For example, the way a young mother upheld her family by her own acceptance of death and how she helped them to trust in the future was one of our joys. The victory was entirely her own, yet she needed much medical and nursing help to make it possible.

Some will, perhaps, find it shocking that we should speak thus of accepting and preparing for death and will think that both patient and doctor should fight for life right to the end. Some may question why we should be satisfied with what sounds like such a negative role. Yet, I believe that to talk of accepting death when its approach is inevitable is not mere resignation or submission on the part of the patient, nor defeat or neglect on the part of the doctor; for each of them accepting death's coming is the very opposite of doing nothing.

The way between too much and too little treatment for the patient with terminal malignant disease is found only by the most careful looking at him. The patient who said when asked to describe her pain, "Well, Doctor, it began in my back but now it seems that all of me is wrong," was describing a situation with which we deal continually. To bring comfort and peace to her and to many others calls for much skill, and for an attention to detail that brings many rewards.

The care of the dying demands all that we can do to enable patients to *live* until they die. It includes the care of the family, the mind, and the spirit as well as the care of the body. All these are so interwoven that it is hard to consider them separately. I believe, however, that the most important factor of all is an atmosphere of such welcome and confidence that a patient can end her talk with me by saying, "But it's so wonderful to begin to feel safe again."

Many students who have come to us to learn have tried to describe this atmosphere. And one group wrote, "It would be tedious to put down what everyone said so we will enumerate: There is absence of pain and drowsiness; liveliness (in its true sense) and peacefulness; an indefinable atmosphere which left us feeling that death was nothing to be worried about, but rather a sort of homecoming. There was integration—patients, staff, and visitors were all of equal importance; there seemed to be no dividing barriers. We noticed especially how easy it was to talk to the patients and how easily they accepted us. There was simplicity of approach to the problem of pain, and a lack of narrowmindedness which might so easily be prevalent in a place run by a religious order. Agnostics, atheists, or nonthinkers, as well as those with a strong Christian faith, are helped to accept death in the way most suitable to *them*. And, there is the use of a casework approach to each individual."

Every student and visitor who comes to St. Joseph's Hospice remarks on the happiness in the patients' faces and goes on to ask whether the patients know that they have cancer and are dying when they are admitted or whether we tell them these truths. On the whole, patients in England are not told when they have cancer and, although some may well learn their diagnosis in one way or another, they rarely talk about it with us. I believe, more often, that the diagnosis seems irrelevant to them at this stage, rather than too frightening to be discussed.

Still less often are patients told that they are dying and that this is why they have been transferred to St. Joseph's; some may well suspect, but choose not to discuss it. We believe that most patients do not consciously realize what is happening to them when they are admitted, but we know that the truth dawns on most of them by the end and we know that they are not afraid. Death is not frightening when it is near.

I am most fortunate to be able to go around the wards alone and informally in this essentially unhurried setting. I leave the initiative in starting discussion with the patients; rather less than half of them discuss the truth openly with me. When they do, it is they who tell me that they know that they are dying, not the other way around. Often they do so very indirectly or hardly in words at all, for this sort of truth lies more in a relationship than in words.

Most patients who want to talk already know what is happening. They may want to bring out their fears—"Will it be very long? Will it be painful? Will it be in my sleep?"—to talk about their families, or perhaps just to thank us in a simple and sometimes most matter-of-fact way. Sometimes they want to leave the subject immediately. It is important that we find out afresh on each visit whether the patient wishes to go on talking about death or whether he prefers to talk as if he were going to live forever, to complain about a minor symptom, or to talk about the weather. Jokes are not at all inappropriate and, like all families, we have many.

I know that a patient is not afraid if he finds himself in a climate of safety and is allowed to come to insight in his own way and time. Relatives, doctors, and nurses often are far more afraid to think about death than are dying patients. There are some patients, however, who show by their denial of illness, or by their demands for reassurance, that for the moment, at least, they want such truths as, "I am pleased with you so far because your pain is better," "We are doing our best and I am going to give you a new drug which I think will suit you better," or "It is too soon for me to be sure, but if you ask me again in a week or two I promise I will never run away." They find their own way and it seems abundantly clear to me that one does not necessarily have to know that death is imminent to be well prepared to meet it. In life and in death, trust and faith are not so very different.

Very occasionally, I am asked a direct question. I remember such a question from Mr. Martin whom I knew well and who really wanted a direct answer. When I gave it to him, he said, "Was it hard for you to tell me that?" When I said, "Well—yes—it was," he said simply, "Thank you. It is hard to be told, but it is hard to tell, too. Thank you."

This sums up so much about the dying. They are not self-centered, but have a great regard and courtesy for those around them. They are direct and meet us with great simplicity, one person to another, when the complications of ordinary life fall away. As in the example above, telling should be hard; if it is not, we should hesitate. The situation demands all that we can bring of understanding and compassion, and we must know the right moment and the right way. We must care very much that each person do well with what we are able to give him. Mr. Martin, and so very many others I have known, made such achievements of their dying that it was indeed a "good end."

Nurses do not have the taxing responsibility of telling or not telling, but because they often are nearer to the patient than anyone else they may be faced with searching or ambiguous questions without warning. The nurse will have to say something. How she can try to deal helpfully with such patients was considered in an article by Baker and Sorensen in the [American] Journal [of Nursing] in July 1963. Fortunately, we are more often faced with confidences that require no comment. Patients usually do not want our judgments or our explanations but rather our understanding, and often just our silent listening. They do not want to know what we think. They do want to know that we are interested in what they think. In no situation is it more true that "In quietness and in confidence shall be your strength."

I asked Mr. Martin what he looked for above all in those who were caring for him. He said, "For someone to look as if she is trying to understand me." We can never really understand another person any more than we can alter the hard thing that is happening, or take away the weariness and the partings. We can help the patient mobilize his own resources and come to his own personal victory. I always remember that Mr. Martin did not ask for good words, nor indeed even for success in understanding him, but only that someone should care enough to try.

We should never look on such patients with mere pity or indulgence. So often it is they who make us feel humble. Nothing is more corroding to their morale than sentimental sympathy. Nothing is more helpful than a compassionate matter-of-factness coupled with expectation and appreciation of achievement and a quickness to see the practical help needed.

We do not always realize how much relief from pain and anxiety can be given the patient by treatment based on careful assessment of his symptoms coupled with a positive approach toward his care. Not only the patient, but his family and, indeed, even the doctor, benefit. Pain is the chief complaint of over 70 percent of our patients, but it is rarely seen or treated alone. Patients do not overrate their pain, certainly not when we have been able to gain their confidence. Most important, though, is that we hear what they are trying to say.

Three patients who recently died illustrate something of what I have tried to express. Mrs. Kraft was deaf and dumb. Forty-eight hours before her death, she told me that she knew she was dying by quietly shaking her head. Miss Frances, a retired headmistress, who, too, was dying, talked to me about her a few days afterward. "Mrs. Kraft didn't suffer," she said. "They don't here. I think the motto of this place is 'There shall be no pain here.' It makes you feel very safe."

Miss Frances had talked with me a great deal during the three months she was with us, and she often had met students on rounds in the Hospice. She died very quietly. Given narcotics regularly so that pain never intruded, and so that she never had to lose her independence and ask for help, she was enabled to carry on with all she wanted to do.

Miss Walker was in the bed opposite Miss Frances for over two months and they became close friends. Like Miss Frances, she had a firm religious faith, though she belonged to a different denomination. When we talked one afternoon, neither of us was careless concerning the fact that Miss Frances was dying, for we both were very attached to her; yet we were certain that all was well with her.

Some weeks earlier Miss Walker had asked me a direct question. She waited until she considered that she really knew me and then put it like this: "Doctor, I have to decide whether I should give up my flat. I know I can be rather emotional at times, but that doesn't mean that I'm not all right underneath, and I really want to know. I already know what was the matter with me the time I was sick before."

Curtains and an examination can always exclude the rest of the ward, and, feeling my way gradually, I told her of her grave prognosis and that in her position I would give up the flat. She appeared to take my answer very calmly; it was obviously no great surprise to her. On my next visit two days later she said, "I do feel so much more settled now that I know, and I am very grateful to you. But you did take a bit of a risk for me, didn't you? As I look around the ward I realize that every one of us is different. Some wouldn't really want to know, in spite of what they said to you, and you could never be quite certain what would turn out to be right for them." She never lost her calmness and objectivity (nor her love of color and clothes), and she died in quiet faith two months later. She did not need to have her dose of narcotic changed, receiving by injection the dosage of medication we had begun orally two and one-half months before.

Each of these patients, in turn, handed on strength and confidence to the others and to all who had the privilege of knowing them. It has been important during these years at St. Joseph's Hospice to learn something of the need such people have for skilled nursing and medical care, for the right handling of drugs, and for the confident understanding of their mental as well as their physical distress. Through these three patients, and countless others, we have been given something still more important—the heritage of a philosophy concerning death which has helped all of us to see death as an essential part of life and as life's fulfillment.

# Bibliography

Baker, J. M., & Sorensen, K. C., "A Patient's Concern with Death," *American Journal of Nursing*, 1963, *63*, 90–92.

Hinton, J. M., "The Physical and Mental Distress of the Dying," *Quarterly Journal of Medicine*, 1963, *32*, 1–21.

LeShan, L., "The World of the Patient in Severe Pain of Long Duration," *Journal of Chronic Diseases*, 1964, *17*, 119–125. [See Chapter 3 of this volume.]

Kasley, V., "As Life Ebbs," *American Journal of Nursing*, 1948, *48*, 170–173.

Saunders, C. M., *Care of the Dying*. London: Macmillan, 1960.

Worcester, A., *The Care of the Aged, the Dying, and the Dead* (2nd ed.). Springfield, IL: Charles C Thomas, 1940.

# 2

# The Dying Role: Its Relevance to Improved Patient Care

*Russell Noyes, Jr. and John Clancy*

Society is failing to meet the obligation it has to its dying members. Persons with terminal illnesses suffer isolation and neglect in hospitals, receive overzealous treatment by physicians, and are kept in ignorance of their situation by families and medical personnel. Evidence for these statements has come from observers of the medical care system and from dying patients themselves (Kübler-Ross, 1969; Reynolds & Kalish, 1974; Sudnow, 1967). In the nineteenth century it was common for persons to die in the familiar environs of their homes, surrounded by grieving families from whom they parted in a meaningful manner (Blauner, 1966). Dying persons of today no longer fill a well-defined social role. Instead, the distinction between the roles of sick and dying persons has been lost and, in the resulting confusion, the care of dying people has suffered. The purpose of this article is to clarify the distinction between the dying and sick roles, identify the signs of existing role confusion, suggest ways in which this confusion may be corrected, and show how reestablishment of the dying role can result in improved care of dying people. The important part physicians play in defining sick and dying roles will be emphasized.

*From:* Russell Noyes, Jr., and John Clancy, "The Dying Role: Its Relevance to Improved Patient Care," *Psychiatry,* 1977, *40,* 41–47. Copyright 1977 by The William Alanson White Psychiatric Foundation, Inc. Reprinted by special permission of The William Alanson White Psychiatric Foundation, Inc. and Russell Noyes, Jr.

## Sick Role

The social role accompanying illness was first described by Parsons (1951). Like other roles, it is a constellation of expectations involving both rights and duties. In the case of the sick role, there are two of each. Within this role a patient is, first of all, exempt from the responsibilities of his usual social role. Important business or social obligations may be broken without fear of censure. The second right is that of being cared for. The sick person is not responsible for becoming ill, and consequently, members of society become obligated to him. This obligation falls primarily upon the family, and, of course, the physician.

The duties of the sick person are twofold, as well. Because society regards illness as an undesirable state, the patient must wish to get well. A person lacking this desire is not favorably regarded by his fellows and may be denied the rights of the sick role. Secondly, the sick person is obligated to obtain competent help in an effort to regain his health and is expected to cooperate with the treatment prescribed. A person who does not seek professional help is regarded as a drag on society.

Like other social roles, the sick role determines how a person perceives his situation. When sick he adopts a new set of expectations relative to his behavior, his obligations toward others, and their duties toward him. At the same time family members, physicians, and others in the social system are made to see their role in caring for the sick person. Both sick and well perceive a set of reciprocal obligations.

## Dying Role

The social role of the fatally ill person is, like that of the sick person, time-limited. However, while the one terminates in the restoration of health, the other ends in death. Both are conferred by medical authority via the diagnosis, which for the dying person carries an unfavorable prognosis. The expected duration of life is important in assigning this role, and the physician therefore has an obligation to the parties concerned to estimate this in terms that reflect the limitations of his knowledge.

As a person enters the dying role, it is important for him to desire to remain alive. By so doing he assures his family and community that he is without responsibility for his approaching death. If he too readily accepted his fate, he might appear to "give up" and reject loved ones or social obligations. The obligation appears to continue, in some degree, as long as family and friends maintain meaningful attachments to the dying person. He may relinquish unrealistic hope of recovery but must retain the "will to live," a motivational set commonly attributed to dying persons. Later appreciation and acceptance of death's reality do not mean that the final parting is willful. Only suffering or disability justifies a wish to die.

When an individual becomes ill, he temporarily vacates healthy social roles. For a period of time they are held open in anticipation of his return. The dying person is obliged to transfer them to others on a more permanent basis. It is, therefore, a second duty of a person in the dying role to exercise the prerogatives he may have and arrange for an orderly transfer of property and authority. The person who fails to execute a will or participate in decisions regarding the future of his business or family may become an object of disapproval. The social disruption consequent to his death can be great. On the other hand, timely decisions and transfer of responsibility make a smooth transition possible.

The dying person has an obligation to avail himself of the necessary supports to life and to cooperate in their administration. If he fails to do so, he may impose a burden upon his family and overload those on whom he has grown dependent. He is not expected to remain dependent upon the physician, who has already, in the process of diagnosing a fatal illness, transferred him from the sick to the dying role. Having done so, the doctor no longer holds a position of primary importance in the person's care, although he may oversee supportive and palliative treatments. Society reserves the physician's role for the more important restorative function and, in so doing, jealously guards against inroads upon the physician's time and energy.

Another of the important aspects of the dying person's cooperation is his acceptance of the curtailment of freedom and loss of privileges imposed by caregivers. If institutional care is required, he is expected to abide by the rules and routines which enable the facility to deliver that care efficiently. Such routines are, in large measure, supportive and permit a higher level of functioning within a limited range.

Lastly, dependency is encouraged in the sick role, whereas independence, within the limits of an individual's declining resources, is encouraged in the dying role (Twaddle, 1972). In this regard it appears to resemble the impaired role described by Gordon (1966). The dying person is expected to limit his claim on others for attention and rely upon himself to a greater degree. Cooperation with caretakers especially calls for independence. The dying person who appears capable but unwilling to feed himself is often viewed with irritation by those looking after him. He is regarded as imposing an unnecessary burden upon the caretaking system. Attendant to this expectation of greater independence, dying persons are encouraged to keep certain complaints to themselves, use a minimum of medication, remain active, and care for themselves to the extent possible.

The dying person has a right to exemption from social role responsibilities and commitments. As he undergoes physiologic decline, he is free to withdraw from active engagement in the social system of which he has been a part (Cumming & Henry, 1961). Ultimately the dying person may be freed from every expectation save that of cooperation in the maintenance of physiologic functions—e.g., eating and elimination. As an individual dies, his attachment to and interest in the world around him diminishes, and his need, or even ability, to respond to the attachments of those about him is reduced. The emotional demand upon his family declines as he moves toward final disengagement.

A second right of the dying person is to be taken care of. Because his plight is not of his own making, society feels obligated toward him. Again, the duty falls primarily on his family or on whatever nursing care the family secures to assist it. And the family's obligation usually extends beyond the provision of physical care to decisions regarding that care and the general welfare and well-being of its dying member. No family is obligated to respond to its detriment, however, or beyond the limits of its physical, emotional, or economic resources.

Finally, the dying person is entitled to continuing respect and status, despite his loss of health and function. His dignity is maintained by those caring for him so long as he meets the obligations of the dying role. The dying man makes room in social order for others. In the process he is expected to do what he can to make a smooth transition and to impose as little burden as possible. If he does so, he is entitled to the continuing care and concern of his family and community.

To summarize, both the sick and dying roles are time-limited and defined by physician authority. In addition, both maintain for the individuals occupying them the continued respect and status of their community. Beyond this point there appear to be important differences. The duty of the sick person is to desire to get well; that of the dying person is to desire to live as long as he can. The sick person is obliged to cooperate with a physician for the purpose of getting well. The dying person must cooperate with nonphysician caretakers in the hope of functioning at a high level, with minimal distress, for as long as possible. Important differences also appear to exist as far as rights are concerned. The sick person has the right to be cared for and is encouraged to become dependent. The dying person is also entitled to care but is encouraged to become independent within limits. While both sick and dying persons are exempt from social responsibilities, the dying person is permanently freed from them and allowed to disengage from family and community.

## Role Confusion

In recent years dying persons have been assigned to the sick role. Signs of this confusion of roles are not difficult to identify. The trend toward more vigorous and active treatment of terminal patients by physicians is one manifestation. Technological advances have given the physician increased control over physiologic aberrations, which he has naturally exercised with enthusiasm. In so doing he has often lost sight of the fact that he has done little to alter the fatal course of an illness. And, caught up in temporary treatment successes, both doctor and patient have tended to indulge in false hopes. It is, of course, natural for the physician to be energetic in his treatment. Within his professional role the life-saving cure of disease has first priority. Confronted, in an emotionally charged atmosphere, with a patient having high expectations and a family wishing "everything to be done," the doctor responds in an active manner. What we have begun to realize is that such treatment is often more appropriate to acutely ill persons and may unnecessarily prolong the suffering and disability of dying people.

Dying persons are treated as acutely sick ones with respect to the information they are given about their disease and prognosis. In fact a "conspiracy of silence" often surrounds the dying person, maintained by the family, community, and patient himself. Early denial is supported by those who judge the person too frail or vulnerable to cope with the anticipation of his death. It is common practice to withhold bad news from acutely ill persons lest their weakened system be overloaded and their condition aggravated. Our approach to chronically impaired persons is quite different, however. We strive to provide information which, for them, is a source of independence and a foundation for adjustment to physical limitations. Clearly a person needs knowledge of his illness and prognosis if he is to fulfill the obligations of the dying role. The behavior of a dying patient who clings to the sick role, long after the diagnosis of a fatal illness, places inordinate demands upon his family and care givers. His false hopes, insistence upon restorative treatment, and dependent behavior often lead to a deterioration of relationships with family and physician.

Another sign of confusion between the dying and the sick roles is the increasing tendency to care for dying persons in hospitals. These institutions are primarily oriented toward diagnosis and treatment. Chronic support of function and rehabilitation are, in fact, looked upon by personnel as a drain on the hospital caregiving system. Persons in need of such services are viewed with annoyance as occupying beds needed for the acutely ill. It is hardly surprising that dying patients are neglected on acute medical and surgical floors. Which of their needs competes with falling blood

pressures, rising temperatures, and other matters of life-or-death consequence? Yet, are they truly neglected? Or, do the observers who make this
accusation—including some patients—harbor the mistaken notion that
dying persons should receive the same kind of attention that sick persons
receive? The hospital is a relatively authoritarian community where privacy and autonomy are limited. Such a setting is optimal for the diagnosis
and treatment of acute illness but may encourage dependency among the
chronically ill or dying.

## Reestablishment of the Dying Role

Open communication with persons suffering from fatal disease appears
essential to reestablishment of the dying role. The notion that dying persons may be overwhelmed by learning about their prognosis remains unsupported, and unilateral decisions to withhold information ignore a person's right to it and the likelihood that he is already aware of it. Significant
tasks may be completed by the dying person providing he knows what lies
ahead of him. A will insures that property shall be distributed according to
his wishes and in a gift-like manner. Timely decisions regarding business
or household affairs allow a smooth transfer of authority. Participation
in decisions regarding treatment increases the dying person's sense of
mastery and reduces the possibility of his becoming a burden to his family.
Awareness of a fatal illness may be spiritually meaningful to a religious
person. And, finally, a dying person may draw together a variety of loose
ends as he seeks a sense of completion.

Open communication does not imply insensitivity on the part of the
physician who must share his understanding of a fatal illness. It does imply
a common or shared awareness between the dying person and significant
others such that family members or friends may aid that person in carrying
out the aforementioned tasks. As a part of the growing consumerism, dying persons can be expected to insist upon a larger say in how they are
cared for. And many, as a part of this movement, are already making arrangements for funerals and medical care well in advance of a final illness.
The attitude reflected in such actions will, no doubt, contribute to greater
independent cooperation on the part of dying persons.

The doctor has an important part to play in reestablishing the dying
role. It must be clear to him that once he has made the diagnosis of a fatal
illness and exhausted possible curative treatments, his obligation to the
dying person changes. He must follow the course of his patient's illness,
respond in the event of complications, see to the patient's comfort, and
counsel the family and patient regarding his care. Though his role contin-

ues to be one of importance, it is no longer primary. Other professionals, in charge of supporting function and controlling symptoms, must assume major responsibility when care is needed.

The physician should begin to modify the relationship he has with his dying patient. While assuring him of his continuing availability, he should encourage the patient to assume more responsibility for his care, e.g., medications, diet, and exercise. In contrast to the parent-child mode of interaction that may have characterized the relationship during the acute or undiagnosed phase of the patient's illness, the doctor should strive for one of mutual cooperation (Szasz & Hollender, 1956). While in acute illness he may order analgesic medication according to the need he observes, in chronic illness the physician should rely to a greater extent on the patient's observations and opinions, sharing with him responsibility for safe administration of the drug. When he does so, the dying person may gain a greater sense of control and experience less anxiety.

Persons with fatal illnesses should be cared for in an appropriate setting by personnel who regard their needs as having high priority. As has been pointed out, in most hospitals the needs of dying persons are overshadowed by more urgent affairs unless special programs or units are set up to meet them. Home care is ideal in many ways, but the community at large must be prepared to support families and furnish institutional placement when the burden exceeds their resources. The requirements of the chronically ill, whether convalescing or deteriorating, appear sufficiently similar to the needs of dying persons that they may be cared for together, thereby avoiding the stigma of the "death house."

Those who care for the dying must be mindful of three important privileges or rights granted to persons meeting the obligations of the dying role. The first of these is the right of disengagement. As the dying person's energy declines, he withdraws his investment in the world around him and shifts his remaining interest to his body and its disordered function. The process is, of course, stimulated by his anticipated separation. Such disengagement is complicated by a family or community that resists it and clings to him. Inordinate demands are then placed upon the dying person. Too often his emotional needs are assessed by health persons, who judge them to be like their own. Sentimentalism is an impediment to solving the problems of dying persons; what is needed are practical answers to difficult questions.

The dying role carries with it the right of unchanging status or valuation within the community. The fact that dying persons have not been held in high esteem by our society may be another reason why the role has been avoided in favor of the sick role. If these persons are to assume the role described, attitudes must begin to change. Of course, appropriate behavior by persons occupying the dying role should result in increased respect for them from families and community.

Finally, the dying role confers the right of protection from abuse. Too many dying persons are exposed to inadequate or neglectful care. Consequently their care must become a matter of higher priority. Unfortunately, it, like the care of chronically ill persons in general, will probably remain a matter of lesser importance regardless of changing attitudes. Still, the vocal concern currently focused on another issue—the rights and status of aged persons—may bring with it constructive change in the approach to dying people.

## Implementation

The dying role, if properly established, should clarify the expectations a dying person and his community might reasonably have of one another. But if community leaders and administrators become more aware of an obligation to their dying members, how should they act? What type of programs should they develop? There is, of course, no final solution, and simply shifting dying people from one setting to another is not the answer. The plight of chronic mental patients is an example of how a variety of relocations have, in the end, only recreated the poor conditions they were designed to correct (Siegler & Osmond, 1974). Most recently such patients have been moved from crowded and poorly staffed hospitals to the community. Now, however, it has become clear that programs to care for them there are inadequate, and they are neglected in the community as they were in the hospital.

Any new programs to improve the care of the dying should be undertaken with caution, lest they make matters worse instead of better. At this time, guiding principles are more to be relied upon than uncertain, action-oriented objectives. Foremost is a need to clarify the confusion surrounding the sick and dying roles through public education. Much of the current emphasis on death and dying is backed by emotionalism and based on individual experience. Such a thrust makes the public aware and ready for change, but does not point to the direction that change should take. Improved care for dying persons can begin within the existing health system through the application of proven practices of care and delivery.

Continuity of care is a high priority. It allows persons to move about in the care system without major disruptions or abrupt transitions in the services delivered. The needs of the dying are not static, and the provision of adequate care may require a high degree of professional expertise. Flexibility in a program goes hand in hand with continuity and helps to individualize the services required. Essential to coordination of activities within the system is communication. In many instances, particularly in smaller communities, communication among a dying person, family, and health personnel may be an easy matter. In larger communities, public hospitals, multiple clinics, rotating personnel, and geographical isolation from families all combine to fragment communication. Special services and personnel may be required to prevent this from occurring.

In a time of increasing consumer awareness, health professions are being called upon to account for the quality of care delivered. Utilization reviews, medical audits, and federal standards are all designed to improve care and provide for consumer satisfaction. It may also be appropriate for institutions to set standards for and examine the care given dying persons in a manner similar to their monitoring of care provided the sick. Ultimately, high-quality care rests upon continuing public awareness and support of the needs of dying people.

## Conclusion

The dying role appears to be a distinct and useful concept. It helps clarify what dying persons and those caring for them can reasonably expect of one another. If these expectations can be met, the care of dying persons will be improved and their status in the community enhanced. And, because they occupy an important, life-affirming role, their improved position can only serve the betterment of their communities. The care given dying persons reflects the value placed on life and, in turn, has an influence upon it.

## References

Blauner, R., "Death and Social Structure," *Psychiatry*, 1966, *29*, 378–394.

Cumming, E., & Henry, W., *Growing Old: The Process of Disengagement.* New York: Basic Books, 1961.

Gordon, G., *Role Theory and Illness: A Sociological Perspective.* New Haven, CT: College and University Press, 1966.

Kübler-Ross, E., *On Death and Dying.* New York: Macmillan, 1969.

Parsons, T., *The Social System.* New York: The Free Press, 1951.

Reynolds, D. K., & Kalish, R. A., "The Social Ecology of Dying: Observations of Wards for the Terminally Ill," *Hospital and Community Psychiatry*, 1974, *25*, 147–152.

Siegler, M., & Osmond, H., *Models of Madness, Models of Medicine*. New York: Macmillan, 1974.

Sudnow, D., *Passing On: The Social Organization of Dying*. Englewood Cliffs, NJ: Prentice-Hall, 1967.

Szasz, T. S., & Hollender, M. H., "A Contribution to the Philosophy of Medicine: The Basic Models of the Doctor-Patient Relationship," *Archives of Internal Medicine*, 1956, 97, 585–592.

Twaddle, A. C., "The Concepts of the Sick Role and Illness Behavior," *Advances in Psychosomatic Medicine*, 1972, 8, 162–179.

# 3

# The World of the Patient in Severe Pain of Long Duration

*Lawrence LeShan*

In physical illness there are many situations in which the patient has severe pain of long duration which is impossible or inadvisable to control by chemical or surgical means. The psychotherapist has only very rarely seen this as an area in which his skills may be of use. Only in the use of hypnosis (particularly since its major scientific advances of the past few years) has he worked in this field on any large scale. Outside of this, such psychological help as has been given in an attempt to aid the patient in pain has been left usually to the clergyman or to the physician. The intuitive understanding they provided has often been of great depth and efficacy, but the time and energy they could bring to bear on the problem has been limited. It would appear that the insights of modern psychology and psychiatry might make worthwhile contributions if applied to the problem.

In the course of a 10-year research program on the psychosomatic aspects of neoplastic disease (LeShan 1957, 1959, 1960, 1962; LeShan & Gassmann, 1958; LeShan & LeShan, 1961; LeShan et al., 1959; LeShan & Resnikoff, 1960; LeShan & Worthington, 1956a, 1956b) a good deal of time was spent by the writer with patients in severe pain, or facing the threat of severe pain. Certain impressions gained and observations made during this work may, perhaps, be worth presenting. This paper is an attempt to describe these observations and to provide a tentative philosophical basis for future work in this area by psychotherapists.

Our understanding of pain is usually taken from our experience with acute pain—the toothache, the burn, the cut or bruise. This type of pain is conducted very rapidly in the nervous system, causes the defensive reflexes, and usually passes quite quickly. We are taught from childhood to regard this as a good and useful warning. We generalize from this to the severe, chronic pain causing genuine suffering which we see in an advanced cancer, a trigeminal neuralgia or a severe arthritis. This generalization leaves much to be desired, and its validity is extremely doubtful. There are qualitative differences between the two types. They are apparently discontinuous. In this paper I shall be discussing the second type of pain, the severe, chronic type which does not provoke defensive reflexes and which gives the patient no clue at all as to how to lessen it.

The amount of published material on the subject of the situation of the patient in chronic pain is surprisingly small. Buytendjick (1962, p. 15), in one of the few serious works on the subject, has commented on this. "Modern man regards pain merely as an unpleasant fact which, like every other evil, he must do his best to get rid of. To do this, it is generally held, there is no need for any reflection on the phenomenon itself."

We shall here be concerned with some aspects of the phenomenon and then attempt to draw some implications from these for the psychotherapist.

## The Person in Pain

If we observe the world with which we are concerned here—the *universe* of the patient in chronic pain—we can perceive a similarity to the universe of the nightmare. If we look at the terror dream, and ask what are its structural components, we see that there are three basic ones: (1) Terrible things are being done to the person and worse are threatened; (2) others, or outside forces, are in control and the will is helpless; (3) there is no time limit set, [and] one cannot predict when it will be over. The person in pain is in the same formal situation: Terrible things are being done to him and he does not know if worse will happen; he has no control and is helpless to take effective action; no time limit is given. This aspect of the psychic assault upon the integrity of the ego that accompanies severe, chronic pain is a major one: The patient lives during the waking state in the cosmos of the nightmare.

This is further emphasized by the meaninglessness and inexplicability of pain. Mental suffering seems to follow naturally from our thoughts and actions; with the possible exception of some of the obsessive-compulsive states, it is somehow organic to us, syntonic to our views of ourselves. Chronic pain is alien; it seems to indicate an utter senselessness. It appears to be meaningless and so, since it is very hard for man to accept that real experience may be unreasonable, we attempt to give it meaning. Our ancient guilts and anxieties are aroused, and we try to assign our pain to these insufficient causes. Although this is a frequent reaction, is rarely leads, for individuals of our society, to a useful sense of meaning. Not only does the lack of a time limit militate against this, but the concept of purgatory (in this world or the next) is not a part of the Zeitgeist. This attempt, however, further weakens the ego, as is done even more by the returning concept that there *is no sense* to the pain. The meaning of pain has been approached by every great religion and philosophy. In our own antimetaphysical culture it is largely ignored. This lack of a perceived meaning, of a culturally understood context, makes it much harder for the individual to deal with chronic pain. As the Nazis well understood and demonstrated, meaningless and purposeless torture is much harder for the person to accept and resist than is torture which the subject can place in a coherent frame of reference. A perceived senselessness in the universe weakens our belief that our efforts have validity and point. They appear to be essentially futile. This makes it much harder to continue these efforts, including those of coping with pain and stress.

It is common, in our generalization from acute to chronic pain, to assign to pain the idea of a warning—a signal that something is wrong and that we should do something about it. This orientation often makes it more difficult for the therapist to be clear about the problems involved. Scheler (1923, p. 41) points out that the sensation of weariness says "rest," dizziness at the edge of an abyss says "step back," and hunger [says] that one should eat. Chronic pain, however, indicates only a state of existence. It does not warn or tell us what to do. It does not help us act and may be so severe as to disrupt potentially useful activities and habits. The adequate expression of thirst is to drink. The adequate expression of this kind of pain is only a scream.

Another aspect of the psychic assault made by severe pain is implied in this. It is related to the fact that it is important to ourselves that we respond to strong stimuli—that we are connected to and react to the environment. With pain this is much more difficult; we are constantly pushed towards suffering rather than interacting. We cannot act, we can only bear. Time and space are the basic framework for our exchanging energy with the cosmos and thus replenishing the strength of our psychic coherence. Pain weakens our relationship with this framework. There is a pulling to the center, a centripetal force that brings our energies and our consciousness into ourselves and away from all else and all others. "It is a peculiarity of man," says Victor Frankl (1959, p. 74), "that he can only live by looking to the future—*sub specie aeternitatis.*" When he has no real goals in time, the inner life decays. There is a real loss of time perspective in pain—we are pulled to the immediate. The intensity and duration of the stimulus binds us to it. Our libidinal energy is pulled back from its objects and used as a defensive wall against the pain. However, this shift of the libido increases our focusing of attention on the pain and thereby makes it fill our life space to a greater degree and reduces our ability to deal with it. The lost objects can no longer sustain us and help us maintain our inner integrity and sense of being, purpose and meaning. Pain permits personal existence to continue with little assistance from our usual orientations, defenses, safeguards and associations. It attenuates our relationships with the outer world at the same time that it weakens the inner structure. In painless consciousness we are filled with images, association, thoughts. In the loud loneliness of pain, only our existence is real. We float alone in space, conscious only of the suffering.

These reactions and the passive, helpless quality of being in chronic pain tend to press us strongly towards a psychic regression. Our dignity and our hard-won adult status is weakened. The body image—our sense of our physical aspects and a basis of our sense of being, our *persona*—is blurred as the pain seems to obliterate the rest of the body. We are conscious only of the area that is providing the overwhelming sensations. The ego strength is further weakened by this reduction of the complexity of the organization of the adult perception of the body. It returns us to the body image (and, with this, the feelings, the helplessness and dependency) of childhood. This is further added to by the fact that when we are in severe pain we, as in childhood, have to depend on others to take the important actions in our lives.

This is one reason that pity for the person in pain is an extremely corrosive emotion and—when perceived by the patient—further makes less his ability to deal with the situation. The pity reinforces the regression through its implication of a lower status. The strivings to retain dignity and adulthood can be reinforced through empathy, emotional contact, and respect. Pity only weakens them.

It is usual to view pain as an event. As the above comments indicate, it may sometimes be more usefully viewed as a situation, a Weltanschauung, a position in the universe. Its quality is determined by the total context. As E. Strauss puts it, "There are no such things as sensations in themselves, there are only sensitive beings" (quoted by Buytendjick, 1962, p. 122). Hebb (1957) has pointed out that pain is felt when C-fiber nervous impulses disrupt a well-organized pattern of activity. However when these same impulses are assimilated into a well-organized neural action pattern no pain is felt. In discussing pain in cancer, Gotthard Booth has stated that "pain is frequently more dependent on the morale than on the physical condition of the patient" (1962, p. 317). The football player who does not feel the pain of his bone fracture, the schizophrenic who severely mutilates himself with little or no pain sensation, the flagellant in ecstasy, are all too well known to need exposition here. There can be no pain without involvement of the higher nervous centers and it is how these centers handle, absorb, and integrate the pain that will determine its perception and the ability to resist it. In Tolstoi's magnificent existential novel, *The Death of Ivan Illych* (1960), it was only when Ivan realized the total meaninglessness of his life that he was overwhelmed by the pain of his cancer. As long as there seemed to him to be a valid meaning to his existence, he could resist it and retain control and dignity. Once he lost the sense of the meaning of his life, he could only start screaming and continue to scream until he died. The emotional state, the "Lebensgefühl," determines in large part the perception of pain, and its power over a person. One woman who had had terribly severe pain for many years from an inner ear disorder, but who had continued her active, useful, and ebullient life in spite of this, responded to the question of how she did it by saying, "When the pain is severe, I rise above it and look at it from a higher level." To dismiss this remark and technique as "hysteroid" would be missing the entire point. She retained command over herself and the pain and so was not overwhelmed as a person by it. Her psychic structure remained intact and master of her fate.

We have discussed here the general situation of the person in pain. It may be worthwhile also to be aware of some specific aspects which may play a part in the total situation.

These special aspects are possibilities that it appears advisable to keep in mind before action against the pain is taken by means of drugs, suggestion, hypnosis, or other methods.

### Pain as Communication

Szasz (1957) in his discussion of this area has pointed out that pain may be used as an attempt at communicating with another person. It can be a way of stating a psychic situation—an aggression or a cry for help. In studying the specific person who is in pain, it may be important to ask oneself, "Is he saying something by this?" "Is there a message in it?"

### Pain as an Answer to Psychic Needs

Engel (1959), Cangello (1962), and others have discussed in some detail the use of pain to fill an inner need—to maintain the psychodynamic structure of the person. We understand this in mental suffering. One patient, on being reassured that she had not hurt others, cried out in real anguish, "Don't take away my guilt." An experienced psychotherapist will recognize the cry and the needs behind it. However, our cultural orientation towards pain that it is evil and must be immediately relieved is so strong that, in spite of our knowledge of the cases where chronic pain has been relieved, [only] to be followed immediately by emotional breakdown or suicide, we often ignore this problem.

One patient, who had suffered severe pain for several months and was now free of it, spoke of her fear that she would not be able to maintain the "real" feeling and relationships which had arisen during the pain. "I am afraid," she added, "that if I feel good, I'll go back to my phony ways of living again."

"I have discovered by experience," wrote Girolamo Cardano in 1575, "that I cannot be long without bodily pain, for if once the circumstance arises, a certain mental anguish overcomes me, so grievous that nothing could be more distressing" (1930/1958).

The questions should be asked: "Is there a purpose behind this pain in this particular patient?" "Does it hold off guilt?" "Does it provide him with a sense of being 'real' that he desperately needs?" "Is it a conversion symptom and, if so, of what?" One ignores these questions at the risk of successfully answering the patient's conscious plea for relief and destroying his adjustment.

## Some Guidelines for the Therapist

We have discussed briefly some general and some special aspects of the problem of pain. We now proceed to some of the implications these concepts may hold for the therapist who must help the patient with pain that cannot be relieved by physical means.

The hardest task for the therapist, and yet perhaps the most basic, is to help the patient arrive at a meaning, a making some sense out of what is happening to him. Here there can be no rules as to how this is done, only an orientation as to its importance. Each patient must be helped to the path most syntonic to *him*, to his own sense of meaning, not the meaning that makes sense to the therapist. His uniqueness is crucial and the knowledge of this, in itself, may be helpful. To know—to be reinforced in the knowledge—that one is unique and irreplaceable, as a loved one or one who loves, as one with special tasks, or in some other manner—gives much support to the psychic structure and the ability to handle the situation. (This is one reason why experiments with pain-relieving agents often have such positive effects on the control subjects who are receiving only placebos. Their participation in the experiment itself reinforces their status as individual persons, increases their ability to deal with the pain and thus decreases their perception of it.) One patient was able to understand the connection between her pain and the healing process—that the pain was an inexorable part of treatment. She said, "Now that I know there is a reason, I feel it much less and can keep doing things when it comes. It's like the difference between childbirth and the other pains. In labor you know something will be produced at the end. It's never as bad as when the pain doesn't produce anything."

It is perhaps important for the therapist first to be clear about his own feelings in this area before he can effectively help the sufferer. If he believes that there *is* a meaning, even if he cannot find it, he is in a much better position to help. Out of his great experience with pain, Victor Frankl wrote, "If there is a meaning in life at all, then there is a meaning in suffering. Suffering is an ineradicable part of life, even as fate and death" (1959, p. 67). Just as it is important that the psychotherapist who works with the dying patient has to come to terms with his own feelings about death (LeShan & Gassmann, 1958; LeShan & LeShan, 1961), so too, it is important for the psychotherapist who works with the patient in severe pain to have come to terms with his feelings about pain.

Some patients may be able to make sense of the perception that this experience has brought them fully face to face with themselves and their universe—that they are no longer "metaphysically heedless"; that their knowledge of their own existence has been deeply increased. (Indeed, Buytendjick (1962) and others have theorized that it is this very increase of self-consciousness that is the basic "function" of chronic pain.) "Your pain," said Kahlil Gibran (1936) in *The Prophet*, "is the breaking of the shell that encloses your understanding."

One patient who had suffered very severe pain for a long period, and still was in acute physical distress, said, "Sometimes with a lot of pain, a person becomes 'verklart' (clarified) and all the trivial unimportant things become unimportant. You stop spending your life worrying about them."

Other patients can understand that the experience they have had can never be taken from them; that after it is over they will never need to fear anything again; and that, as Nietzsche put it, "That which does not kill me, makes me stronger." Other patients may see the pain they have as *existing in itself*, and *their* experiencing it saves someone else from the experience. Each patient must be helped to his own solution. The effectiveness of the psychotherapist depends, in large part, on his ingenuity in helping the patient to the best answer for him as an individual. It is the knowledge of the importance of this that is central for the therapist. Dostoievsky said, "There is only one thing I dread, not to be worthy of my sufferings." In this dark and wise sentence we see the need for the emergence and maintenance of the self in the welter of pain.

A second major guideline for the therapist is to help the patient find ways to act and react to the situation—to help the patient take some semblance of control over his situation. In the act of control, much strength is given to the inner being: The person is strengthened. Sometimes the patient must be helped to understand that for certain tasks, the action that is called for is to do nothing but to wait and bear and that this can be an active, not a passive, process. This can be a very valuable insight to some patients.

Frequently the patient feels he can only "be brave and heroic" or surrender. This can be an impasse which demands more than the patient has to give. The value of "a stiff upper lip" is often vastly overestimated by both the patient and those around him. Sometimes just permission to cry ("some things are worth a few tears") reduces the rigidity and makes it possible for other responses to take place. This should not be done, however, with the patient with a rigid, brittle ego which may be overwhelmed and drowned by a passive-dependent flood. In these patients it is necessary rather to reinforce the rigid defenses (often with obsessive-compulsive techniques) than to weaken them.

One can also help some patients to understand the concept that the facts, including the facts of our inner life, are not as important as our attitude toward them. In the old story where one soldier was reproached and ridiculed by another for feeling fear under shellfire, the first answered: "It shows we are different, but it does not show I am inferior. If you were one-half as frightened as I am, you would have run away long ago." The "fact" of pain impulses is also less important to the person's ability to deal with them than his attitude toward them.

A third lead for the therapist sometimes may be to make the "nightmare" conditions conscious. To understand clearly the psychic pressures on a person sometimes makes them much easier to resist. Not only do we understand that the pressures and our reactions are "natural," "expected," but also that they are universal and not special and secret to us. Further, the more an emotion and its causes are looked at clearly and objectively, the weaker it tends to become. Booth (1963) quotes Spinoza that "Suffering ceases to be suffering as soon as we form a clear and precise picture of it."

One major way of helping the patient in pain is to help him remove the focus of concentration from the pain to outside events. The pain is felt to be worse when it occupies the entire life field. Work, occupational therapy, relating to others—these things do much more than just "pass the time." They also diminish the pain. Both "attention" and "consciousness" are essential to the perception of pain. We can reduce one or the other, but the reduction of "attention" can often be surprisingly effective.

In the demand the psychotherapist makes that the patient turn his energies outward from the pain and that he function as a person, the therapist should avoid being too "soft" and gentle. He can make high demands; this indicates far more respect and consequently strengthens the person far more than overconcern. The same orientation that we have toward mental anguish in psychotherapy is called for here. To be loving and demanding is a difficult road to walk, but it is the road that gives the greatest support and help to the patient. Sometimes the therapist can be aided in this if he asks himself whether his goal for the patient is painlessness or if it is composure, dignity, and mastery.

## Conclusion

Each of us lives in a unique, existential universe. The effectiveness of the psychotherapist who would relieve suffering is related to his understanding of, and empathy with, the universe of the sufferer. This is as true for the person with severe chronic pain as it is for those whose anguish is felt in the emotional sphere. It is also true, however, that the universes of those in pain tend to have common trends and pressures which appear to have implications for the therapist. This chapter has been an attempt to describe some of these commonalities.

## References

Booth, G., "Disease as a Message," *Journal of Religion and Health*, 1962, *1*, 309–318.

Booth, G., "Values in Nature and in Psychotherapy," *Archives of General Psychiatry*, 1963, *8*, 22–32.

Buytendjick, F. J. J., *Pain: Its Modes and Functions*. Chicago: University of Chicago Press, 1962.

Cangello, V. W., "Hypnosis for the Patient with Cancer," *American Journal of Clinical Hypnosis*, 1962, *4*, 215–226.

Cardano, G., *De Vita Propria Libra* (1575) (J. Stoner, trans.). New York: Dutton, 1930. Quoted in *The Portable Renais Reader* (J. B. Ross & M. M. McLaughlin, Eds.). New York: Viking Press, 1958.

Engel, G. L., " 'Psychogenic' Pain and the Pain-Prone Patient," *American Journal of Medicine*, 1959, *26*, 899–918.

Frankl, V., *From Death Camp to Existentialism*. Boston: Beacon Press, 1959.

Gibran, K., *The Prophet*. New York: Knopf, 1936.

Hebb, D. O., *Organization of Behavior*. New York: Wiley, 1957.

LeShan, L., " A Psychosomatic Hypothesis Concerning the Etiology of Hodgkin's Disease," *Psychological Reports*, 1957, 3, 565–575.

LeShan, L., "Personality States as Factors in the Development of Malignant Disease: A Critical Review," *Journal of the National Cancer Institute*, 1959, 22, 1–18.

LeShan, L., "Some Methodological Problems in the Study of the Psychosomatic Aspect of Cancer," *Journal of General Psychology*, 1960, 63, 309–317.

LeShan, L., "Cancer Mortality Rate: Some Statistical Evidence of the Effect of Psychological Factors," *Archives of General Psychiatry*, 1962, 6, 333–335.

LeShan, L., & Gassmann, M. L., "Some Observations on Psychotherapy with Patients with Neoplastic Disease," *American Journal of Psychotherapy*, 1958, 12, 723–734.

LeShan, L., & LeShan, E., "Psychotherapy and the Patient with a Limited Life Span," *Psychiatry*, 1961, 24, 318–323.

LeShan, L., Marvin, S., & Lyerly, O., "Some Evidence of a Relationship Between Hodgkin's Disease and Intelligence," *Archives of General Psychiatry*, 1959, 1, 477–479.

LeShan, L., & Reznikoff, M., "A Psychological Factor Apparently Associated with Neoplastic Disease," *Journal of Abnormal and Social Psychology*, 1960, 60, 439–440.

LeShan, L., & Worthington, R. E., "Loss of Cathexes as a Common Psychodynamic Characteristic of Cancer Patients: An Attempt at Statistical Validation of a Clinical Hypothesis," *Psychological Reports*, 1956, 2, 183–193. (a)

LeShan, L., & Worthington, R. E., "Some Recurrent Life History Patterns Observed in Patients with Malignant Disease," *Journal of Nervous and Mental Disorders*, 1956, 124, 460–465. (b)

Scheler, M., *Vom Sinn des Leides*. Leipzig: Moralia, 1923.

Szasz, R., *Pain and Pleasure*. New York: Basic Books, 1957.

Tolstoi, L., *The Death of Ivan Illych and Other Stories*. New York: New Library of World Literature, 1960.

# 4

# The Emotional Impact of Cancer of Ear, Nose, and Throat on Patients and Their Families

*Colin Murray Parkes*

Cancer invades a family in much the same way that it invades a human body. At first, locally, there are signs that all is not well but little general reaction; then, as the tumour grows and the diagnosis becomes more obvious, there is a general mobilization of resources, [and] the family focuses attention upon the damaged part; sacrifices are made, a man may sacrifice a limb in the hope that this will save his life, his wife gives up her job or neglects the children to ensure that she can do everything to preserve him. If the sacrifices pay off he may recover, but if not there follows a period of deterioration when reserves of strength are used up, the patient's body grows thinner and weaker, and the family find that their reserves are also drained. With the patient's death the family occasionally disintegrates, but more often it begins a lengthy and painful process of restructuring whose outcome is always uncertain and sometimes disastrous to the lives of its members.

Cancers of the ear, nose, and throat are not essentially different from cancers arising in other parts of the body, although there are some problems which arise more frequently in association with these tumours than they do when the primary tumour is elsewhere. In a series of 31 patients who died from cancers of the ear, nose, and throat at St. Christopher's

*From:* Colin Murray Parkes, "The Emotional Impact of Cancer of Ear, Nose and Throat on Patients and Their Families," *Journal of Laryngology and Otology,* 1975, *89,* 1271–1278. Reprinted by permission of Headley Brothers, Ltd., Invicta Press.

Hospice, the majority had some visible deformity or some difficulty in swallowing, and there were sizeable minorities who suffered defects in communication, most often loss of speech.

Other symptoms which were frequently complained of but which were no more frequent in ear, nose, and throat patients than in those with other forms of cancer were pain, complained of by 84 per cent; anorexia, 77 per cent (usually with considerable loss of weight); dyspnoea (in 42 per cent); and, no surprise to nurses, constipation (61 per cent).

Let us look first at the overall course of events as they impinge upon the patient. In particular, let us consider the situation of the patient whose illness will end fatally. This has become the subject of a sizeable literature in recent years, and I shall not attempt to review this. In some respects the literature is confusing—thus we find some writers claiming that denial is the rule and that no patient is able to confront the prospect of his own death. On the other hand, writers such as Hinton [1967] have shown that a half of the patients whom he interviewed before death "were neither ignorant nor evasive of the fact that their illness might be fatal."

Our own figures, for what they are worth, are not much different from Hinton's. Among the 31 successive cancers of the ear, nose and throat, a third were recorded as having had full insight into diagnosis and prognosis, a third had partial insight into the diagnosis but not necessarily the prognosis, and in the remaining third there was no evidence recorded in the notes of what the patient thought. This was usually because the patient had not disclosed his ideas on the matter or asked questions which indicated a wish to know. (The case notes at St. Christopher's Hospice contain a special pink sheet on which doctors, nurses, or others are expected to record any disclosure which the patient makes about the nature of his illness.) Taken overall, only 6 per cent of all patients expressed a belief that they did not have a terminal illness or were getting better, but there were no ear, nose, and throat cases who said this, perhaps because it is difficult to deny the existence of a tumour that is usually visible to the naked eye in its later stages.

In the earlier stages, of course, denial is much easier, and most of these patients had gone through a stage when they had fully expected their treatment to be successful. Fifty-three per cent had undergone some form of surgical excision, 90 per cent had had a course of radiotherapy, and 13 per cent [had had] cytotoxic drugs.

Nobody wants to believe that they have a terminal illness, and it is not surprising to find both patient and family placing the most optimistic possible interpretation on the information which they are given by the doctor and on the outcome of the treatment which they receive. Some doctors adopt a deliberate policy of concealing the nature of the illness from the patient, though not, usually, from the family.

Despite this, it seems to me that both patients and family members are faced with the need to undergo a process of realization. By this I mean that they need to abandon one view of the world, a view which has been built up and elaborated over many years of their lives, and to substitute another, more appropriate view. This is no easy task. A man's view of his world is determined by the totality of his life experience up to the present moment, and it is not possible for him to change his basic assumptions in a moment.

Changes of this type have been termed psychosocial transitions, and they take time and energy. Several studies now indicate that psychosocial transitions follow a pattern which is not completely predictable but which is sufficiently consistent for us to be able to begin to plot its course (Parkes, 1972). If the change is relatively sudden or if it has not been expected, the most immediate reaction is likely to be one of numbness or disbelief. "I just can't take it in. It can't be true." If the situation is ambiguous, as it usually is in the early stages of cancer, then it may be possible to avoid confronting the reality of what is happening for a considerable length of time; the patient will overlook evidence that his physical state is worsening. Eventually the evidence of deterioration becomes too obvious to ignore, and he will then enter a phase of restless anxiety and pining. Having recognized that there is a major discrepancy between the world that is and the world that had been taken for granted up to now, the individual tries every way to get back the world he has lost. He goes over in his mind the events which led up to the present situation in an attempt to find what went wrong as if, even at this stage, things could be put right. He may become aggressive or angry with people whom he sees as standing in his way or blame the treatments or drugs which he has received for the symptoms which he now has. Often there is an element of what Elisabeth Kübler-Ross (1970) calls "bargaining"—"I only want to get well enough to go home once more, if I can do that, I shall be happy to come back here to die." But we should not expect the patient to keep his side of the bargain if we do enable him to get home "once more." There is always room for more bargains. Alternatively, the dying patient may seek various kinds of magical cures from unorthodox practitioners, or he may invent his own magic—"I have a theory that cancer is all psychological and that a man only has to want to get better strongly enough for it to come about," said one of my patients. Any relief of symptoms which is achieved by palliative means is then taken as evidence that the magic is working. Another patient was discharged home after being admitted for pain control. But he continued to come up to the hospital to attend my patients' group. He assured the patients in the group, "I prayed to God every day again and again, 'God cure me. God cure me,' and he's done it." Then he added as an afterthought, "Of course I'm not quite right yet, but he has cured me of the cancer." The group, at this time, had been talking about the plan of two of their members to visit Lourdes and had made a distinction between two types of miracle, the miracle of cure and the miracle of acceptance. When, subsequently, this patient's symptoms again got worse, he started thinking hard about the second type of miracle and indicated that he was now beginning to realize that he was not cured. But he still swung back to his former view when he began to get anxious.

Despite this type of oscillation there is a greater and greater tendency, as the disease progresses, for the patient to give up, a few at a time, many of the assumptions about himself which have been invalidated by the illness. He may, for instance, decide that he is not going to walk again. But that does not necessarily mean that he expects to die. And even when he decides that a fatal termination is likely, he can always place this event at some remote time in the future. Realization, therefore, tends to occur in fits and starts which often correspond to a fresh incident in the course of the illness—a new symptom appears, hospital admission is decided upon, or the patient is finally compelled to take to his bed. Events of this kind are often followed by a period of depression or "giving up." For a while he becomes apathetic, withdraws from human company, and loses interest in the world around him. But given time, and gentle encouragement, he will usually emerge from this depressive phase into a phase of quiet acceptance which will last until the next setback occurs. And if circumstances of care are good and the disease slowly progressive and not complicated by particularly unpleasant or frightening symptoms, there is every chance that the final phase of life will be peaceful and associated with a great deal of quiet enjoyment of the love and care which the family are pleased to give if only the doctors and nurses will let them.

To recapitulate, the patient, in passing from a state of relative fitness to final decline, tends to pass through four phases—(1) numbness or denial, (2) pining or struggle, (3) depression or giving up, and (4) acceptance. These phases are by no means clear-cut; he may pass backwards and forwards between them, he may be predisposed by temperament or other reasons to "get stuck" at any phase, or the disease may progress so rapidly that he dies before the sequence is completed. Nevertheless the delineation of the sequence is of some value, since it allows us some kind of a yardstick by which we can assess progress and evaluate the consequences of our care. We should not feel, for instance, that our patients should never be allowed to become depressed. This seems to be a necessary phase for most people and, provided it does not go on too long, people are best left alone to come through it.

For the family members too there is a process of realization to be gone through, and, like that of the patient, this tends to proceed in fits and starts. Because they are usually given more information at an early stage in the illness, close family members start the process sooner than the patient, and we tend to assume that they will always be one jump ahead of the patient and able to support him through the successive disappointments of the illness. But I think there is another factor operating here which helps close family members to support the patient—this is our capacity to postpone grief. You are no doubt aware of the way so many family members reply to any concern which we show for their welfare, "Don't you worry about me, Doctor, I'll be all right. He's the one you should be worrying about." By focusing all their attention on the needs of the patient and by denying that they have any needs of their own, family members usually succeed in pushing out of their minds all thoughts of the future. They are bound to do this, not only out of fear that such thoughts will cause them to "break down" and betray their feelings to the patient, but also because there are good psychological reasons why it is dangerous to anticipate and plan for one's own life after the patient's death. We don't, for instance, buy the coffin until the patient is dead for fear that such an act will hasten or bring about the death. This taboo seems to derive from the association between a plan and a wish—if we plan for something we may come to wish it, and in terms of mental dynamics a wish is akin to the acts which bring it about. Hence the woman who plans what she will do when her husband dies may end up feeling that it was her plans which killed him—she will be the murderer.

It seems, then, that however drawn out the patient's death may be, there is still a process of realization to be undertaken after his death. The death itself may be a relief. Even so, within a short time those who are closest to the patient will usually find themselves grieving.

If the death was rapid or in any way unexpected, there will usually be an immediate reaction of numbness or disbelief. But since death is such an unambiguous event, this will not normally last for more than a few hours to a few days. The survivor will then enter a phase of pining or struggle in which he or she finds herself going over in her mind the events leading up to the loss, bitterly seeking for something or someone to blame, and restlessly searching as if she could somehow recover the person who is now lost to her. So strong is her need to search that she may even misidentify sights and sounds around her as indicating the return of the lost person. She may think she sees her husband's car approaching along the road or catch sight of him in the street. But such misapprehensions are fleeting and soon disproved by experience. Nevertheless, a strong sense of the unseen presence of the dead person is less easily disproved and may persist for many years as a normal accompaniment of grief.

As time passes, however, the intensity and duration of these episodes of pining, the so-called "pangs of grief" tends to diminish and the bereaved person becomes apathetic and withdrawn, feeling that there is now no hope of recovering the person who has died and no future left worth living for. Only slowly and intermittently does he or she emerge from this depressive phase to accept the loss and to find new directions and new purposes in life. The total process of grieving after a major bereavement, say the loss of a husband by a woman of 50, will probably take several years, and even then it is possible for events which bring back the memory of the lost person to initiate yet another episode of pining. This is surprising when we compare it with the grief of the dying patient, for this is often completed within a few weeks or months. I would hazard a guess that there are two factors which hasten the process of transition in the patient —one is the progression of the illness itself which, in the case of most cancers, gradually seems to reduce a person's appetite for life or *vis a tergo*. The other is the fact that, since there are no realistic plans which a person can make for living after his death, there is no need for him to begin the struggle to rehabilitate himself. All that he needs to do is to accept the "here and now" situation.

Interestingly, the way a person reacts to his illness may affect the duration of his life. Thus Weisman and Worden (1975) have shown in a recent paper that patients with cancer who subsequently died sooner than had been expected (from statistical studies of the particular form of cancer from which they were suffering), were significantly more likely than other patients to have reacted to their illness by becoming lastingly pessimistic, depressed and wishing for death. They were also likely to have been people who had suffered childhood losses and to have had lasting difficulties in making social relationships. On the other hand patients who had good relations with others, received close and intimate support from family and friends, accepted the seriousness of their illness, cooperated in treatment but in the end, accepted their fate, particularly if they were Jewish and of low socioeconomic status, tended to survive longer than predicted.

The implications of this are clear. If we can help the patient and his family to come to terms with the illness, to stay close to each other, and to develop the type of closeness with the medical and nursing staff which reassures them that they will not be allowed to suffer and that we can be relied upon to stay close whatever happens, we shall not only make patient and family more contented, but we may even prolong life.

We need to show them by our behaviour (and nonverbal behaviour is much more important than words) that we feel secure and confident— not by making unrealistic promises but by trying to create an atmosphere in which, as one patient put it to me, "It is safe to die here." This does not mean that we have to force every patient to face facts which he is frightened to face. But once we have created such an environment, we shall often find that the patient will himself tell us the diagnosis or the prognosis—all we have to do is to confirm what he already knows.

Problems will arise, and there are some which are especially difficult for patients with a cancer of the ear, nose, or throat. The most difficult to handle are, perhaps, the communication defects. The patient who can no longer speak is not only disabled himself, but he disables every one of us who tries to communicate with him. We too feel frustrated and annoyed by his inability to talk, and it is only too easy for us to withdraw, to stop trying to understand. I was recently asked to see just such a patient who had become very depressed after losing her speech. I suggested that she bring out a news sheet for her fellow patients. Her reply reads, "Patients don't want four-letter words"—which is all she felt like uttering. Only great patience on the part of the nursing staff, with, perhaps, the judicious use of a tranquilizer or antidepressant when needed to enable the withdrawn patient to feel secure enough to make the effort to communicate, will succeed in a case like this.

Fears are not always justified. We should enquire about any family members who have died from cancer, because a person who has seen someone else die will tend to expect the same end if they have a similar disease. This may be reassuring if the circumstances of care are good and the death a peaceful one. But one woman of 55 was terrified when I first went to see her. She lay with her head one inch above the pillow and edged away from me in the bed. It transpired that her sister had also had a cancer of the throat and had had a bad time during the six months she took to die. She had been tube-fed and our patient said she would rather "get it over now" than go through all that. Her thyroid tumour was hurting her whenever she swallowed, and before we could do anything else to help her it was essential to relieve her pain. Once that was done she gradually relaxed and allowed the staff to come closer. With their support she expressed appropriate grief for the loss of the home she loved and her husband and 13-year-old son. She seemed to be coming through this when she died suddenly and unexpectedly from a pulmonary embolus.

Pain was also a problem in a man of 60 with a huge invasive growth affecting the left mandible and lower part of the face. He was deeply depressed and asking for euthanasia when first admitted, but even if we had not been opposed to giving this in his own account it was clear that his wife was not yet ready for him to die. She had the idea that we could simply relieve his pain and he would then be fit to return home again. In fact the patient was very ill indeed and there was never any prospect of him returning home. It was possible, however, to relieve his pain and to give him the kind of attention which made life tolerable for him again though it was never pleasant. His wife then found it possible to relax and to find security to prepare herself for his death. Two weeks after his admission she said to me for the first time, "I'm ready for him to go now." He died quietly the following day.

For the person who has suffered a lot of pain, the fear of pain is almost as much of a problem as the pain itself. We need to convince the patient both by our words and our actions that we understand this and that we shall never allow him to suffer severe pain again. To fulfill this promise we tend to give four-hourly doses of narcotic drugs in whatever dosage is necessary to prevent pain. In the majority of cases it is possible to achieve relief from pain without seriously impairing the patient's mental faculties. In our series of 31 deaths from cancer of the ear, nose, and throat, only 10 per cent were said to have been unconscious during the period preceding death; consciousness was blurred in another 13 per cent; 74 per cent were classed as "peaceful." There were only two patients (6 per cent) who were said to have been "distressed" at the time of death.

The surprising thing is the fact that, despite the awful forms which terminal cancers of the ear, nose, and throat can take, so many patients do eventually seem to come to terms with it. Let me give one more example. Mrs. Harris, a woman of 46, was dying from a carcinoma of the oral cavity of five years' duration. She had undergone, successively, a hemiglossectomy, a hemimandibulectomy, and, after a severe haemorrhage from the tongue, a ligation of the internal carotid artery which had caused the remaining half of her tongue to slough and left her in severe pain. Her husband, who attempted to care for her at home, later regretted that this operation had ever been carried out and claimed that it would have been kinder to have let her die. By the time she came to us, the tumour had extended into her cranial cavity and produced diplopia. She was unable to speak and had dysphagia which was so severe that she had to stand up in order to swallow fluids.

Despite all this Mrs. Harris, once her pain was relieved, became amazingly cheerful. She enchanted the nurses, who became quite devoted to her, and the brief periods of depression which she suffered were quite appropriately associated with further deterioration in her condition and soon passed. Three days before her death her husband, who had at first felt that he was of no more use to her, admitted, and I quote, "It's like heaven here"—by which remark he seemed to be expressing his awareness of the contrast between her present condition and her former state when he had struggled to care for her at home.

During the last six days of her life it was necessary to increase Mrs. Harris' diamorphine dosage to 60 mg by intramuscular injection four-hourly, but although this made her drowsy she remained in touch until she died peacefully in her husband's arms.

Because of the nature of their symptoms, a large proportion of patients with ear, nose, and throat cancers will probably need to be cared for in hospital. But that does not mean that they may not also be able to spend much time at home provided the circumstances of care are good and the family are properly supported. To do this we make use of a team of three visiting nurses who provide a very efficient consulting service for families, GPs [general practitioners], and district nurses.

Unfortunately there is no time to describe that work in detail. Nor is there time for me to describe the two major research projects which have now demonstrated the efficacy of the type of inpatient care which is provided at St. Christopher's Hospice from the viewpoint of patients and families.

In conclusion I must point out that terminal care does not necessarily end with the death of a patient. At that point the patient's troubles are, we hope, at an end, but those of the surviving family members may just be beginning.

At St. Christopher's Hospice we rely upon assessments made by the ward staff to identify any family members who are likely to get into difficulties after bereavement. At the present time we are visiting about 20 per cent of bereaved families in their homes 10 to 14 days after the funeral and giving whatever help seems to be needed in succeeding weeks to see the family through the psychosocial transition of bereavement. The visits are made by someone who is already known to the family; this is usually a nurse. The visitors meet with me once a month to discuss any problems which have arisen.

In a random-allocation trial, which will be reported in detail elsewhere, 19 "high-risk" family members who had been supported in this way have been compared with 22 who had received no such support. The supported group 20 months after bereavement were distinguished from the control group in having significantly less depression, fewer psychosomatic symptoms reflecting persisting anxiety and autonomic symptoms, and less inclination to increase in their consumption of alcohol, tobacco, and tranquilizers.

We conclude that a little support given to a family before the patient's death and during the first few weeks of bereavement can go a very long way.

## References

Hinton, J., *Dying*. Harmondsworth: Penguin Books, 1967.

Kübler-Ross, E., *On Death and Dying*. London: Tavistock, 1970.

Parkes, C. M., "Components of the Reaction to Loss of a Limb, Spouse or Home," *Journal of Psychosomatic Research*, 1972, *16*, 343–349.

Weisman, A. D., & Worden, J. W., "Psychosocial Analysis of Cancer Deaths," *Omega*, 1975, *6*, 61–75.

# 5

# The Hospice Concept— The Adult with Advanced Cancer

*Sylvia A. Lack*

The hospice programs which exist in Britain and in New Haven, Connecticut have grown out of the needs of patients and families in the communities they serve. Emergent hospices must first assess the needs of people in their own area, survey the available resources, and tailor a program to meet the situation. It is possible that such a study will reveal that a hospice is not needed in certain communities. However, if a decision is made to start a hospice, it must be realized that this involves a commitment to provide all the necessary elements of care now recognized. These include symptom control, emotional and spiritual support, home care, a follow-up bereavement program, and an informal, relaxed approach to the patient and family.

It is not only the patients who need help. Chronic illness, a death in the family, each has wide repercussions; it is thus the whole family, and not just the patient, who must be the unit of care.

The major goals of Hospice in New Haven are to

1. Provide physical and psychological care for the patient suffering from an illness diagnosed as terminal.
2. Care for the families of dying patients during illness and bereavement.

From: Sylvia A. Lack, "The Hospice Concept—The Adult with Advanced Cancer," in *Proceedings of the American Cancer Society Second National Conference on Human Values and Cancer* (Chicago: American Cancer Society 1977), pp. 160–166. Reprinted by permission of the American Cancer Society, Inc.

3. Provide a support system to help people live effectively in the face of impending death.
4. Be a center for the teaching and study of terminal care in the United States.

St. Christopher's Hospice in London, England, cares for people suffering from cancer or other long-term illness. Many of them die in the Hospice, though about 12 percent are able to go home after their pain and other symptoms have been controlled. Patients with a terminal illness need more personal care than do those whose sickness can be cured. This care must be the best that skilled nursing and medicine can provide, and must keep abreast of every modern development. Such care is provided under a total program embodying the following essential characteristics:

1. Coordinated home care–inpatient beds under a central autonomous hospice administration.
2. Physician-directed services.
3. Control of symptoms (physical, sociological, psychological, spiritual).
4. Provision of care by an interdisciplinary team.
5. Services available on a 24-hour-a-day/7-day-a-week/on-call basis with emphasis on availability of medical and nursing skills.
6. Patient/family regarded as the unit of care.
7. Bereavement follow-up.
8. Utilization of volunteers as an integral part of the interdisciplinary team.
9. Structured staff support and communications system.
10. Patients should be accepted to the program on the basis of health needs, not ability to pay.

## Coordinated Home Care–Inpatient Beds under a Central Autonomous Hospice Administration

The hospice concept—as brought from Britain to the United States—implies a separate free-standing facility for care of patients with a terminal illness. Indeed, Saunders (1973) has written that "those patients who do not need the manifold resources of a large hospital and who cannot be cared for at home are frequently better cared for and happier in a smaller, specialized unit." Lawrence Burke, Program Director for NCI [the National Cancer Institute], has emphatically stated (1977) that there will be no grant funds available to any hospice facility which is not separate and free-standing. It is not difficult to argue that a free-standing hospice with all the necessary elements of care is needed as a focal point for the nation, a demonstration of the total program.

However, any new program must be examined carefully to determine who it will fit within the locale, recognizing that each geographic area is a separate entity with unique characteristics. The Palliative Care Unit at the Royal Victoria Hospital in Montreal and the Symptom Control Team in St. Luke's Hospital of New York have pioneered in exploring other ways of providing hospice care. There is no doubt that establishing free-standing facilities is time-consuming. In the United States it involves certificate-of-need approval from a planning agency; in view of the over-bedding of facilities in many states, this is a laborious process. We must explore all possibilities to bring relief to suffering patients and families as soon as possible, but this urgency must not force us into accepting substandard care. Any group planning a hospice unit within a hospital or nursing home must ensure that elements of the program not usually available in these settings are provided. Extra funds will be needed for adequate medical direction, recruitment of volunteers, education of staff, and 24-hour-a-day/7-day-a-week availability of a home care service.

Many patients want to stay at home if there is nothing more that the hospital can offer them. Most cannot stay at home because the care they need in terms of symptom control, medical attention, nursing expertise, and social work help, is all hospital-based. If this care is taken into the home, families do the most amazing things! They want to help, and they ask for support to enable them to do what they are willing to do. The consistent pattern which I have seen in Britain and in New Haven is that a large number of families desire to care for their dying relatives at home, and that a large number of dying people wish to stay at home. What they need is the support to enable them to do that. What is such support? A lady whose father had just died defined it thus: "Hospice was my backbone; they held me up so that my hands were free to care for my father" (Lack, 1977).

## Physician-Directed Services

Patients and families consistently report feelings of medical abandonment. All too frequent is the sad comment, "Well, I seem to have lost Dr. Q. somewhere along the way." There is a time in a patient's illness when the health care professionals begin to feel that there is nothing more they can do, and it is this loss of their doctor's interest that patients fear most. When a patient elects to remain home for his last weeks, this decision frequently cuts him off from effective medical care because many physicians do not make home visits. We see many patients seriously ill, suffering from vomiting, pain, and other controllable symptoms, bedfast at home, who have not seen a doctor for many weeks. Others find that if they do struggle to the office or a hospital clinic, they see a resident while the person they regard as their doctor is with patients who can be cured. It is vital to the psychological well-being of the patient with terminal illness that the physician is a key figure in the care he receives. This is not only psychologically important; it is also essential to his physical well-being.

In existing hospices the doctors are focal points because of their medical skills and because they provide inspiration, leadership, and a link with the powerful medical community. In each hospice the physician is very involved as a member of the caring team. His essential contribution is reviewing the diagnosis and thereafter relieving troublesome symptoms. The "last straw" at home is often disturbed nights when relatives fail to secure adequate rest. After eliminating common causes for the patient's restlessness (pain, constipation leading to confusion, etc.), the most natural way to secure a quiet night is to ensure activity during the day. Families need practical advice on how to provide daytime stimulation and activity for the patient. Physical, recreational, or dance therapy may be very helpful.

Management is a good term to use when working with the dying, because it suggests attention to all aspects of care, while treatment tends to be more restrictive, often referring only to disease-specific therapy. Successful management means accurate diagnosis, psychological and material support for hardpressed families, and more practical items such as day care, hospital beds, and "family respite" admissions.

## Symptom Control

There is far too much talk in thanatology circles in this country about psychological and emotional problems, and far too little about making the patient comfortable. Any group concerned with service to the dying should be talking about smoothing sheets, rubbing bottoms, relieving constipation, and sitting up at night. Counseling a dying person who is lying in a wet bed is ineffective. Such concerns loom large in the lives of critically ill patients and must be of importance to the physician if the physician is to treat the whole person. A certain amount of interdisciplinary role blurring may be necessary to ensure patient comfort at all times.

If people are cared for with common sense and basic professional skills, with detailed attention to self-evident problems and physical needs, then patients and families themselves can cope with many of their emotional crises. Without pain, well-nursed, with bowels controlled, with mouth clean, and with a caring friend available, the psychological problems fall into manageable perspective.

Any physician who is dealing with a number of patients with terminal illness must become interested in symptom control and skilled in the management of the various types of physical distress. Sadly, the terminal stage has been defined by some as beginning at the moment when the doctor says, "There is nothing more to be done," and then begins to withdraw subtly from the patient. Patients, of course, are very well aware when this happens. There is never a time when "nothing more can be done." There may indeed be nothing more that can be done to cure the disease, but there are always further measures to be taken for the comfort of the patient and family.

I will illustrate this approach by a discussion of the problem of pain. The pain of a terminal illness is not just a physical pain. By the time the patient has reached the terminal stage of his disease, he is suffering from many other types of pain, including mental, financial, interpersonal, and spiritual. One needs to pay attention to the whole person if one is to affect the complaint of pain.

The aims of treatment are

1. To identify the etiology.
2. To prevent pain.
3. To help the patient be alert.
4. To maintain normal affect.
5. To maintain easy administration.

Identification of the etiology is a clinical diagnosis, and investigations should be limited to a basic few; however, it must be remembered that not all pain suffered by the cancer patient is due to the cancer.

The pain should be controlled so that it will not return; continual pain control is the aim. When the blood sugar of diabetics is controlled, the physician does not wait for coma to develop before giving insulin. Instead, it is determined what insulin dose prevents acute manifestations of the disease. This dose is then administered on a regular basis. The same principle of regular dosage is used in chronic pain control.

An alert patient with normal affect relates normally with his family and friends; drugs are not used to produce euphoria.

Finally, a treatment is needed which is easy to administer. If pain control is achieved with continuous IV [intravenous] morphine infusion, patient options in terms of locale are limited. Ideally, a treatment is sought that gives greatest ease and freedom of movement. Forty percent of all cancer patients can be expected to have severe pain. Such pain must be thought of in terms of anxiety, depression, and insomnia as well as physical pain [Figure 5.1]. Unless pain is reviewed with all of these components in mind, control will not be achieved. Anxiety and depression are part of the chronic nature of pain. The patient is anxious about the pain returning; she or he is anxious because of the meaning of the pain. This is not the acute pain that we think of as pain. It is not like the pain of toothache or childbirth or appendicitis, pains which have a foreseeable end. Such pain is serving a purpose by warning of a malfunction. Pain for the cancer patient has a sinister meaning. If I wake up in the morning with a stiff neck, I assume I slept in a draft. The cancer patient wakes up in the morning with a stiff neck and assumes she or he has metastases. The degree of perceived pain is totally different in these two situations. One must take into account the anxiety that these patients are suffering, along with the chronic depression caused by chronic pain.

Narcotics should be reserved for severe physical pain. Narcotics should be started when non-narcotic medication, used correctly, has failed

Figure 5.1.　Pharmacologic Management of Chronic Terminal Pain

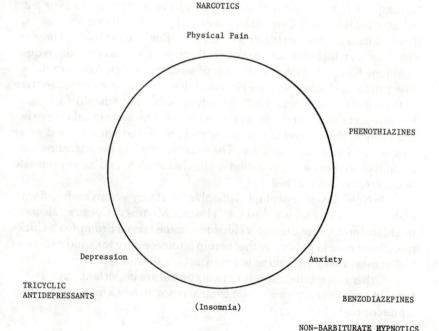

NARCOTICS

Physical Pain

PHENOTHIAZINES

Depression

Anxiety

TRICYCLIC
ANTIDEPRESSANTS

(Insomnia)

BENZODIAZEPINES

NON-BARBITURATE HYPNOTICS

to control the pain. Patients should not be required to wait until they have only hours or days to live. Narcotics are used when medications and pain control measures, such as spinal block or traction, have failed. At Hospice, narcotics are almost always combined with a phenothiazine, routinely Compazine (or prochlorperazine). A phenothiazine is used with the narcotic for several reasons. First, it potentiates the narcotic so that a lower dosage of narcotic can be used. Second, it is an antiemetic. (Since narcotics are taken orally, the phenothiazine is utilized as an antiemetic.) Finally, it is a tranquilizer, which helps with the anxiety component of pain. Other anxiolytic drugs such as the benzodiazepines—Valium and Librium—may be used in combination with a phenothiazine, or, very rarely, alone with the narcotics. Tricyclics are used as antidepressants. Amitriptyline is probably the best known. One needs judgment and experience to treat the depression of terminal illness. Depression may be a perfectly appropriate and necessary reaction or stage—a response to the realization of death. Because somebody is depressed, one does not automatically rush in with an antidepressant. But if depression is an identifiable component of perceived pain, one may find that the addition of a tricyclic antidepressant gets rid of that last vestige of pain.

We look for the dose that controls pain but does not sedate the patient. This may be within a very fine dosage range. If a narcotic is increased in jumps of 10 mg, the optimum dose may be missed because a 1- or 2-mg adjustment is needed. One of the reasons why we give narcotics as an oral liquid is because one can titrate a liquid more finely than tablets. There are two ways in which this can be done: If the patient is in severe pain, requiring immediate relief, even at the cost of sedation, a high dose is initiated. The patient and the family are informed that sedation is expected for two or three days. The dose is gradually reduced until the pain returns; a small increase and the pain-free interval is achieved. The more usual way of accomplishing this, especially on home care, is to start with a low dose of narcotic and build up gradually. The sedative effect of the narcotic wears off in two to three days, sedation is largely avoided, and an appropriate dosage regimen is reached.

In New Haven, morphine is dissolved in cherry syrup combined with a phenothiazine. This is called the "Hospice Mixture." Cocaine, alcohol, or chloroform water are not included as in the classic Brompton's Cocktail. Please note in particular that heroin is unnecessary for good pain control in most cases. Morphine is a satisfactory substitute.

Other less specific aspects of pain control are important, such as distraction and other activities. Pain control is not merely a matter of writing a prescription.

# Twenty-Four-Hour-a-Day / Seven-Day-a-Week Availability

Emergencies all too often occur at night and on weekends when help is scarce. A husband who reluctantly placed his wife in a convalescent home for the last three months of her life described the kind of stress that forced her admission. He remembered, with vivid horror, the time her gastrostomy tube fell out at 3:00 A.M. and he tried to replace it according to phone instructions from an unknown emergency room physician.

The fear and anxiety engendered by even the thought of such a crisis causes many families to give up home care. Having emergency care available in the home from medical and nursing staff gives families and patients the security and support they need to continue.

# Interdisciplinary Team

Individuals often have a limited view of patients with a terminal illness and fail to address the complexity of the problems they present.

The management of the dying must be a team concern. The team includes the patient, his immediate family or friends, his doctor, clergyman, nurses, social worker, volunteers, and other health workers. Continuity of management forms an important element of the total care. Interdisciplinary care must not be a synonym for fragmented care in which the bewildered patient does not know who is in charge or who is dealing with which problem. Real teamwork mandates that interdisciplinary personnel sit down together at regular conferences to work out a plan of care for the patient and family and to learn each other's languages.

# The Family as the Unit of Care and Bereavement Follow-Up

The main burden of home care falls on families and friends. These caregivers must receive adequate help and advice. The sympathetic listener who indicates understanding of the tension and frustration is an essential member of any effective team. Families must be made aware of the help that is available and be assured of its arrival when needed. Nothing contributes to the "end of the tether" syndrome as much as the sense of being hopelessly beleaguered when nobody cares or wants to know. When inpatient admission is required it should be made possible within 24 hours, preferably immediately. Failure to provide timely aid leads to admission to a long-stay facility earlier in the illness. Such an admission often indicates too little help at home, but is commonly construed as yet another manifestation of uncaring relatives and disintegrating family systems.

After the death the dismembered family lives on and may need ongoing aid to prevent the morbidity and mortality of grief described by Parkes (1972). Indeed the health care staff also live on, and attention to their need to grieve is essential if this demanding work is to continue.

## Volunteers

St. Christopher's and St. Luke's in England have demonstrated that in-facility volunteers can be, and should be, effectively utilized as an integral part of an interdisciplinary team. Hospice in New Haven has extended this principle by taking volunteers into the home, where they play an indispensable role in keeping the patient at home.

### Example 1

An exhausted wife was in tears because she could not continue her husband's 24-hour care, and admission to hospital seemed unavoidable. Emergency introduction of two volunteers to "patient-sit" enabled her to spend a full 24 hours in a neighbor's home and return refreshed with long-term help promised from her church congregation.

### Example 2

A 67-year-old man died at home; his wife carried the full brunt of his care while he was bedridden for the last two months of his life. The highlight of her week was the weekly car drive with one of our male volunteers. Sometimes they did errands, but more often they would take a scenic drive. The evening before the trip Mrs. G. would be smartly dressed with makeup on. This well-groomed turnout would last for two or three days after the trip, then she would gradually slip back into the dowdiness characteristic of the essentially homebound—but right on schedule, the day before her next trip, she would be all spruced up again. On other days, volunteers were also in the home helping with the housework or sitting with Mr. G. while his wife popped out to do the shopping. There is no doubt that without them, Mr. G. would not have died at home.

The volunteer is also uniquely able to help the patient maintain or reestablish his sense of self-worth. The dependency and reduction in functioning created by a disability eats away at self-esteem. Withdrawal of professionals as they try to cope with their own feelings of inadequacy reinforces the patient's diminishing sense of personhood. The volunteer, by forming a close, friendly relationship, can counteract this demeaning process. We give our volunteers basic orientation to the program but do not attempt to turn them into "counselors" for the dying. Their special value is as a person with whom the patient can identify. He sees them as "people like myself." He discusses many areas with the lay volunteer that he does not discuss with the professionals.

For one of our low-income families, the volunteer who took the patient fishing was the only person able to provide any meaningful aid. Doctors, nurses, social workers, psychiatric services had all been employed in attempts to help him and his family deal with their multiple problems. All had been consistently rejected. The only person who was accepted was the man who took him fishing, and in the course of those trips discussed, on a person-to-person basis, the philosophies and fears the patient was encountering. It is important to meet the patient on his own ground.

## Patients Should Be Accepted to the Program on the Basis of Health Needs, Not Ability to Pay

Patients are accepted on the basis of health care need, not on ability to pay. No British hospice discriminates against patients because of their financial status, and American hospices must also strive to uphold this high standard of care. We cannot avoid our responsibility in this area by reference to socialized medicine. Most of the hospices in Britain are not under the National Health Service. They are financed by a combination of charitable donations, patient contributions, and government reimbursement.

Increasingly effective therapies which slow down but do not cure the disease make it inevitable that persons with chronic degenerative diseases will live longer in a dependent state. We have to take a much more positive interest in their problems, and realize the satisfaction of successfully meeting the management challenge presented by these patients and their families.

## References

Burke, L., Lecture for the Washington Hospice Committee, Washington, D.C., April 16, 1977.

Lack, S. A., "I Want to Die While I'm Still Alive," *Death Education*, 1977, 1, 165–176.

Parkes, C. M., *Bereavement: Studies of Grief in Adult Life*. New York: International Universities Press, 1972.

Rose, M. A., & Pories, W. J., "Some Additional Notes on Hospice," *The Ohio State Medical Journal*, 1977, 73, 379–382.

Saunders, C., "The Need for In-Patient Care for the Patient with Terminal Cancer," *Middlesex Hospital Journal*, 1973, 72, 125–130.

Twycross, R. G., "Relief of Terminal Pain," *British Medical Journal*, 1975, 4, 212–214.

# II

# Analgesics
# and Polypharmacy

We have already noted in Part I the difference between acute and
chronic pain. The latter, especially in its severe forms, is a complex and
multidimensional entity. As such, it has rightly been called "total pain."
Management of such pain must respect its uniqueness and address its
many aspects. A comprehensive program of caregiving will involve
much more than just medication. Nevertheless, drug regimes for terminal illness are in many cases a prerequisite for other forms of intervention and for successful caregiving. Other responses are addressed in
Part III; here we confine ourselves to analgesics and polypharmacy.

Although the basic goals of drug therapy should be similar in both
cure- and care-oriented contexts, distinctive aspects of the situation of
dying persons call for distinctive responses. For example, the aim of
clinical pharmacology in terminal illness is not simply that of responding to pain, but its prevention and (ideally) erasure of the very memory
of pain. In the first two selections here, Robert Twycross and Arthur
Lipman describe both the practice and the underlying principles for
achieving this aim. A high level of sensitivity, understanding, and professional expertise is required for both assessment and management of
pain in dying persons. Physicians must use the analgesic that is required, determine the proper dose, and administer it regularly. What is
needed is the right drug, in the right amount, given in the right way and
at the right time—that is, on a schedule planned to match individual
needs.

Many misperceptions and a good deal of misinformation bedevil
this area of the hospice philosophy. Twycross and Lipman strive to dismiss fears of addiction, insistence upon heroin as a uniquely valuable
analgesic, and adherence to the Brompton's Cocktail or similar complex
mixtures. At the same time, they also seek to encourage therapeutic

*dosages, oral administration, regular scheduling, the use of morphine, and a general confidence that analgesia can be achieved in most cases without undue side effects. With the availability of commercial morphine solutions and the prospect of new morphine compounds whose solubility will match the advantage of heroin for small volume in injections, there is every reason to look for widespread improvements in pain management in terminal illness. In this area, advanced hospice units which deal with a particularly severe range of patient problems have demonstrated what can be achieved. The resources are at hand and careful hospice management has shown the way to their proper use.*

 *Of course, pain is not the only source of distress to dying persons. Hospice care anticipates side effects from narcotic analgesics and simultaneously addresses other symptoms that can be relieved by a comprehensive program of polypharmacy. This is especially well represented here by the latest edition of St. Christopher's brochure,* Drug Control of Common Symptoms, *edited by Mary Baines. This document outlines a simple, practical approach to relieving common problems, and one that has been demonstrated by the premier hospice unit over the years to be effective.*

# 6

# Principles and Practice of Pain Relief in Terminal Cancer

*Robert G. Twycross*

Many patients dying of cancer do so only after weeks or months of uncontrolled pain, so perpetuating the belief that death from cancer is inevitably a painful, sordid business. In fact, published reports suggest that no more than 60% of patients with far-advanced cancer experience pain. Data concerning the incidence of unrelieved pain are harder to come by. By means of postbereavement visits to the surviving spouse of patients under 65 years of age, Parkes (1976) concluded that 20% of cancer patients dying in hospital and almost a third of those dying at home do so with their "severe and mostly continuous pain" unrelieved. By contrast, at St. Christopher's Hospice—a hospital specialising in the care of patients with terminal disease—the percentage of patients with severe pain fell after admission from 36% to 8%.

There are many reasons for failure to control pain in far-advanced cancer (Table 6.1). There is undoubtedly a tendency for a doctor to allow his or her objectivity to become submerged under a shower of negative emotion. The first step therefore is to recognise this and to discipline oneself to maintain an analytical approach in this area as in other areas of clinical practice.

Table 6.1
Common Reasons for Unrelieved Pain

I.  Fault with patient and/or family

    1.  Patient believes that pain in cancer is inevitable and untreatable.
    2.  Patient fails to contact family practitioner.
    3.  Patient misleads doctor by "putting on a brave face."
    4.  Patient fails to accept or take prescribed medication and does not
        "believe in" tablets.
    5.  Patient believes that one should only take analgesics "if absolutely
        necessary."
    6.  Patient or family fears "addiction."
    7.  Patient believes that tolerance will rapidly develop, leaving nothing
        "for when things get really bad."
    8.  Patient stops medication because of side effects and fails to notify
        doctor.

II. Fault with doctor and/or nurse

    1.  Doctor ignores patient's pain because he or she believes that it is
        inevitable and intractable.
    2.  Doctor does not appreciate the intensity of patient's pain; fails to
        get behind the "brave face."
    3.  Doctor prescribes an analgesic that is too weak to relieve much or any
        of the pain.
    4.  Doctor prescribes an analgesic to be taken "as required" (prn).
    5.  Doctor fails to appreciate that standard doses (derived from post-
        operative studies) have no relevance in the management of cancer pain.
    6.  Doctor fails to give patient adequate instructions about optimal use
        of the analgesic prescribed.
    7.  Due to lack of knowledge about relative analgesic potency, doctor
        either reduces or fails to increase the absolute analgesic dose when
        transferring from one preparation to another.
    8.  Doctor fears that patient will become "addicted" if a narcotic analgesic
        is prescribed.
    9.  Doctor regards morphine/diamorphine as drugs to be reserved until the
        patient is "really terminal" (moribund), and continues to prescribe
        inadequate doses of less efficacious drugs.
    10. Doctor fails to institute adequate follow-up arrangements in order
        to monitor patient's progress.
    11. Doctor does not know about "coanalgesics" and other drugs that are of
        value in situations where narcotics are only partially effective.
    12. Doctor fails to use nondrug measures when appropriate.
    13. Doctor fails to give adequate emotional support to the patient and
        family.

1.  *Thou shalt not assume that the patient's pain is caused by the malignant
    process.*

As always, diagnosis must precede treatment. Careful assessment is
much helped by the use of a body image on which to record pain data (Figure 6.1). Not only is it of value as a baseline for future reference, but it
helps in the consideration of underlying pain mechanisms. In a survey of
100 terminal cancer patients experiencing pain, 80 had more than one
pain; 34 had four or more pains (Figure 6.2). About half the patients had
pain associated with both malignant and coexistent nonmalignant disease,
and 14 had pain relating to current or past anticancer treatment (Table

Figure 6.1. Pain Chart of 65-Year-Old Male with Carcinoma of Prostate

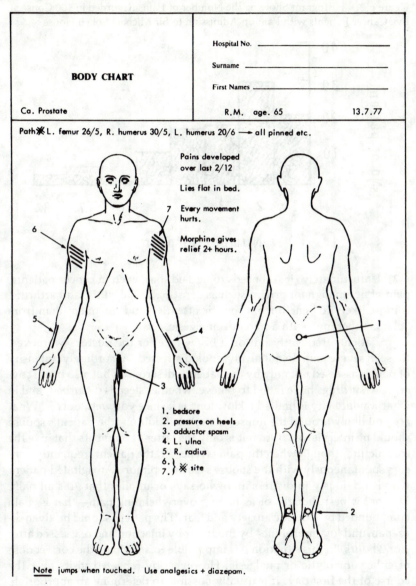

From: R. G. Twycross, "Bone Pain in Advanced Cancer," in D. W. Vere (Ed.), *Topics in Therapeutics, 4* (Turnbridge Wells, England: Pitman Medical Publishing, 1978), 94–110. Reproduced by permission of Pitman Medical Publishing.

*Note:* Adductor spasm is usually protective (i.e., secondary to involvement of the pubis); treatment is as for bone pain, though sometimes diazepam may also be necessary.

Figure 6.2.   Histogram Showing the Number of Pains Recorded in 100 Consecutive Cancer Patients with Pain on Admission to Sir Michael Sobell House

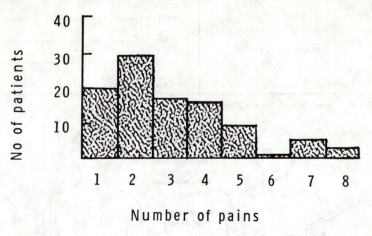

Number of pains

6.2). Unfortunately, it still needs to be said that, even in cancer patients, pain of nonmalignant origin, such as constipation, cystitis, and arthritis, is more likely to benefit from specific attention and treatment than from "blanket therapy" with a narcotic analgesic.

Patients frequently put on a brave face for the doctor. Moreover, those in severe pain do not always look distressed. Accordingly, intensity of pain is assessed not only by the patient's description but also by discovering what drugs have failed to relieve, whether sleep is disturbed, and in what way activity is limited ("How long is it since you went out?", "What are you doing around the house?", etc.). In addition, the patient's spouse should be interviewed. Often it is only the latter's comments that give the true picture, though when the pain is relieved, the patient frequently concurs spontaneously with the spouse's earlier opinion. An agitated patient who is obviously in distress and who says or implies that "It's all pain, Doctor" is best thought of as having overwhelming pain—that is, pain compounded by extreme anxiety and fear. The patient should be given diazepam and (dia)morphine* by mouth or by injection and reassessed after 1 or 2 hours. In this situation it is impossible to anticipate the correct dose of either anxiolytic or analgesic. However, by repeated visits over the course of the first day, it is usually possible to determine an appropriate combination of doses to ensure that the patient has a reasonable rest that night.

*Diamorphine (diacetylmorphine, heroin) is available only in a few countries, notably Britain; it is *not* available in the United States.

Table 6.2
Pain in Terminal Cancer

| 1. Caused by cancer: | 2. Related to cancer: | 3. Related to therapy: | 4. Unrelated to cancer or therapy: |
|---|---|---|---|
| Soft tissue infiltration | Constipation | Post-operative neuralgia | Migraine |
| Visceral involvement | Bedsore | Post-radiation fibrosis | Tension headache |
| Bone ± muscle spasm | Lymphoedema | Post-chemotherapy neuropathy | Osteoarthritis |
| Nerve compression | Candidosis | Phantom limb pain | Rheumatoid arthritis |
| Raised intra-cranial pressure | Herpetic neuralgia | Post-radiation myelopathy | Musculo-skeletal |
| Ulceration ± infection | Deep vein thrombosis | | |
| | Pulmonary embolus | | |

**2.** *Thou shalt take into consideration the patient's feelings.*

It is not so much a lack of knowledge or of means that is responsible for much of today's unrelieved pain, but rather a failure by doctors and nurses to appreciate fully that pain is not simply a physical sensation. Pain is, in fact, a dual phenomenon, one part being the perception of the sensation and the other the patient's psychological reaction to it. It follows then that a person's pain threshold will vary according to mood and morale. For any given noxious stimulus, the pain experienced varies from ache to agony and depends on the psychological reaction of the sufferer to his or her discomfort. Attention must be paid, therefore, to factors that modulate pain threshold, such as anxiety, depression, and fatigue (Table 6.3). Much can be done to alleviate pain by explaining the mechanism underlying the pain (this reduces anxiety) and by continuing concern for the patient (this raises morale).

It is perhaps in cancer pain that the interaction of the physical and the psychological is most apparent. Whatever patients may know and have accepted about diagnosis and prognosis, the course of the illness—

Table 6.3
Factors Affecting Pain Threshold

| Threshold lowered | Threshold raised |
|---|---|
| Discomfort | Relief of symptoms |
| Insomnia | Sleep |
| Fatigue | Rest |
| Anxiety | Sympathy |
| Fear | Understanding |
| Anger | Companionship |
| Sadness | Diversional activity |
| Depression | Reduction in anxiety |
| Boredom | Elevation of mood |
| Introversion | ----------------- |
| Mental isolation | Analgesics |
| Social abandonment | Anxiolytics |
| | Antidepressants |

loss of appetite and weight, less energy, more symptoms, more time off work, increasing visits to the hospital, and more frequent periods of in-patient treatment—means that any pain will be seen not as a useful (posi-tive) warning but as a (negative) threat both to their way of life and to their very existence. The lack of positive meaning tends to intensify the patients' pain. Most patients fear the process of dying—"Will it hurt?" "Will I suffo-cate?"—and many fear death itself. Many of these fears remain unspoken unless the patients are given the opportunity to express them and to talk about their progress or lack of it.

Many doctors find that as the doctor-patient relationship improves, it is possible to reduce the amount of drugs given. As the true diagnosis of a patient's pain becomes clear and the patient is helped to deal with the pain of dying, less medication is needed. A good example of this appears in an article describing a vocational training course for family practitioners (Special Correspondent, 1971). At a weekly seminar the trainees talked about patients encountered in their work in order to demonstrate that psy-chological factors exist even in an apparently straightforward physical ill-ness and vice versa. On one occasion, discussion centered on the problem of a patient with metastases in bone from disseminated breast cancer whose pain remained unrelieved by narcotic analgesics. During the semi-nar it was suggested that the pain was intractable because the woman was angry that her doctors and relatives would neither admit that she was dy-ing nor discuss the problems this created. This proved to be the right ex-planation; a full and frank discussion resulted in immediate improvement in her mental state and the resolution of her pain.

### 3. *Thou shalt not use the abbreviation prn.*

To allow pain to reemerge before administering the next dose not on-ly causes unnecessary suffering but encourages tolerance. "As required" (*pro re nata*, or prn) medication has no place in the treatment of persistent pain; whatever its aetiology, continuous pain requires regular preventive therapy. The aim is to balance the dose of the analgesic against the patient's pain, gradually increasing the dose until the patient is pain-free. The next dose is given before the effect of the previous one has worn off and, therefore, before the patient may think it necessary (Figure 6.3). In this way it is possible to erase the memory and fear of pain.

As patients do not like constantly taking tablets or receiving injec-tions, a 4-hour interval between doses should be regarded as the norm, though sometimes more frequent administration may be necessary. With a larger dose at bedtime (plus or minus a hypnotic), some patients do not need a middle-of-the-night dose, though if necessary they should be wak-

Figure 6.3.   Diagram to Illustrate the Result of "As Required" (prn) and Over-
spaced Time-Contingent Medication Compared with Regular 4-Hourly Morphine
Sulphate

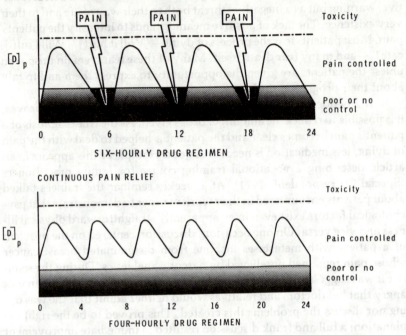

ened to take it (or have their alarm set) rather than let them wake later
complaining of pain.

**4.** *Thou shalt not prescribe inadequate amounts of any analgesic.*

The effective analgesic dose of a narcotic analgesic varies considerably from patient to patient; the right dose is that which gives adequate relief for at least 3, preferably 4 or more hours. Patients will usually accept
two, sometimes three, analgesic tablets per administration together with
additional medication; four or more tablets of the same preparation are
not often acceptable. Generally, if two tablets are not adequate, the patient should be transferred to a more potent alternative. Pain unrelieved
by other measures, not short life expectancy, is the primary criterion for
prescription of morphine or other strong narcotic analgesic. "Maximum"
or "recommended" doses, derived mainly from postoperative parenteral
single-dose studies, are not applicable in advanced cancer. For example,
the effective dose of oral morphine ranges from less than 5 mg to more
than 100 mg every 4 hours (Figure 6.4).

5. *Thou shalt try non-narcotic analgesics in the first instance.*

The use of aspirin or paracetamol (acetaminophen) regularly every 4 to 6 hours may be sufficient to relieve mild to moderate pain. By and large, however, most hospice pain patients present with more intense discomfort. Aspirin is also important in the relief of malignant bone pain, even when severe. Many metastases in bone produce a prostaglandin that causes bone resorption and that also lowers the "peripheral pain threshold" by sensitizing free nerve endings (Twycross, 1978). Aspirin (3 to 4gm

Figure 6.4. Histogram of Maximum 4-Hourly Doses of Orally Administered Morphine Sulphate in 955 Patients at St. Christopher's Hospice (1978–1979)

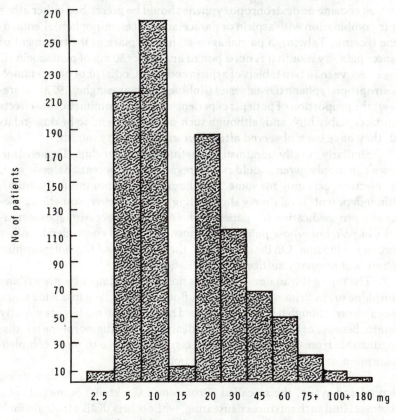

Maximum dose of oral morphine sulphate

We gratefully acknowledge the assistance of Dame Cicely M. Saunders.

*Note:* Median dose = 10 mg. "75 +" means 75, 80, or 90 mg, and "100 +" means 100, 110, or 120 mg.

a day) and other aspirin-like anti-inflamatory drugs inhibit the synthesis of prostaglandins and by so doing alleviate pain. This suggests that, compared with morphine, these drugs should be relatively more efficacious in bone pain than in pain caused by soft tissue infiltration. Response is variable but, even so, aspirin or an alternative anti-inflammatory agent should always be tried (usually in combination with a narcotic analgesic) when seeking to relieve bone pain by pharmacological means. Of the newer drugs, 50 to 100 mg of flurbiprofen every 8 hours appears particularly promising.

**6. *Thou shalt not be afraid of narcotic analgesics.***

When the non-narcotic analgesics fail to relieve, a weak narcotic such as codeine or dextropropoxyphene should be prescribed either alone or in combination with aspirin or paracetamol (acetaminophen). Pentazocine (Fortral, Talwin), a partial agonist, has no place in the treatment of cancer pain. By mouth it is not a potent analgesic; 50 mg of pentazocine is less effective than two tablets of aspirin codeine (Codis) or of paracetamol-dextropropoxyphene (Distalgesic) (Robbie & Samarasinghe, 1973). Moreover, the proportion of patients experiencing psychotomimetic side effects is unacceptably high and, although such side effects tend to be dose-related, they have been observed after even small doses by mouth.

Similarly, orally administered pethidine (meperidine; Demerol) in doses commonly given should not be regarded as a potent analgesic and, by injection, acts only for some 2 to 3 hours. Dextromoramide (Palfium), although potent, is relatively short-acting; it is, however, sometimes useful as a prn medication for patients who experience occasional exacerbations of pain but whose pain for the most part is well controlled by other regular medication. On the other hand, the use of prn *additional* morphine sulfate will normally suffice in this situation.

The top of the analgesic ladder is not reached simply by prescribing morphine or, in Britain, diamorphine. Both may be given in a wide range of oral doses, though it is unusual to need more than 60 mg (Figure 6.4). By mouth, because of fairly rapid *in vivo* deacetylation, diamorphine is indistinguishable from morphine in its effects; though, due to more complete absorption, it is about 1.5 times more potent.

Both are commonly dispensed with cocaine in a vehicle containing alcohol and syrup, the so-called "Brompton's Cocktail." Some patients, however, find such mixtures nauseating, while others dislike their alcoholic "bite." Moreover, the benefit of a small fixed dose of cocaine is negligible and has, on occasions, caused restlessness and hallucinations in the elderly. It is my practice, despite the recent inclusion of a convenient formulation in the British National Formulary, to dispense morphine sulphate in water alone, the patient adding milk, fruit juice, or a favourite tipple as desired. If given with prochlorperazine (Stemetil, Compazine) or chlorpromazine (Largactil, Thorazine), use of a flavoured proprietary syrup circumvents the need for additional flavouring.

When regular injections are required, I use diamorphine hydrochloride, available in ampoules as freeze-dried pellets (Figure 6.5). It is considerably more soluble than morphine sulphate—100 mg will dissolve in 0.2 ml. This means that the volume injected need never be large, an important consideration when repeated injections have to be given to a cachectic patient. It should be emphasized that most patients can be maintained on oral medication. The main indication for parenteral administration, apart from the last few hours of life, is intractable nausea and vomiting despite the prescription of antiemetic.

Levorphanol (Dromoran, Levo-dromoran) and phenazocine (Narphen) should be regarded as alternatives to morphine and diamorphine. By mouth on a weight-for-weight basis, both are approximately four to five times more potent than morphine and tend to have a longer duration of action (Table 6.4). Methadone (Physeptone) may also be useful in these circumstances but, because of its prolonged plasma half-life, is best not used in the elderly or extremely debilitated.

Many doctors are reluctant to use narcotic analgesics, particularly diamorphine or morphine, because they assume that tolerance will result in the medication becoming ineffective. This is understandable, as little information has been available concerning the long-term effects of narcotic analgesics when administered regularly to relieve persistent pain. Recent studies have, however, shown that, in patients receiving diamorphine regularly for periods ranging from 1 to 2 years, the longer the duration of treatment, the slower the rate of rise in dose. Moreover, the longer a patient's survival after prescription of diamorphine, the greater the likelihood of a reduction in dose (Twycross & Wald, 1976). It has been concluded that, when used as part of a pattern of total care, diamorphine may be used for long periods without concern about tolerance. Moreover, although physical dependence probably develops in most patients after several weeks of continuous treatment, this does not prevent the downward adjustment of dose if considered clinically feasible. Experience with methadone, levorphanol, and phenazocine suggests that the "natural history" of their long-term use in patients in pain is similar to that of diamorphine and morphine.

7. *Thou shalt not limit thy approach simply to the use of analgesics.*

Most patients with terminal cancer have more than one symptom. Nausea and vomiting are both common, and the use of a narcotic analge-

Figure 6.5. Histogram of Maximum 4-Hourly Doses of Intramuscular or Subcutaneous Diamorphine Hydrochloride in 1,064 Patients at St. Christopher's Hospice (1978–1979)

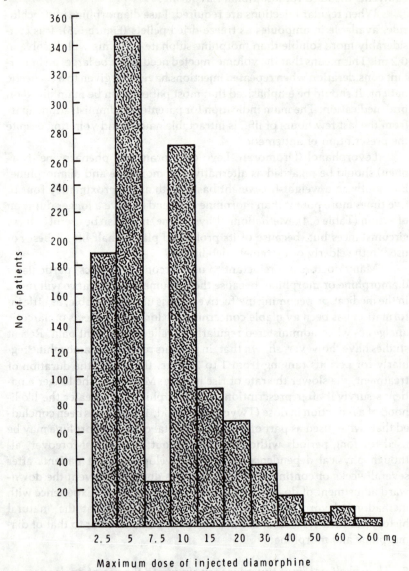

We gratefully acknowledge the assistance of Dame Cicely M. Saunders.

*Note:* Median dose = 7.5 mg.

sic tends to precipitate or exacerbate these symptoms, particularly if the patient is ambulant. Patients prescribed a narcotic analgesic should be questioned about nausea and vomiting and should either have an anti-emetic prescribed simultaneously or have the need for one reviewed after a day or so (Table 6.5). Constipation almost always occurs when a narcotic is taken regularly, but generally responds to the *regular* use of an appropriate aperient—for example, Dorbanex capsules or syrup (danthron plus softener)—together with suppositories and enemas as indicated.

The value of diversional activity should not be forgotten. It ranges from back rubs to craft work, talking books, access to radio and television, someone to talk to, and dayroom activities. Pain is worse when it occupies the patient's whole attention. Diversional activity does more than just "pass the time"; it also diminishes the pain.

Some patients continue to experience pain on movement despite analgesics, other drugs, radiotherapy, and nerve blocks. In these, the situation may be improved by suggesting commonsense modifications to daily activity. For example, a man may continue to struggle to stand when shaving unless the doctor suggests that sitting would be a good idea. Such a suggestion is accepted more readily if accompanied by a simple explanation of why weight bearing precipitates or exacerbates the pain.

**8.** *Thou shalt not be afraid to ask a colleague's advice.*

The occasion will arise when even the most skilled doctor will find that a patient's pain is failing to respond to whatever measures he or she introduces. In this situation, consultation with a colleague is obligatory. It is the patient's pain and not the doctor's pride that matters. Having said that, it is up to individual doctors to build up their own systems of contacts to help in cases of difficulty. Who they turn to will depend on the local situation.

Radiation therapy gives partial or even complete relief in 90% of patients experiencing bone pain, and frequently may be administered in a single, nonfractionated dose. However, the fact that the patient is receiving radiotherapy or has started hormone treatment does not mean that analgesics should be withheld. A combined approach should be employed. If relief is obtained and there are no complaints of pain "breaking through," then the analgesic regimen can be modified—a less potent analgesic can be prescribed, or the treatment can be withdrawn completely.

Nerve blocks have an undoubted place in the relief of nerve compression pain, particularly intrathecal phenol, though analgesics alone are effective in perhaps 50% of cases. If the response is poor, the use of prednisolone in addition is recommended, initially 10 mg three times a day. By reducing inflammatory swelling around the growth, the effective tumour

## Table 6.4
### Approximate Oral Narcotic Analgesic Equivalents

| Analgesic | Proprietary Name | Unit Size[1] | Potency Ratio with morphine sulphate | Oral dose (mg) morphine sulphate | Oral dose (mg) diamorphine hydrochloride[2] | Duration of action (hrs)[3] |
|---|---|---|---|---|---|---|
| pethidine/meperidine | Demerol | 50 mg | 1/8[4] | 6 | 4 | 2–3 |
| | | 100 mg | | 12 | 8 | 2–3 |
| Pentazocine | Fortral, Talwin | 25 mg | 1/6[4] | 4 | 3 | 2–3 |
| | | 50 mg (caps) | | 8 | 5 | |
| | | 50 mg (supp) | | 8 | 5 | |
| *dipipanone | Diconal | 10 mg (+ 30 mg cyclizine) | 1/2 | 5 | 5 | 3–5 |
| *papaveretum | Omnopon | 10 mg | 1/2 | 5 | 3 | 3–5 |
| *oxycodone pectinate | Proladone | 30 mg (supp) | 2/3 | 20 | 13 | 6–8 |
| *Nepenthe[5] | | 1 ml (solution) | 1 | 12 | 8 | 3–5 |

| Drug | Trade name[1] | Dose | | | | Duration (h) |
|---|---|---|---|---|---|---|
| *dextromoramide | Palfium | 5 mg | (2)[6] | 10 | 7 | 2–4 |
| | | 10 mg | | 15 | 10 | |
| | | 10 mg (supp) | | 15 | 10 | |
| Methadone | Physeptone, Dolophine | 5 mg | (3–4)[7] | 15–20 | 10–13 | 4–8 |
| Levorphanol | Dromoran, Levo-dromoran | 1.5 mg | 5 | 8 | 5 | 4–6 |
| phenazocine | Narphen, Prinadol | 5 mg | 5 | 25 | 16 | 4–6 |

*Not available in the United States

[1] Tablets unless stated otherwise.

[2] By mouth, diamorphine hydrochloride is 1.5 times more potent than morphine sulphate (i.e., 5 mg is equivalent to 7.5 mg of morphine sulphate).

[3] Dependent to a certain extent on dose, often longer-lasting in very elderly and those with considerable liver dysfunction.

[4] Experience suggests that, compared with *regularly* administered morphine sulphate, these preparations are not as potent as these ratios would indicate.

[5] Nepenthe is a standard solution of morphine (as base). 1 ml contains the equivalent of about 12 mg of morphine *sulphate*, and is usually prescribed as a 10% (1 ml diluted in 10 ml) solution.

[6] A single 5 mg dose of dextromoramide is equivalent to diamorphine 10 mg/morphine 15 mg in terms of *peak* effect but is generally shorter-acting; overall potency rate adjusted accordingly.

[7] A single 5 mg dose of methadone is equivalent to diamorphine 5 mg/morphine 7.5 mg. It has a prolonged plasma half-time, which leads to cumulation when given repeatedly. This means it is several times more potent when given *regularly*.

## Table 6.5
### Controlling Morphine-Induced Emesis

| Drug | Proprietary Name | Preparation | Dose | Frequency | Comment |
|---|---|---|---|---|---|
| haloperidol | Serenace Haldol | capsule or *liquid | 0.5 mg | every 8-12 hours | Routine prophylactic antiemetic at Sobell House, Oxford<br>Non-sedative<br>Usually no unwanted effects at this dose |
| metoclopramide | Maxolon | syrup (10 ml) or tablet | 10 mg | every 4 hours | Useful for troublesome dyspepsia<br>May enhance gastric emptying<br>Non-sedative<br>Does not cause dry mouth |
| Prochlorperazine | Stemetil Compazine | syrup (5 ml) or tablet | 5 mg | every 4-8 hours | Traditional in many hospices<br>Sometimes causes drowsiness<br>Tends to cause drying of mouth |

*Serenace liquid contains 2 mg/ml. For convenience, this should be diluted by the pharmacy to 2 mg/20 ml, given 0.5 mg in each 5 ml. Label "haloperidol" *dilute* liquid 0.5 mg/5 ml.

mass is reduced and the compression alleviated. In patients with a prognosis of only a few weeks, this may be sufficient to circumvent the need for a nerve block. In those with a longer life expectancy, the pain may return as the tumour continues to grow. In patients whose morale is low or precarious, it is advisable to warn that a block may become necessary in order to avoid loss of confidence should the pain return.

**9.** *Thou shalt provide support for the whole family.*

During a terminal illness, the patient's relatives experience a variety of emotions. These will vary according to the depth of relationship between the patient and his or her family, as well as by the duration of the illness and mode of death. Some people feel so repelled by the thought of death that they cannot face the one who is dying and retreat into a world of their own. In consequence, they reassure the patient that all is well, that he or she is getting better and there is nothing to worry about. This sort of behaviour not only isolates the patient but is ultimately harmful to those who indulge in it. The reaction to bereavement is frequently more prolonged and more guilt-ridden in those who have not faced the impending death realistically than in those who have.

When talking with relatives, one learns a lot about family relationships. Sometimes it is possible to encourage reconciliation between a patient and an estranged spouse or other members of the family. Financial problems or need for support in other ways require the help of the medical social worker, who should be kept informed even in situations that appear ideal. Patients often improve generally following admission as a result of the control of pain and other symptoms. They become physically independent again and no longer need to be in hospital. Because they remember what it was like before the patient was admitted for pain control, many relatives fear what might happen if the patient is discharged. A trial day out or weekend at home does much to allay their fears (or confirms that discharge is after all impractical). Clear advice should be given about whom to call—general practitioner or hospital—in the event of a crisis.

**10.** *Thou shalt have an air of quiet confidence and cautious optimism.*

Cancer is a progressive disease. This means that new pains may develop or old pains reemerge. It should not be assumed that a fresh complaint of pain merely calls for an increase in a previously satisfactory analgesic regimen; it demands reassessment, an explanation to the patient, and, only then, modification of drug therapy or other intervention. The probability of the initial prescription being inadequate increases with the intensity of pain. Patients should, therefore, be reassessed within hours if the pain is overwhelming, or after 1 or 2 days if severe or moderate. If troublesome or unacceptable side effects result, treatment may need to be modified. In addition, the relief of the major pain may allow a second, less severe pain to become apparent.

Although in some patients relief may be obtained fairly easily, it is important to bear in mind that with others, particularly those who have pain on movement and those whose pain is compounded by extreme anxiety or depression, it may take 3 to 4 weeks of inpatient treatment to achieve satisfactory control. However, in all patients it should be possible to achieve some improvement within 24 to 48 hours. Although the ultimate aim is always complete freedom from pain, doctors will be less disappointed but, paradoxically, more successful if they aim at "graded relief." Moreover, as some pains respond more readily than others, improvement should be assessed in relation to each pain.

The initial target should be a pain-free, sleep-full night. Many patients have not had a good night's rest for weeks or months. To sleep through the night and wake refreshed is a boost to both the doctor's and the patient's morale. Next, one aims for relief at rest in bed or chair during the day; finally, for freedom from pain on movement. The former is always eventually possible; the latter is not. However, the encouragement that relief at night and when resting during the day brings gives patients new hope and incentive and enables them to begin to live again, despite limited mobility. Freed from the daily burden and nightmare of constant pain, his life takes on a new look. There must, however, be a determination to succeed on the doctor's part and a preparedness to spend much time assessing and reassessing the patient's pain and other distressing symptoms.

## References

Parkes, C. M., "Home or Hospital? Terminal Care as Seen by Surviving Spouses," *Journal of the Royal College of General Practitioners*, 1976, *28*, 19–30.

Robbie, D. S., & Samarasinghe, H., "Comparison of Aspirin-Codeine and Paracetamol-Dextropropoxyphene Compound Tablets with Pentazocine in Relief of Cancer Pain," *Journal of International Medical Research*, 1973, *1*, 246–252.

Special Correspondent, "Vocational Training for General Practice," *British Medical Journal*, 1971, *2*, 704–705.

Twycross, R. G., "Bone Pain in Advanced Cancer," in D. W. Vere (Ed.), *Topics in Therapeutics, 4.* Tunbridge Wells, England: Pitman Medical Publishing, 1978, 94–110.

Twycross, R. G., & Wald, S. J., "Long-Term Use of Diamorphine in Advanced Cancer," in J. J. Bonica & D. G. Albe-Fessard (Eds.), *Advances in Pain and Research Therapy.* New York: Raven Press, 1976, 653–661.

# 7

# Drug Therapy of Chronic Pain

*Arthur G. Lipman*

Chronic pain is one of the most difficult problems that clinicians face. Interpatient differences in the perception of pain, and in the acceptance of pain medications, are great. The variety of drugs and nondrug treatments currently advocated for pain management often produces confusion, and the pain literature is replete with anecdotal reports while sorely lacking in scientific content.

Pain is a highly subjective phenomenon. The admission and acceptance of pain are influenced by the patient's socialization process and cultural mores. Many Scandinavians and Orientals are stoic about pain, while many Mediterranean peoples are more expressive.

Adequate clinical rating scales and measurement instruments for pain are not available. Investigators' attempts to determine objective data on pain are often frustrated by the multiple variables that affect the experience. The clinical experiences and biases of pharmacology instructors may comprise more of some instructors' teaching about pain than do objective data. The data base on pain and pain management of many pharmacists, physicians, and nurses contains previous beliefs that have now been disproven.

Pain management is becoming increasingly multimodal and multidisciplinary. This paper will address the use of drugs in the management of chronic pain.

*From:* Arthur G. Lipman, "Drug Therapy of Chronic Pain," *The Journal of Continuing Education in Hospital and Clinical Pharmacy,* 1979, *1,* 11–20. Reprinted by permission of Arthur G. Lipman.

## Defining Pain

A contemporary clinical definition of *pain* is "a more or less localized sensation of discomfort, distress or agony, resulting from the stimulation of specialized nerve endings" (*Dorland's Illustrated Medical Dictionary*, 1974). But this definition is inadequate to describe the many types of experiences called "pain" for which drug therapy is appropriate. Pain is an important body defense mechanism. It induces an individual to withdraw from the source, and it can serve as an important diagnostic and monitoring parameter. But pain can also become counterproductive.

The etiology and natural history of a pain experience must be known in order for optimal pain therapy to be planned. Low back pain may be entirely physical, entirely psychological, or result from a combination of causes. Pain associated with cancer may be a result more of loneliness and fear than of tumor growth. Intense pain of short duration is often more easily tolerated than chronic low-level pain. Some persons function well with pain, while others do not. Perhaps the only generalization about pain that is appropriate is that its optimal management requires individualization of treatment.

The socialization process of most Americans has included encouragement of brave acceptance of pain. Parental admonitions such as "Be a big girl, don't cry," or "Take it like a man, son," are common in our society. The attitudes thus fostered often result in patients' denying pain and refusing analgesics when the pain is serving no useful purpose and drugs would be of help. Much unnecessary pain is experienced due to health professionals' reluctance to use analgesics when they are indicated. Patients' attempts to withstand severe, chronic pain without drugs may lead to adverse psychological sequelae.

## Acute Versus Chronic Pain

*Acute pain* has been experienced by nearly all persons. The pain associated with trauma, surgery, or childbirth can be significant, but it generally resolves rapidly. The use of analgesics on a "prn" schedule is often the only therapy needed for such pain. Patients generally expect that the pain will resolve, and it does.

Acute pain is commonly classified as mild, moderate, or severe. The more intense the pain, the more potent the analgesic that is indicated. Aspirin for mild pain, aspirin plus codeine for moderate pain, and morphine for severe pain are common and appropriate associations. As the pain resolves, less potent analgesics are indicated, and a physician's orders might well include Percodan$^R$ prn *and* aspirin prn for the same hospitalized patient. The nurse then selects the more potent analgesic when it is needed and the less potent drug as the pain diminishes.

But when pain does not resolve rapidly, management becomes far more complicated. Chronic pain cannot be rationalized as a part of the healing process. Analgesics that are prescribed on a "prn" basis are often demanded more frequently than the orders permit. The patient's anxiety about the pain exacerbates it, and the continual presence of pain increases the anxiety. Patients frequently develop reactive depression, and their sleeping and eating habits become abnormal. Such patient behavior frequently discourages visits by friends and avoidance by health professionals. Loneliness ensues, and this dimension increases the complexity of the patients' misery. Pharmacologic, psychological, and social support is often needed to manage such pain successfully.

Unlike acute pain, *chronic pain* cannot be nicely classified according to severity. A rank order from mild to severe does not apply. Rather, chronic pain might be better expressed as a circular continuum of aching to agony (Figure 7.1) (Lipman, 1975). The agony phase is represented by the severe, chronic pain often associated with cancer, ischemic disease, degenerative organ disease, and neurologic disease. This type of pain becomes the central focus of the patient's existence and precludes normal social interaction. When there is a physical etiology for the pain (e.g., tumor growth), it may be unreasonable to state elimination of the pain as the therapeutic goal. Transition from the agony phase of chronic pain to the aching phase may be a more appropriate objective of therapy. Most indi-

Figure 7.1.   The Continuum of Chronic Pain

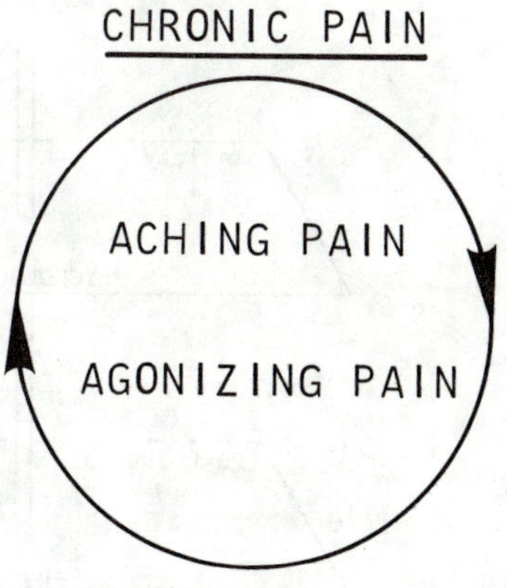

## CHRONIC PAIN

ACHING PAIN

AGONIZING PAIN

*Adapted from:* Arthur G. Lipman, "Drug Therapy in Terminally Ill Patients," *American Journal of Hospital Pharmacy,* 1975, *32,* 270–271.

viduals can function with a dull background ache. The major etiologic difference between tolerable chronic aching and intolerable chronic agony may be that the former is due primarily to a physical cause, while the latter often has physical, psychological, and social dimensions.

## The Dimensions of Severe Chronic Pain

The severe chronic pain experience may have three dimensions—physical, psychological, and social (Figure 7.2). The physical dimension of pain is the initial problem. The pain is due to a pathologic, physiologic process that elicits a pain response. If the physical dimension of pain resolves in a few days, the other dimensions often do not appear. If the pain remains for weeks, the psychological dimension is commonly seen as well. If the pain persists for an extended period, the social dimension may further complicate the problem. Each of these dimensions requires therapeutic intervention.

The clinical presentation of severe chronic pain may therefore be quite complex. Commonly, physical pain produces anxiety, which exacerbates the pain. The anxiety also produces depression, which in turn

Figure 7.2.   Dimensions of Severe Chronic Pain

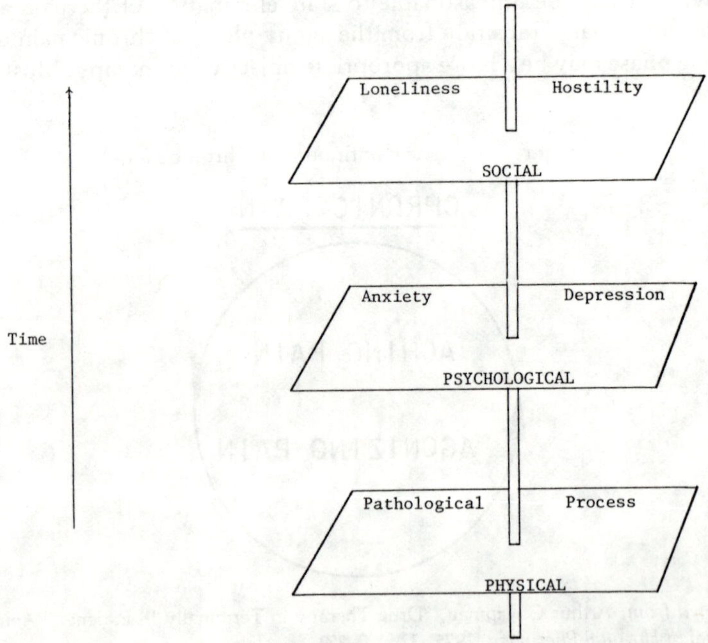

Figure 7.3. The Symptom Complex of Severe Chronic Pain

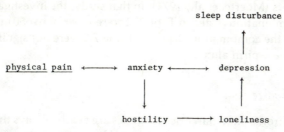

worsens the anxiety. The anxiety also produces hostility, which frequently results in loneliness. The loneliness reinforces the depression. And the
depression causes insomnia and eating disturbances. The interrelationship
of the problems must be recognized to avoid initiating an inappropriate
polydrug approach to this complex problem. The presentation of chronic
severe pain is presented graphically in Figure 7.3.

Psychosocial intervention for severe chronic pain due to physiologic
processes is of limited usefulness without appropriate drug therapy. Conversely, optimal pharmacologic management may be ineffective if appropriate psychosocial support is not provided. Reports of the efficacy of psychological or psychotherapeutic drug therapy without analgesics have appeared.
Such regimens may be highly effective in the management of pain due primarily to psychological causes. When the pain is due principally to physiologic events, appropriate analgesic drugs are nearly always an essential
component of therapy.

## Treatment of Pain

### Non-Narcotic Analgesics

Non-narcotic analgesics are useful in mild to moderate acute pain, and in
the aching phase of chronic pain. They are of minimal value in severe pain
and generally should not be used when maximal analgesia is needed.

Few good controlled comparative studies of non-narcotic analgesics
have been reported. One double-blind, crossover, single-dose comparative study of commercially available analgesics documented that aspirin
(650 mg) was superior to mefenamic acid (250 mg), pentazocine (60 mg),
acetaminophen (650 mg), phenacetin (650 mg), and codeine (60 mg), all of
which were superior to placebo (Moertel et al., 1972). In the same study,
propoxyphene (65 mg), ethoheptazine (75 mg), and promazine (25 mg)
showed no evidence of analgesic efficacy. A later double-blind, crossover,
single-dose study of the efficacy of analgesic combinations in 100 patients

with chronic or recurring pain due to cancer was conducted by the same investigators (Moertel et al., 1974). In that study, the investigators found that the combinations listed in Table 7.1 were superior to 650 mg of aspirin alone, and the combinations listed in Table 7.2 were not significantly superior to the aspirin alone.

*Narcotic Analgesics*

In severe chronic pain, narcotic analgesics are nearly always the preferred drugs. Although there are advertising and literature claims of differences between the commercially available narcotics, most appear to be similarly useful if given in appropriate doses and at appropriate time intervals. Codeine and oxycodone (in Percodan[R], Percocet-5[R], Percobarb[R]) are useful drugs in moderate acute pain and in the aching phase of chronic pain. These two narcotics are *not* advocated in severe chronic pain. While analgesia similar to that achieved with low-dose morphine can be achieved with codeine and oxycodone, the latter drugs do not provide the increasing analgesia with increasing doses that occurs with morphine and most other narcotic analgesics. Approximate equianalgesic doses of some commonly used narcotics are described in Table 7.3.

Narcotics, and especially the more lipophilic narcotics, i.e., levorphanol and methadone, may produce accumulation after several days of therapy if they are administered too frequently. This effect may occur more commonly in the elderly (Symonds, 1977). It is generally safer to adjust the dose upward rather than to shorten the dosage interval below the times listed in Table 7.3. Published reports on narcotic analgesic equipotent doses and dosing intervals are inconsistent. Single-dose pharmacokinetic study data may also differ from data collected in patients with steady-state serum levels (Beaver et al., 1967). The data in Table 7.3 are derived from both published reports and the author's clinical experience.

Table 7.1
Analgesic Combinations Found Superior to Aspirin, 650 mg

---

Codeine sulfate, 65 mg, plus aspirin, 650 mg.

Pentazocine hydrochloride, 25 mg, plus aspirin, 650 mg.

Oxycodone, 9 mg, plus aspirin, 650 mg.

---

Table 7.2
Analgesic Combinations That Produced
No Significant Difference from Aspirin, 650 mg

---

Propoxyphene napsylate, 100 mg, plus aspirin, 650 mg.

Ethoheptazine citrate, 75 mg, plus aspirin, 650 mg.

Promazine hydrochloride, 75 mg, plus aspirin, 650 mg.

Pentobarbital sodium, 32 mg, plus aspirin, 650 mg.

Caffeine, 65 mg, plus aspirin, 650 mg.

---

*Adapted from:* C. G. Moertel et al., "Relief of Pain by Oral Medications," *Journal of the American Medical Association,* 1974, *229,* 55–59. Copyright © 1974 by the American Medical Association. Used by permission of the Association.

Narcotic analgesics are commonly used in suboptimal doses (Marks & Sachar, 1973). This is particularly true of meperidine, which is also commonly administered on an every-four-hour rather than every-three-hour schedule. Inappropriate fear of induction of tolerance or dependence often is the reason for the drugs being given in too low doses and not frequently enough to maintain pain control. Patients who have physiologic pain etiologies respond differently to narcotics than do individuals seeking euphoric effects. When there is physical pain, high-dose narcotic therapy does not induce the tolerance or dependence that sometimes occurs when narcotics are used for extended periods for pain of a psychological origin. These findings are consistent with the new findings of endogenous opioid receptors and of enkephalins and endorphins (Snyder, 1977).

There are three important principles in the dosing of narcotic analgesics in severe chronic pain. The first is that the optimal dose is determined through titration for effect. The second is that it is better to start with a dose that is initially a little too high than one that is too low. And the third, and most important, principle is that the narcotic be administered on a regularly scheduled basis, not a "prn" schedule.

The optimal dose of narcotic is the lowest dose that provides prevention of return of pain which cannot be tolerated. It is not always possible to eliminate the pain totally. It is usually preferable to diminish the pain to a level that the patient considers tolerable. It is useful to discuss this objective with the patient once initial pain relief is established. Some patients think that they should endure the maximum pain possible, while others think that therapy should eliminate all sensation of discomfort. Neither perception is appropriate, but the patient is usually the best person to determine the level of pain relief to be sought. It is important to realize that

Table 7.3
Narcotic Analgesics: Approximate Equianalgesic Doses
of Selected Commercially Available Dosage Forms

| Drug | Route | Dose | Average Duration of Action (hr.) |
|------|-------|------|----------------------------------|
| Hydromorphone | PO[a] | 3–4 mg. | 3–4 |
| (Dilaudid[R]) | PR[b] | 3–6 mg. | 3–4 |
| | IM [c], SC[d] | 2–3 mg. | 3–4 |
| Levorphanol | PO | 2–3 mg. | 6–8 |
| (Levo-Dromoran[R]) | SC | 2 mg. | 6–8 |
| Meperidine | PO | 100–150 mg. | 3 |
| | IM, SC | 75–100 mg. | 3 |
| Methadone | PO | 12.5 mg. | 6–8 |
| (Dolophine[R]) | IM, SC | 10 mg. | 4–6 |
| Morphine Sulfate | PO | 15 mg. | 3–4 |
| | IM, SC | 10 mg. | 4–6 |
| Oxymorphone (Numorphan[R]) | PR | 2–5 mg. | 4 |
| | IM | 1–1.5 mg. | 4 |

[a]Per os (orally).
[b]Per rectum (rectally).
[c]Intramuscularly.
[d]Subcutaneously.

the amount of analgesia a patient will require does not remain constant throughout the course of the pain experience. Some etiologies will progress; others will remit. For example, bony metastases of cancer produce excruciating pain for a short time until the metastatic site is destroyed, after which the pain will resolve. Pain of an origin different from the primary etiology may also complicate management. For example, pain from a severe headache may be superimposed over that of peripheral vascular disease, resulting in an increased analgesic requirement until the headache resolves. Dosing flexibility should be maintained with the option to increase the dose as needed, but always with subsequent periodic attempts to lower the dose.

The starting dose of narcotic analgesic is selected by considering the patient's pain intensity, prior analgesic drug use, body weight, and metabolic and excretory capabilities. Parenteral therapy is not indicated in most patients who are capable of taking [an] oral drug and absorbing it. Generally, patients capable of taking nourishment orally are also capable of taking analgesics orally. Parenteral therapy produces higher initial body levels. But with regularly scheduled doses, oral doses maintain the level as effectively as do injections. Furthermore, parenteral drugs create a feeling of patient dependence on others and an intimation of heroic measures that are better avoided. Morphine, which was once thought to be less effective orally than parenterally, has now been shown to be an effective oral analgesic if administered in sufficient doses (Twycross, Fry, & Wills, 1974). The drug is only about two-thirds absorbed. Therefore, 15 mg orally produces activity similar to a 10 mg parenteral dose.*

The effectiveness of the initial doses of drug greatly influences the perceived efficacy of subsequent doses. If the clinician starts with a low dose of narcotic with the intention of increasing the dose until an effective one is reached, the patient may rapidly lose confidence in the drug's ability to produce pain relief, and this perception may significantly decrease the efficacy of higher doses of the drug. Patients experiencing the agony phase of chronic pain may require high initial doses of narcotics to break the pain-anxiety cycle. Therefore, a high initial dose of narcotic is indicated.

The clinician should also recognize that severe pain is exhausting and usually precludes restful sleep. Thus it is common for a patient to sleep for many hours after an initial effective dose of analgesic. Such sleep alone is not indicative of overdose; the patient's respiration and pulse are more useful indicators of that.

After the pain is initially controlled, the dose of narcotic can often be reduced without diminished efficacy. Continued control of the pain results in decreased anxiety about it. The dose of narcotic frequently can be reduced several times until lessened pain control necessitates raising it. The optimal dose is usually between the lowest effective one and that at which an increase in pain was noted, as illustrated in Figure 7.4.

Admininistering the drug on a regularly scheduled basis is of great importance in the management of chronic pain of physical origin. Saunders has described pain as the strongest antagonist to analgesia, and has long advocated regularly scheduled administration of analgesia to prevent pain recurrence, rather than attempting to treat pain after it has recurred (Saunders, 1967). The recurrence of pain produces anxiety resulting in an increased perception of pain. In the author's experience, total daily doses

*Editors' note: Lipman reports that recent clinical experience suggests that the oral to intramuscular dose ratio for morphine sulfate should be changed from 1.5 to 1 to 2 or 2.5 to 1.

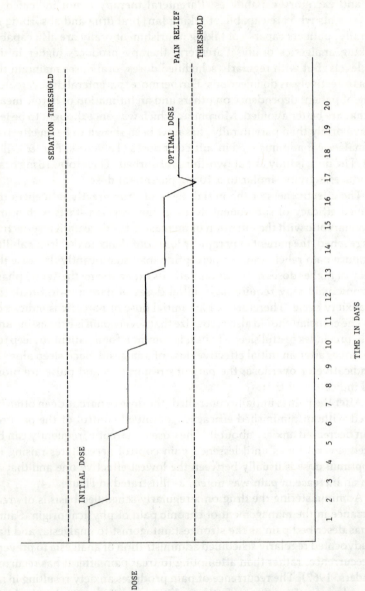

Figure 7.4. Narcotic Dose Titration in Chronic Pain

SEDATION THRESHOLD

PAIN RELIEF
THRESHOLD

OPTIMAL DOSE

INITIAL DOSE

DOSE

TIME IN DAYS

1 2 3 4 5 6 7 8 9 10 11 12 13 14 15 16 17 18 19 20

*Adapted from: Arthur G. Lipman, "Drug Therapy in Terminally Ill Patients," American Journal of Hospital Pharmacy, 1975, 32, 270-271.*

of regularly scheduled narcotics needed to prevent the recurrence of pain successfully are often lower than doses necessary to treat the pain, sometimes without success, after it recurs.

## Brompton's Cocktail and Other Multidrug Analgesic Formulations

Scientific study of the efficacy of highly touted narcotic mixtures and of heroin have only begun in earnest in this decade. As recently as [the] 1970[s], leading European (Twycross, 1974a) and North American (Mount, Ajemian, & Scott, 1976) clinicians were advocating the use of Brompton's Cocktail as the preferred analgesic in advanced cancer pain, and a noted political columnist (Alsop, 1974) was demanding that heroin be legalized as an analgesic in this country. There is no scientific foundation to the claims of the superior efficacy of these drugs. Recent controlled studies have shown that neither Brompton's Cocktail nor heroin has any advantage over morphine as an analgesic (Twycross 1977a, 1977b).

The use of narcotic-adjunct cocktails in the management of severe pain can be traced to the late nineteenth century when Snow, a surgeon at the Cancer Hospital, London (now the Royal Marsden Hospital), reported the use of morphine and cocaine in advanced cancer (Snow, 1896). He later deleted the cocaine due to cost. In the 1920s, Roberts, a surgeon at the Brompton Hospital, London, reintroduced a morphine-cocaine mixture for analgesia following thoracotomy. Several similar combinations became popular in the following years, and in 1952 the Brompton Hospital published a pharmacopeial supplement containing the following formulation entitled Haustas E (*Martindale*, 1973):

| | |
|---|---|
| Morphine HCl | 15 mg |
| Cocaine HCl | 10 mg |
| Alcohol 90% | 2 ml |
| Syrup | 4 ml |
| Chloroform water | qs [sufficient quantity] ad [up to] 15 ml. |

Several similar formulations have been described in the succeeding 25 years. Many of these have substituted diamorphine for the morphine. The names of such formulations include Hospice Mix, Saunders Solution, Euphoriant Solution, and Brompton's Mixture. It should be noted that Brompton's Mixture is a cough preparation containing morphine, hydrocyanic acid, syrup of tolu, and flavoring (*Martindale*, 1973). It is not an analgesic preparation.

In 1973 the British Pharmacopeial Codex included a diamorphine and cocaine elixir in an effort to standardize the many opiate-cocaine formulations that were then being used throughout the United Kingdom (Twycross, 1973, 1974b). A wide variety of opiate combination formulations has come into use in this country in recent years. Most are irrational, expensive, and unnecessary.

A controlled, double-blind study has now demonstrated that morphine is as effective as heroin as an analgesic (Twycross, 1977b). It is unfortunate that public groups, and state and federal legislatures, are attempting to legalize heroin for use as an analgesic in this country. Heroin offers no therapeutic advantage over commercially available narcotic analgesics. But because of its ability to produce a euphoric "rush" following administration, the abuse of heroin and the potential for the diversion of a legitimized drug into illicit channels is great.

Cocaine has also been shown not to be additive to the analgesic effect of either morphine or heroin in a controlled, double-blind study reported in 1977 (Twycross, 1977a). Cocaine is believed to have been added to the original Brompton's Cocktail as a local analgesic for the throat and/or to relieve some of the sedation produced by the narcotic. The former suggested indication may apply in some pulmonary disease patients (the Brompton Hospital is an institution primarily for chest disease), but is not applicable to most pain patients. The latter indication is not appropriate because titration of the narcotic dose, as described above, results in minimal sedation from the analgesic.

A third component of many opiate cocktails is alcohol. While it is true that alcohol is an additive central nervous system depressant to the narcotic, the addition of the alcohol offers no pharmacologic or therapeutic advantage. Because the narcotic dose is titrated to effect, the addition of alcohol may allow the use of a few less milligrams of narcotic, but it provides no advantage in safety or efficacy.

The fourth common ingredient of many British opiate mixtures in the past has been chloroform water. This agent was added to impart a medicinal taste. Chloroform has been implicated as a carcinogen and has been removed from the American GRAS list (agents generally regarded as safe for use in drugs, foods, and cosmetics).

A common expectation of Englishmen is that drugs be in bitter-tasting liquids (Lipman, 1975). The opiate cocktails fulfill these expectations. The common American expectation is that drugs be in oral, solid-dosage forms or contained in sweet-tasting liquids. The attempts of many Americans to adapt British formulations in this country have simply led to decreased patient acceptance of the drugs.

Other narcotic combinations (e.g., Schlesinger's Solution) may similarly be shown to be irrational. There is no pharmaceutic or therapeutic rationale for administering more than one narcotic analgesic to a patient. Neither decreased toxicity nor potentiation occurs.

Both St. Christopher's Hospice in London, directed by Dr. Cicely Saunders, and Sir Michael Sobell House in Oxford, directed by Dr. Robert Twycross, now use a simple aqueous solution of morphine as their primary narcotic analgesic. Dr. Saunders is a pioneer in symptomatic care for patients with advanced cancer symptoms, and Dr. Twycross is the clinical pharmacologist who has published the most definitive data on advanced cancer pain. Neither of them any longer advocates the use of heroin or Brompton's Cocktail over the simple narcotic analgesics commercially available in this country (Twycross, 1978).

## Adjunctive Drugs

The principal adjunct to narcotics in severe chronic pain is a phenothiazine. There are three reasons for adding this drug. High-dose narcotic therapy often induces nausea. The nausea may become a major problem, but more often it is low-grade and simply adds to the patient's lack of a feeling of well-being. Phenothiazines are among the most effective antiemetics available. The second reason for the phenothiazines is that in low doses they do provide some antianxiety activity. The third reason is that the combining of a phenothiazine with a narcotic allows the use of a lower dose of the narcotic without loss of effectiveness. Some mild reduction in narcotic-induced respiratory depression and constipation may result, but the therapeutic gain is minimal.

Some clinicians have successfully used benzodiazepine adjuncts for the antianxiety activity, but these drugs do not provide antiemetic action.

Commercially available phenothiazines can be classified according to the chemical side chain on the phenothiazine nucleus. The alkylamino side chain phenothiazines, which include chlorpromazine and promethazine, are very sedating. This effect is generally not desired in pain patients, because the narcotics can also be sedating. Occasionally an alkylamino side chain phenothiazine adjunct may be useful in an agitated patient, however. The piperidine side chain phenothiazines may produce more parasympatholytic (anticholinergic) activity than the other types. This effect is also undesirable, because the narcotics are constipating, and additional constipating drugs may result in fecal impaction. The two drugs in this group available in this country are thioridazine and mesoridazine. The piperazine side chain phenothiazines are preferred. These drugs also produce some anticholinergic effects, but the effects are less severe than those caused by the piperidine group and no more severe than those caused by the alkylamino group. In high doses, the piperazine phenothiazines may cause extrapyramidal symptoms and dysphoria. For use as narcotic adjuncts, low doses are indicated. This group of phenothiazines offers the advantages of minimal sedation and maximal antiemetic activity. A typical drug and dose would be prochlorperazine, 5 mg every eight hours.

Reactive depression frequently accompanies chronic pain of extended duration. The depression often resolves when the anxiety diminishes, however, and pharmacologic intervention for depression is not always indicated. Tricyclic antidepressants are not optimally effective in exogenous depression, and the drugs have significant anticholinergic effects. Management of the pain and anxiety usually diminishes the depression. If the depression becomes a major problem in itself, however, antidepressant drug therapy should be considered.

Constipation is a problem for some patients taking narcotics. Adequate oral hydration may minimize this problem, but if laxatives are needed, they should be used. Bulk-producing cathartics (e.g., psyllium) are the safest drugs, but they may not be effective due to diminished peristaltic tone. If bulk producers are not effective, stimulating agents (e.g., bisacodyl) should be used. Stool softeners (e.g., docusate sodium) are generally not effective in patients with diminished peristalsis.

The phenothiazine adjunct is generally sufficient to control narcotic-induced nausea. Occasionally, patients do not respond to the phenothiazines alone. In such cases, one should consider adding an antihistaminic antiemetic (e.g., cyclizine) to the phenothiazine. The antihistamine drug acts on the vestibular source (Gutmer, Gould, & Batterman, 1952) of nausea, while the phenothiazine acts on the medullary source (Byck, 1975). Narcotics may induce nausea through both mechanisms.

## The Pain Control Regimen

Patient convenience and acceptance of the drugs should be considered in planning a pain control regimen. The duration of action of the narcotic should be considered in selecting the drug. Generally, a drug which provides six to eight hours of analgesia is preferred to one which must be administered every three to four hours. Once initial pain control is achieved, morphine is often effective for six hours and methadone for eight. The dosing schedule should be arranged so as not to disturb sleep if a dose is required during normal sleeping hours. It is better to awaken a patient for a dose of drug before pain recurs than to have the patient awaken in pain.

Methadone is now available in the United States as a compressed tablet, but not as an oral liquid. Morphine is available in tablet triturates.

If an oral liquid formulation is needed, it can be prepared easily by dissolving the morphine tablet in a dose of commercially available Compazine$^R$ syrup just prior to administration. Methadone liquid may be prepared from the commercially available Dolophine$^R$ diskets. If an oral solid dosage form is used, many patients prefer to swallow a compressed tablet rather than a tablet triturate, because the latter dissolves rapidly on the tongue and morphine is bitter-tasting. Rectal suppositories are available for the administration of several narcotics. Rectal administration is preferred to injections by many patients who are unable to take their drugs orally.

## Conclusion

Chronic pain is a far more complex phenomenon than acute pain. The several dimensions of chronic pain often necessitate multimodal approaches, including pharmacologic, physical, psychological, and social interventions. Multiple drug therapy is often indicated, resulting in an increased risk of drug interactions and adverse effects. Interdisciplinary evaluation and management of chronic pain through pain management teams is increasing. Pharmacists may play important roles on such teams in the planning, implementation, and monitoring of drug effects.

## References

Alsop, S., *Stay of Execution*. Philadelphia: Lippincott, 1974.

Beaver, W. T., et al., "A Clinical Comparison of the Analgesic Effects of Methadone and Morphine Administered Intramuscularly, and of Orally and Parenterally Administered Methadone," *Clinical Pharmacology and Therapeutics*, 1967, *8*, 415–426.

Byck, R., "Drugs and the Treatment of Psychiatric Disorders," in L. Goodman & A. Gilman (Eds.), *The Pharmacological Basis of Therapeutics* (5th ed.). New York: Macmillan, 1975, p. 166.

*Dorland's Illustrated Medical Dictionary* (25th ed.). Philadelphia: W. B. Saunders, 1974.

Gutmer, L. B., Gould, W. J., & Batterman, R. C., "The Effects of Potent Analgesics on Vestibular Function," *Journal of Clinical Investigation*, 1952, *31*, 259–266.

Lipman, A. G., "Drug Therapy in Terminally Ill Patients," *American Journal of Hospital Pharmacy*, 1975, *32*, 270–276.

Marks, R., & Sachar, E., "Undertreatment of Medical Inpatients with Narcotic

Analgesics," *Annals of Internal Medicine*, 1973, *78*, 173–181.

*Martindale: The Extra Pharmacopeia* (27th ed.) (A. Wade, Ed.). London: Pharmaceutical Press, 1973.

Moertel, C. G., et al., "A Comparative Evaluation of Marketed Analgesic Drugs," *New England Journal of Medicine*, 1972, *286*, 813–815.

Moertel, C. G., et al.; "Relief of Pain by Oral Medications," *Journal of the American Medical Association*, 1974, *229*, 55–59.

Mount, B. M., Ajemian, I., & Scott, J. F., "Use of Brompton Mixture in Treating Chronic Pain of Malignant Disease," *Canadian Medical Association Journal*, 1976, *115*, 122–124.

Saunders, C., *The Management of Terminal Illness*. London: Hospital Medicine, 1967.

Snow, H., "Opium and Cocaine in the Treatment of Cancerous Disease," *British Medical Journal*, 1896, *2*, 718–719.

Snyder, S., "Opiate Receptors and Internal Opiates," *Scientific American*, 1977, *236*, 44–56.

Symonds, P., "Methadone in the Elderly," *British Medical Journal*, 1977, *1*, 512.

Twycross, R. G., "Euphoriant Elixirs," *British Medical Journal*, 1973, *2*, 552.

Twycross, R. G., "Clinical Experience with Diamorphine in Advanced Malignant Pain," *International Journal of Clinical Pharmacology*, 1974, *9*, 184–198. (a)

Twycross, R. G., "Diamorphine and Cocaine Elixir, BPC 1973," *Pharmaceutical Journal*, 1974, *212*, 153ff. (b)

Twycross, R. G., "Value of Cocaine in Opiate Containing Elixirs," *British Medical Journal*, 1977, *2*, 1348. (a)

Twycross, R. G., "Choice of Strong Analgesic in Terminal Cancer: Diamorphine or Morphine," *Pain*, 1977, *3*, 93–104. (b)

Twycross, R. G., personal communication, 1978.

Twycross, R. G., Fry, D. E., & Wills, P. D., "The Alimentary Absorption of Diamorphine and Morphine in Man as Indicated by Urinary Excretion Studies," *British Journal of Clinical Pharmacology*, 1974, *1*, 491–494.

# 8

# Drug Control of Common Symptoms

*Mary Baines*

## Pain Control

More than 60 per cent of patients admitted to St. Christopher's Hospice complain of pain: sometimes mild, often severe, not infrequently overwhelming. All these patients subsequently experience substantial, if not complete, relief.

Perhaps the two most important reasons for inadequate pain control prior to admission are:

An inadequate concept of the nature of pain.

Ill-founded fears and fantasies concerning the "addictive" nature of narcotic analgesics.

Pain due to advancing cancer is usually chronic, constant in nature even if variable in intensity. Chronic pain, unlike acute pain, is a situation rather than an event. It is impossible to predict when it will end; it usually gets worse rather than better and often expands to occupy the patient's whole attention, isolating him from the world around. Depression, anxiety, fear, social isolation, and other unrelieved symptoms will tend to exacerbate the total pain experience. All these factors must be considered in relieving terminal pain.

Addiction—a compulsion or overpowering drive to take a drug in

*From:* Mary Baines (Ed.), *Drug Control of Common Symptoms* (unpublished pamphlet, St. Christopher's Hospice, n.d.). Reprinted by permission of Dame Cicely M. Saunders.

order to experience its psychological effects—does not occur when patients' pain control is part of a pattern of total care. Occasionally a patient admitted to the Hospice appears to be addicted, demanding "an injection" every two or three hours. Such a patient typically has a long history of poor pain control and will, for several weeks, have been receiving somewhat irregular ("four-hourly prn") and often inadequate injection of one or more narcotic analgesics. Given time, it is usually possible to control the pain, prevent clock-watching and demanding behaviour, and sometimes transfer the patient to an oral preparation. But even here, can it be said that the patient is really addicted? Is he craving the narcotic in order to experience its psychological effects? Or is he craving relief from pain, in part if not in full, for at least an hour or two?

Analgesics should be given regularly, usually four-hourly. The aim is to titrate the level of analgesia against the patient's pain, increasing the dose until the patient is pain-free. The next dose must be given before the effect of the previous one has worn off and therefore before the patient may think it necessary. In this way it is possible to erase the memory and fear of pain.

If a rapid increase in narcotics seems to be required to maintain an adequate level of analgesia, additional or alternative measures should be considered; for example, an anti-inflammatory agent, or radiotherapy, or occasionally a nerve block. When the dose has to be increased fairly rapidly the patient may at first feel sleepy, but tolerance to the sedative effect of narcotic analgesics and phenothiazines usually occurs within two or three days.

*Mild Pain*

1. Paracetamol (Panadol): 2 four-hourly.
2. Dextropropoxyphene with paracetamol (Distalgesic): 2 four-hourly.
3. Soluble aspirin: 2 four-hourly, or Codis: 2 four-hourly.

These are also used as adjuncts to stronger analgesics and are especially useful in bone pain and headache.

*Moderate Pain*

1. Dipipanone 10 mg with cyclizine 30 mg (Diconal): 1–2 hourly (tab 1 equivalent to 5 mg morphine). This is a useful analgesic of medium

strength and is especially valuable with outpatients or if the patient prefers a tablet to a mixture.

2. Morphine or diamorphine elixir. A controlled double-blind trial comparing these two drugs, given in an elixir, with a phenothiazine (both at individually optimized doses) showed that there was no clinical observable difference, if given in the ratio of diamorphine : morphine = 1 : 1.5. There were no measurable differences in side effects such as nausea, constipation, or euphoria. (A further controlled trial showed that no sustained benefit was obtained by the addition of cocaine to the opiate, so the use of this drug in the mixtures has been discontinued.)

Because morphine is available world-wide, we now prescribe for moderate pain a morphine elixir, e.g., Rx morphine sulphate 5–10 mg, and chloroform water to 10 ml.

Unless transferring from another potent narcotic analgesic, the initial dose of morphine given is usually 5–10 mg (the lower dose should be used with the frail and elderly). This is given with a phenothiazine, often as a syrup. Prochlorperazine (Stemetil) 5 mg in 5 ml is the one usually added, chlorpromazine (Largactil) 12.5–25 mg in 5 ml if sedation is required. These potentiate the effect of morphine, and also act as antiemetics and tranquilizers. For outpatients, Stemetil or Largactil syrup can be incorporated in the mixture when a stable level of analgesia is obtained; for example:

```
Morphine HCl        20 mg
Stemetil syrup       5 ml
Chloroform water to 10 ml
```

There are four BPC [British Pharmaceutical Codex] preparations, with diamorphine or morphine and cocaine, with and without chlorpromazine. These are not recommended, as the drugs used are in a fixed ratio, and it is most important to prescribe all components individually.

3. Phenazocine (Narphen): 5 mg 1–3 four-hourly (5 mg equivalent to 25 mg morphine). This is a useful strong analgesic, especially if the patient dislikes the morphine elixir or prefers a tablet.

4. Methadone. This is probably equipotent with diamorphine but has a much longer half-life and therefore a cumulative effect which could be dangerous in the very ill. It may be possible to give it less frequently, e.g., 6–8 hourly.

5. Dextromoramide (Palfium). This is twice as potent as diamorphine but is of limited use in the control of chronic pain. It has a short half-life, about one and a half hours, and for effective pain control needs to be

given 2–3 hourly, an undesirable drug regime for the patient. It is occasionally used for rapid relief of an exacerbation of pain.

## Severe Pain

Morphine elixir containing morphine 20–60 mg (or even up to 90 or 120 mg), four-hourly, is usually effective. If this does not control the pain with the use of adjuvants (e.g., Distalgesic 2 four-hourly) the patient should be transferred to four-hourly injections of diamorphine. Very occasionally, for the few patients needing high doses, a three-hourly regime may be required.

Diamorphine remains the drug of choice for injections; it is more soluble than morphine and can, therefore, be given in a smaller volume of solution, and subcutaneously if given alone.

Both morphine and diamorphine are at least twice as potent by injection. Thus, if transferring from the oral route to injections, the dose should be halved and then slowly increased until pain control is achieved.

The phenothiazine should, of course, be continued, either orally or by injection.

## Pain and Vomiting

The morphine elixir with phenothiazine may be tolerated and prove effective. However, it may be necessary to give injections of diamorphine and a phenothiazine for a few days, after which it is often possible to return to the oral route. Injections will be required in intractable vomiting, obstruction, or if the patient cannot swallow. Oxycodone pectinate (Proladone) suppositories (30 mg) 1–2 eight-hourly are occasionally used with outpatients to avoid the regular injection of analgesics.

## Bone Pain

This is a difficult problem, as frequently the pain level varies widely and depends on the patient's activity. It is often useful to add a nonsteroidal anti-inflammatory drug to other analgesics. Aspirin is useful, and phenylbutazone (Butazolidin or Butacote) will help about half these patients. In severe bone pain phenylbutazone may be started in a dosage of 600 mg–800 mg/day reducing after a week to 300 mg/day if possible. The drug should be withdrawn after 5–7 days if there is no improvement. Indomethacin (Indocin) and ibuprofen (Brufen) are probably less potent alternatives.

# Anorexia

This is one of the commonest symptoms in malignant disease. Glucocorticosteroids are frequently used, either prednisone 5 mg tds [three times a day] or prednisolone (enteric-coated) 5 mg tds. In the majority of cases this produces, after about a week, a marked increase in appetite and sense of well-being.

Alcohol before or with meals may help.

# Nausea and Vomiting

The phenothiazines are probably the most useful drugs. Prochlorperazine (Stemetil) 5–10 mg, promazine (Sparine) 25 mg, or chlorpromazine (Largactil) 25 mg are all useful antiemetics and are in ascending order of sedative effect.

They may be given four-hourly in syrup or as a suspension in the case of promazine (Sparine). Alternatively, they may be given in tablet form or by IM [intramuscular] injection. Stemetil suppositories (25 mg) and Largactil suppositories (100 mg) are useful if oral preparations are not tolerated and injections impracticable—for example, if the patient is at home. These are normally given eight-hourly.

If these prove inadequate it is probably better to add a further antiemetic of a different type rather than to increase the dose. Cyclizine (Valoid) 50 mg orally or IM bd (twice daily) is often useful, as is metoclopramide (Maxolon) 10 mg, especially if given orally or IM about one hour before meals.

## Obstructive Vomiting

It is usually possible to control the pain and nausea of malignant bowel obstruction in its terminal phase by the use of adequate analgesics and a combination of antiemetics. In these cases, Dioctyl-forte 1–2 tds is sometimes used until it appears that obstruction is complete. Lomotil 2 qds [four times daily] or prn may have a place in the control of painful colic.

# Dry Mouth

This may be due to one or more of many causes, e.g., local radiotherapy, various drugs, dehydration. Intravenous fluids and nasogastric feeding cannot be justified in dying patients who rarely feel thirsty, and it is perfectly possible to correct the only common symptom of dehydration, namely a dry mouth, by local measures such as frequent small drinks or crushed ice to suck and special attention to mouth care.

## Hiccough

Chlorpromazine (Largactil) 25 mg orally or IM.

Metoclopramide (Maxolon) 10 mg orally or IM.

## Dyspnoea

1. *Bronchodilators.*  Salbutamol (Ventolin) 2–4 mg tds or amino-phylline suppositories 1–2 prn are used for bronchospasm.
2. *Glucocorticosteroids.*  Prednisolone may help considerably when there is diffuse malignant involvement of the lungs and, of course, in bronchospasm. In such circumstances, the recommended starting dose is 10–15 mg tds, reducing to 5 mg tds.
3. *Antibiotics.*  If dyspnoea is associated with a cough productive of purulent sputum, an antibiotic may ease the patient's distress. But the indiscriminate use of antibiotics may merely prolong the terminal phase. Septrin, ampicillin, and chloramphenicol are all used.
4. *Opiates.*  In many cases, e.g., large pleural effusion and extensive carcinoma of bronchus, the above measures are ineffective and then opiates must be used to relieve the distress of continued dyspnoea. The morphine elixir may be adequate, but often injections of diamorphine are used with a phenothiazine or diazepam (Valium) to combat the associated mental distress.
5. *Hyoscine.*  IM hyoscine 0.4–0.6 mg is given with an opiate to dry up the excessive secretions which accumulate when a patient is dying, and eliminates the "death rattle" which is distressing to relatives, if not to the patient. N.B.: IM hyoscine with an opiate may give the quickest relief in a major crisis, e.g., haemorrhage or pulmonary embolus. It also produces some amnesia if the patient survives the crisis.

## Cough

1. Benylin expectorant is often adequate.
2. Linctus methadone 5–10 ml, especially at night.
3. Antibiotics.

4. Bromhexine (Bisolvon) 8 mg tds (tab 1 or 10 ml syrup) is often effective in liquefying tenacious sputum.
5. Morphine elixir or diamorphine injection given for pain or dyspnoea is, of course, also an effective cough suppressant.

## Anxiety, Mental Distress

1. Diazepam (Valium) 2-5 mg tds.
2. Promazine (Sparine) 25 mg tds or chlorpromazine (Largactil) 10-25 mg tds.
3. IM or IV diazepam (Valium) 10 mg is of use in acute panic states or prior to some procedure which distresses the patient, e.g., difficult catheterisation.

## Confusion

In mild confusion oral chlorpromazine (Largactil) 10-25 mg qds may be adequate. In severe restlessness and confusion IM chlorpromazine (Largactil) 25-100 mg may be needed, or IM methotrimeprazine (Veractil) 25-50 mg. These may be given with opiates or in conjunction with diazepam (Valium) if necessary. Thioridazine (Mellaril) 10-25 mg has a place in the elderly.

## Depression

1. Attention to physical and mental distress.
2. Antidepressants: Tricyclic antidepressants, e.g., amitriptyline (Tryptizol), trimipramine (Surmontil), or dothiepin (Prothiaden). Patients with malignant disease should usually be started on a small dose, e.g., 10 mg tds or 25 mg nocte, as larger doses sometimes precipitate confusion. This is possibly due to their potentiation by the phenothiazines. These doses may be gradually increased.

## Insomnia

Unless a patient is already habituated, nonbarbiturate sedatives are preferred, such as dichloralphenazone (Welldorm) or nitrazepam (Mogadon). It is sometimes useful to add chlorpromazine (Largactil) 25-50 mg, either with the hypnotics or in the early evening. Chlormethiazole (Heminevrin) 500 mg-1 gm is useful in the elderly. Night sweats are an occasional cause of insomnia. They can often be relieved by an indomethacin (Indocid) suppository 100 mg on settling, or probably less effectively by caps indomethacin 50 mg.

## Constipation

The majority of terminally ill patients suffer with constipation. This is usually due to a combination of factors: their inactivity, anorexia, low-residue diet, and analgesic drugs.

Dietary bran is a logical treatment but is commonly unacceptable. These patients need a combination of softening and peristalsis-inducing aperients, conveniently given in some dual action proprietary preparation, such as Dorbanex Medo or Forte, or Normax. The aperient should be given regularly, e.g., Dorbanex Medo 5–10 ml bd.

Suppositories or an enema or a manual removal may be needed if a patient presents with a loaded rectum, or if the above aperient regime is not effective.

## Diarrhoea

1. Codeine phosphate 15–60 mg tds, or
2. Lomotil 2 qds.

Some cases of diarrhoea are due to malabsorption from pancreatic insufficiency, and these respond to pancreatic replacements, e.g., caps Pancrex V 1 tds with food.

## Fungating Growths

1. Povidone-iodine 4% (Betadine skin cleanser) has proved most effective in the cleansing and deodorizing of many fungating lesions. It should be well mixed with an equal volume of liquid paraffin; the wound cleansed with this preparation; then gauze, well soaked in it, applied as a dressing. Dilution may need to be 1 in 4.
2. Eusol and paraffin (1 to 4) remains useful, especially for desloughing wounds.
3. Gauze soaked in adrenaline (1 to 1,000) may prevent capillary bleeding.
4. A course of systemic antibiotics may help to reduce sepsis, with its associated offensive discharge.

## [Urinary] Frequency

1. Treatment of urinary infection.
2. Emepronium bromide (Cetiprin) 100 mg tds or 200 mg nocte.

## Catheterisation

1. Septrin 2 bd for two days when catheter is inserted or changed.
2. Maintenance of a urinary antiseptic, e.g., hexamine hippurate (Hiprex) 1 bd.
3. A course of an appropriate antibiotic should frank infection occur, as indicated by a suprapubic pain, or if the catheter is blocked by debris.
4. Catheter changed every four weeks.
5. Regular bladder washouts with Hibitane 1 in 5,000 or Noxyflex bladder washouts bd for two days in patients unable to take urinary antiseptics by mouth or if, in spite of these, the catheter tends to block.

## Itch

1. Antihistamines, e.g., chlorpheniramine (Piriton) 4 mg tds or promethazine (Phenergan) 25 mg at night.
2. Steroids.
3. In the irritation caused by biliary stasis, cholestyramine (Cuemid, Questran) 1 sachet qds is the drug of choice, but patients find it difficult to take.
4. Crotamiton (Eurax) or local anaesthetic creams may be of value.

# III

# Caregiving

*In Part III we explore the principal modes of caregiving that fall within the hospice approach. No summary of a need-oriented program of care can ever claim to provide a complete listing of professional skills and disciplines that might be called upon. Every skill that can be brought to bear on the care of dying persons and their families is valuable precisely to the extent that it is relevant and effective. Our chapters are intended to represent at least the major modes of caregiving that apply. The order in which these selections follow is conventional and is not intended to reflect judgments of relative importance.*

*As one reads through the first eight chapters in Part III—describing contributions to care that can be made by physicians, nurses, social workers, physical therapists (or physiotherapists), occupational therapists, chaplains, psychotherapists, and volunteers—a number of common themes emerge: the development of an interdisciplinary team that includes patients and families; role blurring in the provision of services; the importance of the caregiver's understanding of and attitudes toward hospice care; the insistence that hospice care requires a high level of professional expertise, although skills may be applied in ways that are not typical of acute care programs; the value of imaginative and scrupulous attention to detail; care addressed to the needs of the total patient/family unit as those persons define their needs and desire their care; and positive contributions that can be made by volunteers.*

*The conviction that underlies these themes is that caregiving skills are appropriate for dying persons and family members because all are living human beings. "Rehabilitation" for these and many other people does not consist in cure or restoration of a bygone state; rather, it means obtaining maximum value from existing capabilities and preventing atrophy or increased distress from their neglect. Appropriate care can assist such people to find meaning in life and to retain or regain control even over small aspects that contribute to a sense of individuality and worth. The only qualifier is that some interventions depend upon*

*others; one cannot have intense psychosocial or spiritual interactions
with someone who is severely nauseated or in extreme pain. Further,
just as spiritual care is in part a responsibility of the entire team, so also
individual specialists can teach others to fill in for them in their absence. And every member of the team—including the dying person or
members of the family—can function as a concerned friend ministering
to the burdens of any needy party.*

*For caregivers in traditional settings, perhaps the most distinctive
of these points—one that relates to all of the others—is the nature of
the* inter*disciplinary team.* Multi*disciplinary teams, or those in which
many separate disciplines are represented, are common. But they are
typically plagued by fragmentation and the limits of professional specialization. The* inter*disciplinary team requires of its members a willingness to learn from each other and, within the limits of legal restriction,
to cross disciplinary boundaries where that is required for need-oriented
care. A physician making a home visit alone must be willing to clean up
vomit, just as a social worker will help a patient walk to the toilet, or a
nurse will sit down at the bedside to listen to an urgent sharing of a dying person's understanding of life. Unless we can do these things or just
make a gift of our presence in silence without being ill at ease or experiencing a sense of futility and resentment, we do not have our priorities
in the proper order for giving care to dying persons and their families.*

*Our last two selections in Part III speak to preparation for and
stress within caregiving. Whether as professionals or lay persons, caregivers need introduction to the hospice philosophy of care. It is in orientation sessions that individuals can first test their suitability for this sort
of work. And it is in its initial plan of training that a hospice program
first expresses its own commitment to the value of its staff. As Eve
Kavanagh has said (p. 211), "one does not have to be terminally ill to
be important." Nor does one have to be dying to require support. In
both introductory and ongoing training activities and in attention to
staff stress and support, hospice programs recognize two interrelated
points. First, there are unusual stressors in caring for dying persons and
their families. But that must be kept in a balanced perspective. "Burnout" is a popular term these days, in intensive care units, emergency
rooms, and even elementary school classrooms—as well as in hospice.
Much stress in hospice work comes from newness, novelty, problems of
administration, public attention, role blurring, and the demands of the
interdisciplinary team itself. Death and loss are not the sole sources of
difficulty. Second, support can come from many sources, including
one's own inner strengths, one's family, the interdisciplinary team, the
work situation, and both informal and formal programs of assistance.*

*It has been said that one never receives so much as when one is giving to others. Thus, hospice caregiving and the hospice approach address the full spectrum of human needs in a community of concern that includes staff, as well as families and persons with chronic or life-threatening illness. In other words, in its broadest sense the hospice philosophy orients itself to the living, with special attention to difficulties faced by living persons as they encounter dying, death, and bereavement.*

# 9

# Physician Roles
# in Hospice Care

*Daniel C. Hadlock*

During the past 10 to 15 years there has been a remarkable maturing in concepts of appropriate care for the dying patient. At the time when Elisabeth Kübler-Ross began her pioneering work, subsequently reported in her book, *On Death and Dying* (1969), there were no "dying" patients in a local hospital for her to associate with. The issue of "terminality" is still hotly debated in medical circles, but the focus of discussion has shifted from whether or not such patients exist to the more practical questions of how they should be appropriately cared for. The validity of the concept of hospice palliative care seems to be generally accepted at this point. The issues being discussed are, rather, these: How does such care compare with and relate to more standard modes of health care in our society? Does hospice care have anything unique to offer? Is it a special kind of care in its own right? Or is it only a new perspective on how to use standard medical skills and practices that we already have? I believe this is a very healthy development. The debate is now focusing on how we can make a practical reality—a relatively predictable and expected result—out of the emotionally appealing idea of humane and effective care for the terminally ill.

Part of the reason why the concept of effective palliative care has become increasingly acceptable is that a number of pioneer hospice programs in England, Canada, and the United States have demonstrated that it can be done. Care for the terminally ill *can* be competent and effective in both the professional and the humane sense. We also have reason to believe that such care can be provided at costs comparable to those of more usual forms of health care (albeit forms of questionable appropriateness) previously available for the terminally ill. Committees of the National Hospice Organization have spent several years analyzing the characteristics of these pioneer programs. The *Standards of a Hospice Program of Care* (National Hospice Organization, 1979) that have resulted are a first step in identifying those characteristics of structure and organization that do the most toward providing the "efficient loving care" that characterizes hospice.

Because such care is being given and because such criteria can be identified, society's expectations concerning care for dying persons and their families are becoming more demanding. Such expectations impose increasing responsibilities on those who seek to provide hospice care and on the general health care system. Quite rightly, they constitute a challenge for professional competency, and for fiscal and ethical responsibility. This chapter describes some of the elements that are necessary to meet that challenge, with special attention to physician roles in hospice care.

## Hospice Palliative Care

The existing health care system in our society exhibits a heavy bias toward a cure orientation. As physicians, we are taught to diagnose and treat disease, and to expect cure rates as a consequence. Not much emphasis is placed on the management of patients who have diseases that cannot be cured. As patients, we go to the physician to be cured, and comedians evoke much bitter laughter with wry comments about how the therapy was a success but the patient died. Even payments from insurance companies and Medicare are limited to services, places, and durations of care based on the presupposition that the only appropriate therapies are those that result in cure or control of disease. Against this, we need to remember the fuller definition of medical care which has been with us at least since the 15th century: to cure sometimes, to relieve often, to comfort always. From this broader perspective, we must remind ourselves that cure is not always possible—even for a highly advanced and skilled medical system. But "if cure is perceived as the only acceptable goal of medical care, then chronic, degenerative, eventually fatal disease is a fact that cannot be acknowledged" (Hadlock, 1980, p. 134). That is intolerable for a realistic and humane health care system. Even where cure, arrest, or control of disease are beyond our capabilities, it is never true that "there is nothing more that we can do." Palliative care historically and at present constitutes a major part of medical treatment; nevertheless, in the form of hospice care for dying persons and their families, it must be newly understood and carefully defined.

The goal of all medical therapy should be to provide *appropriate treatment*. The definition of "appropriate" in this context has been well described as follows:

*appropriate treatment*

> Treatment is appropriate if patients benefit from application of one of two complementary systems at the correct time: one concerned with eliminating a controllable disease, the other with relieving the symptoms of an incurable disease. Either must be available when needed; no patient should be "locked into" a system directed in what is, at a particular stage of illness, the wrong course. . . . When it becomes appropriate not to extend a patient's life the emphasis should be on improving the quality of the life remaining. (Shephard, 1977, p. 522)

The basic purpose of hospice care is best summarized in the response a terminally ill patient gave to Cicely Saunders when asked that question. The answer was, "I am a traveler on the journey from one life to the next, and I need a place where I can be welcomed and looked after and cared for and be myself on that journey." The National Hospice Organization *Standards* (1979) express the philosophy of hospice care more formally:

> Hospice affirms life. Hospice exists to provide support and care for persons in the last phases of incurable disease so that they might live as fully and comfortably as possible. Hospice recognizes dying as a normal process whether or not resulting from disease. Hospice neither hastens nor postpones death. Hospice exists in the hope and belief that, through appropriate care and the promotion of a caring community sensitive to their needs, patients and families may be free to attain a degree of mental and spiritual preparation for death that is satisfactory to them. (p. 3)

In short, hospice is a program of care oriented to meeting the needs of those patients who cannot realistically expect to be cured and whose needs are primarily for comfort and relief for the limited time of life they are expected to have. It is focusing on the quality of living remaining for those who have minimal quantities of time left.

Since quality is such a personal matter when one is talking of life style, hospice is very much *a need-oriented program of care* in which the dominant priority is that the patient and the family have a primary role both in defining their needs and in being participants in the process by which they will be treated. What is appropriate in such circumstances is what the patient and the family find comforting and supportive in all areas of existence—physical, emotional, social, spiritual, financial. Because patients and families under stress cannot be expected to exercise the best judgment, and because families who may be facing the most serious illness they have ever experienced cannot be expected to be knowledgeable in how to handle it, hospice programs must be prepared to provide the professional and personal resources necessary to meet needs in all these areas. Hospice programs also must have the patience and insight to apply those resources in a manner that the family sees as responsive, supportive, and caring.

The focus of such care is not simply symptom control (i.e., keeping the patient physically comfortable). The focus of such care is *palliation* (i.e., assisting the patient to live until the day he or she dies).

> We should aim for the relief that enables a patient not only to die peacefully, but also to *live* until he dies, as himself and not as what has been termed an "uncomplaining residue." (Weismann & Hackett, 1962)

Dying patients are alive. When in distress, they require a broad treatment program with a high level of skilled professional competence.

> People consistently miss the point about Hospice. We're concerned with people who need care for the *symptoms* that make them miserable. We're not zeroing in on death. I don't need someone to help me die. If I were dying, I would hope for concern about the way I live out my life. People don't understand that Hospice is not just a hand-holding place. . . . We work with pain, nausea, weakness, breathing difficulty—as well as with emotional pain and spiritual distress. (Edward F. Dobihal, as quoted in Kron, 1976, p. 45)

The goal of this sort of care is to help the patient to continue life in as near to a usual manner as possible—at work, being with the family, doing whatever is especially significant before the close of life, feeling a part of ongoing life even as the patient is concluding his or her own. Appropriate treatment of this sort is an active and positive form of caregiving.

> It is clearly imperative for us, the care-givers, to try to help patient and family to make the best use of the time that remains to them. This is the main aim of terminal care and the most important single service which we have to offer. It we fail to recognize the opportunity which terminal care represents in terms of family growth and development we have nothing to offer but palliation, the mitigation of suffering by symptom relief alone. This type of palliative care is purely negative. (Parkes, 1978, p. 46)

As a result, we should not think of "hospice therapies" as being in opposition to "medical therapies." Figure 9.1 illustrates how hospice compares with and complements current concepts of health care. By virtue of this construct, one can see that hospice differs from traditional care not so much in what kind of therapies are utilized, as *how* they are utilized. The intensive care unit and the hospice care program are both, in their own way, forms of highly structured, well-organized therapeutic programs. However, an intensive care unit is oriented toward treating diseases for the sake of achieving a cure. Modern medicine has made major strides in such endeavors in the last 20 years by virtue of many scientific and technological advances that necessitate a much more structured form of care. The

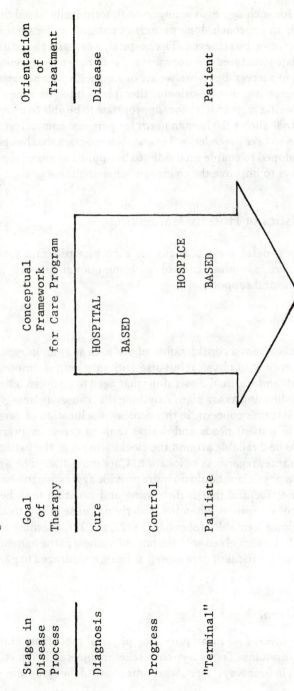

Figure 9.1.   Interface between Curative and Palliative Health Care Systems

| Stage in Disease Process | Goal of Therapy | Conceptual Framework for Care Program | Orientation of Treatment |
|---|---|---|---|
| Diagnosis | Cure | HOSPITAL BASED | Disease |
| Progress | Control | | |
| "Terminal" | Palliate | HOSPICE BASED | Patient |

*From:* Daniel C. Hadlock, "Hospice Care: Implications and Influence on Current Health Care Concepts," *Long-Term Care and Health Services Administration Quarterly,* 1980, *4,* 139. Reproduced by permission of Panel Publishers.

justification for such aggressive, impersonal, technically based therapy is that, by such an approach, long periods of control of disease if not outright cure can often be achieved. The hospital, a caregiver's institution, is the appropriate structured environment for such care to be given with optimal chance of success. But when we are dealing with patients where—despite such aggressive, disease-oriented therapies—it has become apparent that cure is not likely, then it is more appropriate to be able to provide care in a fashion that allows the human needs for personal comfort, relief, and consideration to take precedence. Hospice is a program that has been specifically developed to enable such skills to be applied in more humane settings and ways to improve the chance of achieving these goals.

## Characteristics of Hospice Caregiving

There are six general areas of focus for a hospice program (Shephard, 1977): total care, symptom control, pain, emotional support, families, and staff stress and support.

### Total Care

By *total care* is meant a consideration of the patient as an integrated personality not only with physical but also with intellectual, emotional, social, financial, and spiritual dimensions that need to be taken into consideration in establishing a care plan. Anything that causes distress is worthy of the hospice team's concern. In this context, the location of care should relate more to patient needs and desires than to caregiver preferences. Care needs to be available around the clock, whenever the patient might require assistance, regardless of location. Care must always be appropriate; that is, "a physician should no more provide aggressive treatment that cannot be effective and that is distressing and isolating than he should merely control symptoms when the underlying cause is still treatable or has again become treatable" (Shephard, 1977, p. 522). We must recognize that the family is as involved with the patient's illness as the patient, and so they also become a focus of care as well as being encouraged to participate in caregiving.

### Symptom Control

By *symptom control* we mean providing physical relief from chronically distressing symptoms. To achieve such relief requires skilled medical and nursing input in four ways. First, where the cause of the symptom (i.e., the disease) is recognized to be incurable and/or uncontrollable, then the symptom itself becomes the focus of medical therapy. Good symptom control requires careful and continuing clinical assessment by physicians and nurses to determine the pathophysiology of symptom generation before any treatment decisions can be made. Second, once an appropriate diagnosis has been made, it requires great clinical skill and imaginative medical management to ensure that symptoms are controlled with appropriate therapy without unnecessary side effects. Terminally ill patients have extremely low, if any, physical, physiological, and emotional reserves. Inappropriate therapy—either too little or too much treatment— would complicate patient management rather than simplify it. Third, the concept of symptom control contains within it the concept of symptom prevention. Appropriate therapies are applied routinely at intervals that maintain a continuing beneficial effect without the breakthrough of previous chronic distress. Finally, symptom control is not custodial care. There is a need for careful clinical supervision that responds to changes in patient condition whenever they occur with immediate and appropriate changes in management.

*Pain*

Pain is the most feared symptom in cancer. Reports indicate that pain is actually a problem only 50% of the time (Aitken-Swan, 1959; Turnbull, 1954). Nevertheless, patients often are referred to hospice programs because of uncontrolled pain. Thus, the incidence of pain in a hospice patient population tends to be high. Published reports that pain can be controlled in the majority of patients with an aggressive approach (e.g., Twycross, 1978) are consistent with the clinical experience of many hospice physicians. As more hospice programs become established and more experience is accumulated, we can hope that other symptoms may likewise come to be as readily managed.

*Emotional Support*

Emotional support for the patient is an essential aspect of hospice care. The emotional needs of the dying have been aptly noted to fall in three general categories of request: "Don't leave me," "Listen to me," and "Help me" (Shephard, 1977, p. 525). This is consistent with Davidson's study (1979, p. 169), which found that terminally ill patients ranked their major problems as "abandonment," "loss of self-management," and "intractable pain." A program of hospice care seeks to meet these needs and to achieve not passive resignation, but active acceptance.

Active acceptance is completely different from passive resignation: the former brings something positive and vital to the patient while the latter, being essentially negative, casts a shadow of gloom across the final phase of the patient's illness. (Twycross, 1975, p. 11)

Ideally, a patient should be able to say, as Fry writes (1954), "I have heard illness out, until it has nothing to say to me, and I thank God I have the last word."

### Families

Families as persons in bereavement are at high risk for both physical and emotional illness (Butler, 1975, pp. 372, 383). Hence, there is a definite potential for preventive medicine in this realm of hospice care. Families must be actively supported and assisted in their grieving both before and after a death. Hospice programs generally support families for 1 year following the patient's death; however, preliminary evidence indicates that the period of risk may be longer (Kiely & Hampson, 1980). We must learn how to respond to these real needs within the limits of practical program requirements.

### Staff Stress and Support

It has been well recognized in a variety of clinical settings that the staff that is not self-supportive does not cope well (Beszterczey, 1980; Lyall, Vachon, & Rogers, 1980; Mount & Voyer, 1980). Because of the commitment of those who have initiated hospice programs, staff turnover to date has tended to be low. Nonetheless, a real risk exists for care providers and their programs. It is imperative that a hospice care program, as it opens itself to the stress of patients and families facing death and suffering, address itself to the internal stress within its own team so that it may survive and continue to be supportive. In addition, an external stress for all hospice care programs at the present time is their relationship to standard health care provider systems. Any new health care concept not only has to define what is different about it; it must also justify why it needs to be different. And it needs to demonstrate that by virtue of these differences, it meets a need not previously met.

## The Interdisciplinary Team and Physician Roles

Two aspects of hospice caregiving programs are of particular relevance to medical involvement: the interdisciplinary team and physician roles within the team. The core members of the interdisciplinary patient care team in a hospice program are identified in the National Hospice Organization *Standards* as the patient/family unit, the primary physician, the hospice physician, the hospice nurse, the hospice social worker, the hospice patient care coordinator, hospice volunteers, and hospice clergy. The term *interdisciplinary* refers to the fact that this team has certain basic characteristics in structure and function. First, it has multiple disciplines, and individuals from these disciplines meet together at least weekly to review each patient and family's progress. Thus, they have the chance to share perspectives continually in both assessment and management. Secondly and as a consequence, a phenomenon of "role blurring" takes place (and is encouraged), so that whenever any members of the team are directly involved with a patient or a family, they approach them with a personal as well as a professional awareness of the contributions of all disciplines. A third unique characteristic in this constellation of caregivers is that through such personal and professional interaction, staff support is taking place even as the patient care is being administered. This allows the team to be much more comprehensive and innovative in its caregiving, thereby providing realistic cause for pride in achievement. It also makes the team more resilient and self-sufficient as it seeks to meet the demands and stresses intrinsic to working with the grief and suffering of others.

Physician involvement within the interdisciplinary team is essential to the success or failure of individual hospice programs, as well as to the eventual acceptance or rejection of the hospice concept within our society. In part, this is a consequence of the responsibility and authority, both professional and legal, that physicians have in relation to patient care. For example, physicians are needed to order diagnostic studies and to establish a valid diagnosis, to obtain prescription drugs, to certify legal death, and to secure reimbursement for ancillary health care services. Further, cooperation from physicians and advocacy from physician leaders are required to enable the hospice movement to establish itself as a competent, credible, and appropriate form of health care.

In turn, in order to provide the most effective palliative care, a physician, whether in community practice or on the hospice staff, will find his professional skills and commitment are most effective in the context of a hospice interdisciplinary team. First, by working within a hospice program, a physician would be functioning in association with others of like mind in terms of their *commitment* to this concept of care for those who need it. Such a commitment is both a professional and a personal one with potential satisfactions in each dimension.

Secondly, like any other form of professional and skilled care, there is a continuing need in hospice palliative care to learn and develop one's skills on a daily basis. Participation in a hospice program insures that one is allowed and takes the time to seek out *training* in order to develop the skills especially appropriate for various aspects of this sort of palliative care. This is not to say that palliative care per se is unique, but that exercising one's clinical imagination to apply standard skills effectively to meet a different need does take thought and training. Growth of this sort has positive implications both for hospice caregiving and for general medical practice.

Thirdly, adequate performance in any of these areas requires *time*. This means time not only to do the task at hand, but time to reach the location where the patient may be, time to work through other persons both on the team and in the community, time to educate oneself to become skilled, and time to follow up and make sure the outcome of therapy is satisfactory. It is very difficult, if not an outright conflict of commitment, for physicians primarily committed to office and hospital practice and to learning the skills of cure-oriented medicine to have time to take on the additional responsibilities of a hospice program of care.

Finally, hospice care is not the prerogative of any one person or any one profession. Each individual on the team has to have his or her own commitment to the ideal. But delivery of the care requires an interactive, interdisciplinary, role-blurring type of *team* interaction. There needs to be heavy emphasis on internal communication, both professionally and personally. The team needs to take care of itself even as it takes care of patients and families. As Colin Murray Parkes (1978) has said most eloquently,

> Terminal care is a matter of human relationships. There are skills to be learned and insights which can be gained from reading books but the challenge and the reward of terminal care arises from the fact that it demands that we use the whole of ourselves to relate to fellow human beings who are in trouble. This can only be learned by experience in a community in which relationships are valued and fostered. (p. 64)

There are a number of roles that physicians can fill in relation to the hospice program of care. These roles are defined in the National Hospice Organization *Standards* document (1979). The *primary physician* is

> that licensed medical practitioner whom the patient and family identify as having the most significant role in the determination and delivery of medical care to the patient at the time of referral to and acceptance on the Hospice program. If this physician is not on the Hospice staff, this physician's consent will be necessary for admission of the patient to the Hospice care program. (p. 36)

(*Attending physician* is a synonym for *primary physician*). The *hospice physician* is any licensed medical practitioner on the Hospice staff (salaried or not) who is involved with the determination and delivery (directly or in an advisory capacity) of medical aspects of Hospice care to patients and families on the Hospice program. This individual may or may not be the patient's primary physician. (p. 36)

The hospice *medical director* must be a staff physician on the hospice program. He or she is

that licensed medical practitioner (salaried or not) on the Hospice staff who has been identified by the Hospice team as having ultimate responsibility for medical aspects of Hospice care. This individual can be directly or indirectly involved in actual patient care. This individual will have responsibilities for team support and education as well. (p. 35)

Finally, the *consulting physician* is

any licensed medical practitioner who is asked by medical practitioners already treating a patient and family to provide limited medical advice and therapy for the specific needs of a patient and family. Such care is provided under the coordination of the requesting physician, who may or may not be on the Hospice staff. (p. 36)

## Hospice Staff Physicians

Hospice staff physicians serve four sorts of clientele: the interdisciplinary hospice team, the primary physician, dying persons and their families, and the community at large. In the first place, the hospice interdisciplinary team acts in a consultative capacity to the primary physician and in a service capacity to his or her patients. The primary duty of hospice staff physicians is to ensure that the team satisfies these responsibilities in a medically competent and effective manner. In the light of what we have said above about role blurring, this means that hospice staff physicians must use their skills for interteam support and consultation, for team training and supervision, and for clinical teaching and research. In this way, the skills and influence of the physician are distributed through all the other members of the team, both professional and nonprofessional, paid and volunteer. Further, along with individuals from other disciplines, hospice staff physicians and the medical director need to guide program administration so that the program as a whole retains the capability to provide appropriate care. It must avoid the risk of evolving into a program of care oriented more toward the convenience of the caregiver, one that loses the flexibility and resourcefulness to be able to meet the real needs of patients and families when, where, and how they develop.

If a problem or circumstance requires physician involvement in depth, then the hospice staff physician must be available to offer medical backup—first, to the team, and, second, to the primary physician. It is a sign of an effective and established program when the primary physician is willing to allow the hospice physicians to apply their clinical skills in direct patient care. In such situations, the primary physician often is grateful for additional expertise in symptom control, as well as the expanded ability to provide physician services in the home, especially when the primary physician cannot do so directly. These two points can be explained in the following way. Hospice staff physicians, by virtue of their duties, acquire extensive experience with the special problems of dying persons and their families and with those therapeutic responses that best satisfy such needs. The importance of expert medical judgment in determining the appropriateness of care delivered to the terminally ill patient cannot be overemphasized. As we have suggested above, palliative care and symptom control is far from passive therapy.

> There is a sharp contrast between the clinician who says merely that a patient has advanced disease and requires sedation, and the clinician who says that a patient has advanced disease and requires symptom control—and at the same time recognizes the need for the nature of that symptom to be explored in more detail. (Calman, 1978, p. 36)

Symptom control requires considerable clinical skill in determining the pathophysiology of symptom generation, as well as innovative and detailed medical management in initiating and maintaining a comprehensive therapeutic regimen that blends all the skills of the hospice program in order to establish good physical and emotional comfort for the patient. In other words, as Day (1966) has stated, death

> cannot be denied, but its dignity can be—by thoughtless, underfeeling and overscientific care. Everything that is done for the dying patient should be based on the constant awareness that, although death may be postponed—sometimes dramatically—the master plan cannot be altered. (p. 886)

Nevertheless, as Krakoff (1979) warns,

> In seeking "death with dignity" we may overlook treatable disease and provide patients with the indignity of premature death. . . . It is important both to differentiate and to understand what is truly terminal and what is reversible. (pp. 108–109)

The interaction between the hospice physician and the primary physician will help maintain the balance.

With regard to availability of physician services, hospice staff physicians can be of significant assistance both to primary physicians and to their patients. As we have indicated, hospice care is not custodial care. It may occur in institutions, but it is perhaps even more appropriate for those patients who are able and wish to remain at home. In any context, patient needs are as likely to occur in the middle of the night or weekend as they are during the day and the regular working week. It is difficult for any individual to respond to patient needs on a 24-hour-a-day, 7-day-a-week basis, and that difficulty is compounded when home visits must be made. Physicians who are obligated to keep office appointments or to make rounds in the hospital are constrained by such obligations and thus are not available to patients who cannot accommodate to these schedules. The hospice staff physician, by virtue of working in a team context oriented toward home care, is able to satisfy such needs and to provide backup physician services when the patient's primary physician may be committed elsewhere.

When we turn to patients, it is helpful to bear in mind Abraham Maslow's elucidation of a "hierarchy of human needs" (1943, 1968). The first of these needs is physical (also called physiological), which describes our most basic requirements, such as food, air, water, and shelter. Second comes a need for security (also called safety), the need for protection against danger, accidents, and deprivation. Third is the social need for friendship, community, and home life—that is, the need for love and belonging. Fourth is the need for esteem—that is, having a sense of importance, productiveness, and self-worth. Fifth, is the need for fulfillment (also called self-actualization)—the desire to become all we can, to fulfill our potential. According to Maslow, we are not concerned with higher levels of need until the lower levels are satisfied. For example, we do not worry about meaning in our lives when we are hurting. Patients are referred to hospice because they are physically ill and expected to die within a relatively short period of time. They usually have physical distress. Their first priority is thus for competent medical management, and it is here that hospice staff physicians are of paramount importance.

One very important question the caregiver should ask such patients is this: "If there were one thing I could do for you, what would that thing be?" As a physician, I needed much encouragement to ask such a question the first time. I felt my role was to cure and to cure only, and I was definitely afraid to allow patients the freedom to ask anything of me without reservation, for I feared they would ask me to provide the cure I knew was not attainable. Alternatively, I feared they would ask for death, which was contrary to my personal as well as professional ethics; but I was not trained in how to help them live in the face of death. In fact, however, these are extremes that are rarely encountered. Usually, patients ask for something very practical and attainable, and I have since learned over and over again the truth of something that Cicely Saunders (1978, p. 2) has articulated so well:

> We fail to understand what patients with terminal disease ask of us. They are commonly too realistic to expect that we can take away the whole, hard thing that is happening to them; instead they ask for concern and care for their distress and symptoms. Above all, they ask for our total awareness of them as people. At no time in the total care of the . . . patient is this of greater importance.

A final task for hospice staff physicians is that of educating our society, both professional and lay, concerning the validity and the capabilities of hospice care. In large measure, we are a death-denying society, which means we all tend to have difficulty accepting the idea that care primarily directed toward comfort and relief in terminal illness can be just as appropriate and competent as care that is directed toward cure. It will take physicians who have thought through these issues for themselves and come to terms with them, as well as those who have participated in the process of making the concept work in practice, to be spokespersons to our society at large as well as to other physicians. Such dialogue will need to take place on a patient-by-patient, family-by-family basis, in a hospice-physician-to-primary-physician association, and in the form of presentations to physician and lay groups, as well as in testimony before licensing, reimbursing, and accrediting agencies at the state, regional, and national levels. Such continuing education and understanding will also need to develop within the hospice team, where the hospice physician can act as a liaison between nonphysician members of the team and primary physicians in the community to facilitate continuity of care between programs and professions.

Actually, much of what has been "learned" and is "new" in concepts of hospice care and chronic pain control has been in our medical literature for decades. Yet today, as a society and as a profession, we are not comfortable or familiar enough with palliative care to give sufficient credence to the concept or effort to the practice. This is changing. There is an increasing and continuing need for all health care professionals within hospice to develop the habit of thinking through their therapeutic programs, to reevaluate and reasssess the results of their treatment continually, and to report such observations in the literature so that nationwide health care may benefit. Such continued self-judging efforts will not only give credibility to the hospice concept, but will improve its effectiveness in the delivery of care. There are valid concerns—for example, about the limits of hospice care and about its integration with more familiar forms of health care—which can in this way be addressed in ongoing dialogue and discussion.

## Conclusion

Hospice programs are not the only appropriate way to care for the dying. But they have demonstrated that the hospice philosophy is a valid and reasonable option that many patients and their families desire, one that has important lessons to offer to our health care system as a whole. An old adage reminds us that "nothing is more certain than death; nothing is less certain than the time of its coming." When disease that is neither curable nor controllable distresses dying persons and their families, before death arrives (and continuing afterward in certain respects), they require the most competent skills and humane services that the profession of medicine has to offer. The practice of such medical care enables physicians to identify and in most cases to develop the expertise to satisfy the special physical and personal needs of the terminally ill and their families. Physician roles in hospice care reflect both a new opportunity for medical caregiving and an implementation of the best traditions of our profession. We owe it to our profession, to our fellow human beings, and to ourselves to strike a new and more equitable balance between our duties—to cure sometimes, to relieve often, to comfort always.

## References

Aitken-Swan, J., "Nursing the Late Cancer Patient at Home: The Family's Impressions," *Practitioner*, 1959, *183*, 64–69.

Beszterczey, A., "Staff Stress on a Newly Developed Palliative Care Service: The Psychiatrist's Role," in I. Ajemian & B. Mount (Eds.), *The R. V. H. Manual on Palliative/Hospice Care*. New York: Arno Press, 1980, pp. 489–497.

Butler, R. N., *Why Survive?* New York: Harper & Row, 1975.

Calman, K. C., "Physical Aspects," in C. M. Saunders (Ed.), *The Management of Terminal Disease*. London: Edward Arnold, 1978, pp. 33–43.

Davidson, G., "Hospice Care for the Dying," in H. Wass (Ed.), *Dying: Facing the Facts*. New York: McGraw-Hill/Hemisphere, 1979, pp. 158–181.

Day, E., "The Patient with Cancer and the Family," *New England Journal of Medicine*, 1966, *274*, 883–886.

Fry, C., *The Dark is Light Enough*. London: Oxford University Press, 1954.

Hadlock, D. C., "Hospice Care: Implications and Influence on Current Health Care Concepts," *Long-Term Care and Health Services Administration Quarterly*, 1980, *4*, 132–154.

Kiely, M., & Hampson, A., "Bereavement Follow-Up: The Development and Evaluation of the Royal Victoria Hospital Program." Paper presented at the Third International Seminar on Terminal Care, Montreal, Canada, October 6, 1980.

Krakoff, I. H., "The Case for Active Treatment in Patients with Advanced Cancer: Not Everyone Needs a Hospice." *CA—A Cancer Journal for Clinicians*, 1979, *29*(2), 108–111.

Kron, J., "Designing a Better Place to Die," *New York Magazine*, March 3, 1976, pp. 43–49.

Kübler-Ross, E., *On Death and Dying*. New York: Macmillan, 1969.

Lyall, A., Vachon, M., & Rogers, J., "A Study of the Degree of Stress Experienced by Professionals Caring for Dying Patients," in I. Ajemian & B. Mount (Eds.), *The R. V. H. Manual on Palliative/Hospice Care*. New York: Arno Press, 1980, pp. 498–509.

Maslow, A., "A Theory of Human Motivation," *Psychological Review*, 1943, *50*, 370–396.

Maslow, A., *Toward a Psychology of Being* (2nd ed.). New York: Van Nostrand, 1968.

Mount, B. M., & Voyer, J., "Staff Stress in Palliative/Hospice Care," in I. Ajemian & B. Mount (Eds.), *The R. V. H. Manual on Palliative/Hospice Care*. New York: Arno Press, 1980, pp. 457–488.

National Hospice Organization, *Standards of a Hospice Program of Care* (6th revision). Unpublished booklet, 1979.

Parkes, C. M., "Psychological Aspects," in C. M. Saunders (Ed.), *The Management of Terminal Disease*. London: Edward Arnold, 1978, pp. 44–64.

Saunders, C. M., "Appropriate Treatment, Appropriate Death," in C. M. Saunders (Ed.), *The Management of Terminal Disease*. London: Edward Arnold, 1978, pp. 1–9.

Shephard, D. A. E., "Principles and Practice of Palliative Care," *Canadian Medical Association Journal*, 1977, *116*, 522–526.

Turnbull, F., "Intractable Pain," *Proceedings of the Royal Society of Medicine*. 1954, *47*, 155.

Twycross, R. G., *The Dying Patient*. London: Christian Medical Fellowship, 1975.

Twycross, R. G., "Relief of Pain," in C. M. Saunders (Ed.), *The Management of Terminal Disease*. London: Edward Arnold, 1978, pp. 65–92.

Weisman, A. D., & Hackett, T. P., "The Dying Patient," *Forest Hospital Pub. 1*, 1962, p. 742.

# 10

# Nursing Care of Dying Persons and Their Families

*Marjory Cockburn*

To answer the question, "How long is living?" is not difficult—it is from birth to death. From the moment of birth, living progresses along the road to death, and this road is called "life." What then is dying? Does dying have a fixed time limit? How can dying be defined? It is because these questions have no easy answer that problems of how or where to care for the dying arise. To be dying in today's society is on the whole an unacceptable state of affairs; it is dismissed, not thought about, as if it was the wish of each one to be immortal or to be alive one minute and to be dead the next. But the first is impossible, and the second (even if it really were desirable) is only likely for the minority. Dying, therefore, needs to be seen as part of living, and it is because of its philosophy of allowing the dying to live until they die and to have quality in that living that the work of the hospice movement has been seen to be a necessary part of health care. We need to understand the components of this new form of care—especially the central role of nursing—in order to carry it out more effectively, not only in the hospice setting but elsewhere. Much that is done in hospice programs can also have a place in the care of dying persons and their families in the hospital ward or in the community.

## The Place of Hospice in Caring for the Dying

In the last century, about 95% of deaths occurred in the home, but this is not true today. The number of deaths occurring in hospitals is increasing, and only about one-third of all deaths now take place at home. The terminal or dying patient has been defined as one for whom, following an accurate diagnosis, death appears to be certain and not too distant—and treatment has therefore changed from curative to palliative. The period of the terminal illness may be only a few days, or it may be weeks or months. For the patient suffering from cancer it can be very variable, so that there can never be an accurate answer to the question "How long?" In a short terminal illness, the present resources usually cope well. It is the longer terminal illness that demands special support.

Dame Cicely Saunders pioneered the first modern hospice in answer to a need—the need for the dying person to be allowed to live until he or she dies, and then to be enabled to die in dignity, relatively free of symptoms. *Hospice*, thus, means a place of rest or shelter on the journey from birth to death. Particularly as death approaches and disease may be making the journey more difficult, hospice programs offer care and comfort combined with expert professional services. Many people nowadays think that *hospice* means a place to die because so many of those who enter a hospice program are near the close of their lives, but that is not the proper meaning of the term, and all hospice programs are able to discharge a small proportion of their patients. Indeed, it sometimes happens that the care and refreshment offered enables the patient to take a new lease on life, leave the hospice, and continue further active living.

## The Caregiving Team

The quality of hospice care is to some extent based on relationships: the relationship between the sick person, who in hospital is known as "the patient," and staff members; the relationship between the patient and his or her family; the relationship of all staff members one with another. Teamwork is essential among the caregivers. The team will comprise these members:

Physicians
Nurses
Social workers
Paramedical staff (e.g., physiotherapists
    and occupational therapists)
Clerical staff                                           VOLUNTEERS
Catering staff                                           helping in all
Domestic staff                                           spheres of work
Maintenance staff
Hairdresser and beautician
Chaplain

Each group has its leader; apart from that, there need be little in the way of a hierarchical structure. To enable the team to work together effectively and efficiently, there must be a formal structure of communication between the groups, as well as plenty of opportunity for informal interactions. Poor methods of communication will also mean poor relationships within the team, and this will hinder continuity and quality of care. Each member of the team should see the patient, the sick person, as being the most important unit in the hospice program, with the family group coming a close second. All decisions taken on every aspect of care will be in the interests of the patient and his or her family. Where there is friction among caregivers, the atmosphere will be tense and the patients will be affected.

In order to enable a sick patient to be given individual care, an inpatient hospice unit should usually be small. Twenty-five beds seems to have been recognised as a number large enough to be economically viable and yet small enough to allow for high-quality care, large enough to give a strong team structure for all caregivers and yet small enough to allow staff to relate as a family to the families for whom they are caring. But there are effective units with only a few beds, and some with two or three times the size mentioned. Whatever the size of the unit, the ideal nursing staff/patient ratio should be in a proportion of 1:1 full-time equivalents (i.e., an average of one caregiver per patient over a 24-hour period). That is the equivalent of one caregiver for every three patients on any given shift, although some inpatient units have found it desirable not to distribute staff equally across the three shifts of the day. Instead, staffing ratios are adjusted to patient needs and workload at different times of the day, even while the overall 1:1 ratio is maintained.

Members of home care teams work in much more isolated circumstances than do hospice staff members in an inpatient unit. Therefore, staff/patient ratios for home care are likely to be more variable than for inpatient settings. One can expect, however, that hospice home care nursing, with its broad spectrum of physical, psychosocial, and spiritual concerns, will require more time per patient than traditional district nursing or similar public health services. Furthermore, since home care teams spend much time out on their own, it is even more important for them that there is a strong support structure to allow for good relationships to develop. Periodic meetings and social activities for all team members will help toward good communications and provide a family-like atmosphere in which to share problems and successes. Obviously, each hospice program must act to support the service and local needs of the community in which it is situated.

Cultural differences that exist not only from one community to another but also within different parts of the same community must be recognised, and allowances must be made. Inevitably the cultural background of the local community will affect the way in which the hospice program is run, as will also the community resources, which vary so much from one place to another. In some hospice programs the goal is to make it possible for patients to die at home; in others the emphasis is on the patient being admitted for symptom control and then being discharged back into the community; and in still others the majority will receive terminal inpatient care. But whatever the emphasis, the philosophy will be the same. Patients are allowed to live until they die with as much quality as possible being given for this last part of the journey of life, and they are then allowed to die in dignity. If there is quality of life for the patient, then the quality of life for the family will also be improved, and there will be job satisfaction for the staff.

## Staff Interaction

For a hospice caregiving team to function effectively, convenient structures of communication must be set up. For example, in one hospice inpatient unit, a monthly meeting of department heads for the purpose of discussing interdepartmental problems has been found a helpful way of generating information that is of interest to all. The minutes of this meeting are circulated and are available for all members of the staff to read. Once a quarter, senior staff members meet to share problems and discuss matters of interest. Medical staff and ward sisters (charge nurses) also meet at least once a quarter to discuss and share problems of patient care and related matters. Through the channels of these meetings, staff members are kept reasonably well informed in the total caring for the patients and are also then entitled to make their own comments and contributions to the hospice as a whole. In the clinical area, doctors and senior members of the ward staff meet weekly to discuss each patient in detail. The physiotherapist and social worker are also present so that the "art of the possible" for each one can be worked out in the context of the social background, the physical possibilities, symptom control, and nursing care. After the death of a patient, the ongoing care of the bereaved relatives is discussed by a group consisting of social workers and senior nursing staff.

   Working with the dying brings stresses and strains on the caregivers. Staff members of varying ages, a high percentage of part-timers who will bring in with them the freshness of normal family life to share with the patients, an equal mix of trained and untrained personnel—all of these help to give a family-like structure of staff who are essentially caring for families and help to make a "self-supporting" team. The team is indispensable, especially as not all members of the staff will relate with the same patient in the same way at the same time. Full-time members of staff are of course at greater risk, but this kind of structure seems to avoid the problems of breakdown in anyone. An extended daily handover between the two shifts of the day helps to ensure that, whether nurses and other caregivers are full-time or part-time, they will be fully integrated and informed about total patient care.

## Nursing Care

What the nurse has to offer as a hospice caregiver will depend largely on the condition of the patient—the particular symptoms present in his or her illness and the existing degree of independence. By the very way in which nurses carry out their care of the patient, they can help to give quality to the life that is left, and they can help the patient to go on feeling and being a person until death intervenes.

### Bathing

Even dying persons will enjoy being helped to take a tub bath or shower for as long as possible. Unless there is great pain on movement, one should not resort to the bed bath too soon. To be able to bathe or shower boosts the morale and can also be soothing to an aching, weary body. It should also be remembered that relaxing in the bath with a nurse in attendance can help the individual to be able to talk of matters of concern which may be worrying and which he or she finds difficult to express. This is a very personal, intimate time that patients often appreciate very much and that can be enhanced with simple amenities like bath oil or bubble bath. It may be appropriate to use bathing aids such as hoists or lifts, but for the very frail person just being lifted into the water may bring tremendous pleasure. Showers may be tiring unless the person is able to be seated for this; special shower chairs should be available. Baths and showers have great therapeutic value as regards care of the skin, especially where there may be excessive sweating, discharging wounds, or sores which are often offensive. Talcum powder should be used sparingly.

### Control of Odour

Frequent changes of bed linen are essential. Tub baths or showers, as noted above, are indicated wherever possible. Adequate ventilation should be encouraged. Use of deodorizing antiseptics is often helpful; deodorizing pads may be incorporated into the dressing.

Use of a bidet for offensive vaginal or rectal discharge is desirable—
or the use of a closimatic toilet, as all ambulant patients can use this comfortably. Many patients who would benefit cannot actually sit astride a
bidet.

One example of a simple palliative nursing technique is the use of
yoghourt dressings, which have a soothing as well as a deodorizing effect
when used on fungating lesions. Odour-producing microorganisms in
fungating wounds thrive in an alkaline medium. Yoghourt contains microorganisms that produce lactic acid. When they permit the media to become
acid, then odour-producing organisms are less likely to survive. Yoghourt
acts quickly, and its activity can be enhanced by previously irrigating with
10% lactose solution. Antibiotic therapy may impede and even defeat results because the antibiotics may destroy the lactobacilli. If peroxide is
needed to irrigate the wound, it should be washed out with normal saline
before the yoghourt is applied because hydrogen peroxide ($H_2O_2$) tends to
have an alkaline medium. It is essential even with the above to change the
dressing at least within 24 hours for smelly fungating wounds (in complete
contrast to present-day practice with clean wounds, which are better left
untouched for longer periods). Vaseline gauze (plain Tulle Gras) is helpful
to limit "sticking" of the dressing, because there are many superficial capil-
laries that bleed easily.

## Pressure Areas

The care of skin of persons dying of a malignancy needs scrupulous attention. These individuals are likely to be cachectic; many have had steroid
therapy, which renders the skin more friable; and others will have lost a
great deal of weight. Changing of position every 2 hours for the bedfast
patient is necessary, with skillful use of pillows to help position the individual. For lateral positioning, a firm pillow placed parallel to the spine
and pushed securely against it will provide support and help to prevent the
person from rolling on the back again. A small pillow placed under the
arm may be helpful, and one pillow should be placed between the legs.
Aids to protect the skin may be used (e.g., sheepskins, ripple beds, or
water beds), but no aid replaces frequent repositioning. It should be remembered that the patient who is able to sit out of bed is just as liable to get
pressure sores and should be encouraged to change position or have a walk
at least every 2 hours. Cleanliness of the skin is important, and gentle mas-
saging with an oily preparation is helpful. Where superficial skin breaks
have occurred, the use of the infrared lamp for 10 minutes twice a day may
aid healing.

## Mouth Care

Anorexia is not improved by a foul-tasting, dirty mouth. Oral thrush is a frequent problem in ill patients, and this can be painful and add another burden to the sufferer. Meticulous care of the mouth is essential and must never be neglected, even near death. Where the use of toothbrush and toothpaste is impossible or ineffective, mouthwashes of various flavours can be beneficial. For the patient unable to eat, sips of fluids can be used imaginatively to great effect. Fizzy solutions and flavoured ice cubes all have their place in mouth care. For the patient too ill to use a mouthwash, cleaning with swabs and ending the toilet with swabs soaked in a flavoured rinse may be appreciated. Some patients appreciate sucking an ascorbic acid tablet; this is effervescent and leaves a pleasant taste in the mouth, as well as stimulating the flow of saliva. Dentures should be kept scrupulously clean. A fixative may be helpful where a shrinking jaw has resulted in loose-fitting dentures. The patient should be encouraged to continue the wearing of dentures for as long as possible.

## Care of Hair

Even the most ill patient is very "hair-conscious" and hates to look "messy." The hair should be attractively dressed but so as not to be a burden to the patient. The visit to or by the hairdresser is one of the greatest morale boosters, particularly to women. It is a token of ongoing quality of life even during terminal illness, and it provides occasions for familiar human interactions. Families, too, will appreciate seeing their sick relative looking attractive with well-groomed hair.

## Bladder Care

Independence should be encouraged for as long as possible, even if much assistance is required in journeying to and from the toilet.The bedside commode can be used when trips to the toilet are not possible. Contrary to customary practice in other settings, use of the indwelling urethral catheter has an important place in the care of the very ill patient. For the dyspnoeic patient, the effect of toileting can use up valuable energy as well as being a frightening experience. The use of a catheter can spare the patient and release energy for more positive pursuits, even if it just makes talking more possible. A debilitating condition may mean poor muscle tone, resulting in poor bladder control, "dribbling," and incontinence. The use of the catheter will save embarrassment, increasing dependence, and a wet bed. The catheter should be seen as an aid to improving quality of life in many cases.

## The Care of the Bowels

The patient may be taking drugs that have a constipating effect. General weakness may mean that the patient does not have enough strength to defecate and also that peristaltic action is feeble, so management of the bowel is very important. Constipation can cause or increase symptoms of nausea and vomiting, as well as causing abdominal discomfort and increasing the patient's feeling of wretchedness. Stool softeners and aperients or laxatives should be given regularly, and evacuant suppositories or enemas should be given where needed. Manual evacuation of the rectum two or three times a week is necessary for some patients. It is important that clear nursing records be kept for each patient. Very ill patients are not always reliable witnesses as to their bodily functions, and faecal impaction can occur all too often if sufficient attention to bowel care is not given by nursing staff.

### Diet

Food may remain an important item on the day's programme for many patients. Meals should be attractively served; portions should be small (unless otherwise requested); and adequate time should be given to taking of meals. Patients usually know what foods they can tolerate, so they should be allowed to choose for themselves, bearing in mind the maxim "a little of what you fancy does you good." With good symptom control, the quantity and variety of foods patients can enjoy is surprising. Fresh fruit and foods containing bran should be included as an adjunct to bowel care. A bacon sandwich for breakfast may not seem ideal for the patient dying of primary cancer of the stomach, or fish and chips for an acutely jaundiced patient, but it is not uncommon to see such items being consumed with great enjoyment and no aftereffects! Liquidising foods may be necessary for some patients. It is worth remembering that the meal will be better enjoyed if each item is liquidised separately and served in an individual dish, rather than meat and vegetables, for instance, being liquidised together.

### Fluids

Even when the patient is no longer able to take food, fluids should be encouraged. Trouble should be taken to find out which fluids will be most enjoyed. Avoiding paper, plastic, or styrofoam cups enhances the quality of the drink, and serving in a variety of glasses helps to avoid monotony. The use of flexible straws, spouted feeders, and two-handled cups may help some patients to remain independent for longer. The patient who is well hydrated will not present problems of dehydration during the terminal stages. When it is no longer possible for the patient to swallow, the mouth can be kept moist and comfortable by moistening the lips with swabs soaked in iced water. The use of an intravenous drip is almost never recommended, since it is uncomfortable, heightens dependency, and limits mobility. In the rare case of dehydration causing discomfort (i.e., an intense thirst due to vomiting in a rapidly deteriorating patient), a rectal infusion of a pint of warm tap water administered with a fine catheter during the night is sufficient to remedy the problem.

## Symptom Control

It is the doctor's responsibility to order the medication, but it is the nursing staff who care for the patient. Therefore, close observation of the patient is vital. Accurate observations of the patient's general comfort and pattern of pain will help to ensure good symptom control. Patients are not always good at reporting their pain and discomfort, and often have to be taught to say when pain is present. Good symptom control means that the pain is anticipated and therefore should be obliterated. The correct drug given in the correct doseage regularly should achieve freedom from symptoms and allow the patient to be alert enough to get pleasure from life. In most cases, oral medications can be used right up to the moment of death. There is no place for "prn" drugs except to be used in addition to the regular medication.

Dame Cicely Saunders has offered the following guidelines for good pain control:

> Pain is the chief complaint of over seventy percent of our patients, but it is rarely seen or treated alone. Patients do not overrate their pain, certainly not when we have been able to gain their confidence. Most important, though, is that we hear what they are trying to say. . . .
>
> The art of giving analgesics for continuous pain in terminal illness is to administer such drugs continually at the optimum dose level for each individual. For the majority of patients, this dose will remain low if it is given regularly and if it is supplemented with adjuvants whose effects and side effects are well known, and if those around the patient give him the sense of confidence and security he needs. (Saunders, 1965, pp. 1031–1032)

Coping with pain requires energy; when pain is controlled, energy is released for more positive pursuits, and the visit of the physiotherapist or the occupational therapist can now be welcomed. No one wants to be in a position of always receiving. To be able to give makes life more meaningful, so doing some kind of craft under the direction of the occupational therapist, which results in an object that can be given as a present, helps to bring quality to life. Simple items that need little concentration and that may be finished quickly will give the most satisfaction to the more ill and frail but still alert patient. To see a group of patients at a pottery class is a very rewarding sight, as well as being therapeutically beneficial to those taking part. Even the bedfast patient can gain tremendous satisfaction from kneading a handful of clay into an ashtray or ornament. The physiotherapist's visit is no less important. Exercising weak limbs, helping with the first steps to be taken after a period of immobility, and aiding the paraplegic patient to regain mobility and enter into daily activities are all part of the contribution from physiotherapy.

## Paraplegic Care

The most common site of cancer in the female is the breast, which may be accompanied by metastatic deposits in the spine; in advanced cases, the patient may become paralysed from below the waist. This can be relieved in some cases by a surgical decompression of the spine. In the presence of metastatic deposits in the spine, when symptoms include numbness, "pins and needles," weakness or loss of movement in the lower limbs, and poor bladder or rectal control, a paraplegic nursing regime should be instituted. The patient is nursed recumbent with two head pillows. A long firm pillow is placed in the lumbar region, with a pillow lengthways under each leg. Strict turning from side to side should take place every 2 hours, passive exercise being given at each turn. Continuous bladder drainage must be introduced. Bowels should be evacuated manually two or three times a week. It may be necessary to constipate the bowels to make this more manageable. All general nursing care will be as for a bedfast patient.

If after 4 to 6 weeks there is no improvement in symptoms, strict paraplegic care can be relaxed and the patient can be allowed to do whatever is possible and comfortable, progressing to the wheelchair if appropriate, as no useful purpose will be served by keeping such a person bedfast. If muscle tone improves and movements become possible, a rehabilitative program should be planned, including the following:

1. More pillows.
2. A daily tub bath.
3. Sitting out of bed for increasing periods.
4. Weight bearing.
5. Walking.
6. Reeducation of bladder and bowel control.

Mobility of the paraplegic patient should be carried out under the strict supervision of the physiotherapist. Too often it is assumed that the paralysed patient will never walk again, but many cases are known of those who have been able to go home for an unexpected and reasonable period of living.

## Loneliness

Like birth, death is a lonely experience; it can only be done alone, but there is no reason why the period leading up to death should be lonely. Patients often know intuitively that they are not going to recover. It is not difficult to recognise lack of progress in an illness and to realise that lethargy, weakness, and progressive symptoms are in danger of taking over. In addition, fear may become a strong component in the new situation. Sensitive staff members will recognise and be aware of the patient's thoughts, and should be ready to hear what the patient may be implying but not saying in words during dialogues. The patient can be led gently and realistically to accept what is happening. There are many ways of handling discussions that centre on diagnosis and prognosis, and the patient should usually be allowed to take the lead and should not be pressed to hear what cannot be coped with.

Even more important, the patient should also not be fobbed off with lies, at worst, or hearty negatives, at least. Hope must never be destroyed, but it is important to realize that it may be directed to a variety of ends and that these may change as time passes. Diagnostic honesty is to be encouraged, and in the majority of cases visiting by family and friends will become more relaxed when the main character no longer has to play-act and pretend. "The management of patients who know the situation is often easier" (Wilkes, 1977). It is of the actual dying that many patients are afraid, so reassurance should be given that symptoms will not be allowed to take over, that the patient will not be left alone, and that a peaceful death can be assured with a hand to hold right to the end. Describing death as a "sleeping away" can be helpful to many.

# Family

Care of the dying should always include care of the family or other caregivers. The close relative will usually have been told the diagnosis and
prognosis of their loved one. Thus, even if the patient is ignorant of the
true situation, the family will need plenty of support at visiting times.
Open visiting is usual in the hospice. The close relative should be given the
opportunity to share in nursing duties under supervision and should be
kept involved in the total handling of the dying period. Some patients and
their families like to be included with the medical staff in the control of
symptoms; others prefer to leave it to the professionals. Families need to
be given plenty of opportunity to discuss their feelings as regards the illness and the care being given. Underlying anger or guilt feelings are best
expressed before the death takes place. The work of bereavement is best
commenced during the "dying" period. Many families have expressed
much unexpected happiness and joy during the final period; they have experienced a closeness and peace hitherto unknown in their relationships
with one another. Certainly family frictions have no place at the deathbed, and everything possible should be done to help sort out problems, always taking into account the patient's wishes. Sometimes there is a place
for the deathbed reconciliation, but not just to satisfy the caregivers.

Caring for families is best shared by doctors and nurses, social workers, and pastors or chaplains. It is usually spontaneous interaction that
achieves most. Many families will need to talk out their feelings about
whether to be present at the time of death. Any strong feelings expressed
must be respected, and although attempts to anticipate the future and to
develop plans should be instigated early if possible, decisions made at this
time may not be final, so such discussions should be ongoing. The visits of
children and grandchildren are to be encouraged; they are part of life and
help to give normality to the scene. The majority of children cope far better with being involved and being allowed to see the sick parent or grand-
parent than they do with being kept out. They are quite good at making up
their own minds about whether or not they want to visit. They should be
encouraged but not compelled. The visit from the family pet is also to be
encouraged.

Families may not know what to bring, so suggestions by nursing
staff will usually be welcomed. Sherry for eggnog or as an aperitif, whisky
or brandy for the elderly patient who has always been used to the bedtime
"tot," allowing visitors to arrange their own gifts of flowers so as to make
them more personal—these and other little touches like them can bring
great pleasure both to the giver and the receiver. The drive out or the visit
home will bring delight to the patient; it may be frightening for the family,

but should be encouraged for as long as possible. Remembering a patient's birthday with a card and special cake from the catering staff all bring tremendous pleasure, especially for the lonely ones whose birthdays may have passed unnoticed for some years. Having extra cakes available in a freezer makes such celebrations possible on short notice—even immediately after admission, if necessary.

## As Death Approaches

Families often suffer from feelings of "uselessness" as the illness progresses and the patient begins to drift away from them. It will help if they can be shown that sitting at the bedside, holding a hand, and moistening lips are very positive activities. Professionals must also remember that families can be afraid of being with a dying person. They have fears of what symptoms are likely to present as their relative passes from life to death. Death as portrayed in drama or in the media is usually horrific; in life it seldom is. Whether the death is taking place in a hospice or in the patient's home, time spent by a team member in explaining the probable symptoms leading to death will be time well spent and in fact should be a regular component of hospice programmes. It should be explained that fits, convulsions, and haemorrhages that terminate in death are rare where symptom control is good.

Most people are familiar with the "death rattle"; this, too, can often be controlled by skillful use of drugs. Even when it is present, it is comforting for the family to know that the noise is distracting to them, but not to the patient. Incontinence occurring as death takes place is not common where good nursing practices have been in operation, and on the whole these symptoms are less disturbing to cope with for most families. Emphasis should be placed on the fact that changes in breathing patterns—apnea —and almost inaudible breathing may be the only signs that death is imminent, so that the patient in fact just "sleeps away." When familiar with the possibilities of "how the death is to be," most people will be much less frightened and will feel sufficiently supported to participate in the final hours as their loved one passes from life into death.

## At the Time of Death

If present, the family should not be rushed from the bedside. Family members may appreciate prayers being said, and they should be offered a chance to sit quietly with the body of their relative if they wish to do so.

Some may wish to help wash, dress, or otherwise prepare the body as a concluding expression of love and respect. The formal procedures associated with the death of a patient will vary in different cultures and settings, but never should the event be covered up or treated as abnormal. In an inpatient facility, the death should be shared with other patients in the same unit or ward, who should be encouraged to express any feelings of sorrow, fear, or distress. Quite often families visiting different patients in the same ward will form their own support networks and may wish to be involved with each other at the time of a death. In all of these ways, it is helpful for other patients and their visitors to witness that care continues up to and through the moment of death, that the dying person and his or her family are never abandoned by hospice caregivers, and that death can occur in an atmosphere of peace and reassurance. This respect and security is carried one step further by many inpatient hospice units, which leave the bed empty for 24 hours after a death occurs.

## Home Care

Hospice care aims at caring for individuals in as homelike an atmosphere as possible, so it should be seen as helping families to continue as long as possible the giving of care at home for those who are able and wish to do so. Much hospice care can be given in the home when housing is suitable and when there are caregivers, be they relatives, friends, or volunteers, to share in the nursing. The expertise of the professional in skilled procedures may be required, as well as plenty of advice and the sharing of thoughts and feelings with the home care team. Many families are unaware of their capabilities in the area of home nursing, but, with support, they can achieve a good standard of care. This brings tremendous satisfaction to themselves and to the patient.

Obviously, the success of home care is based on good symptom control, but often it is just fear of the unknown that inhibits the family from caring for the patient in his or her own environment. With the development of home care teams, death in the home is becoming more possible for dying persons. In general, it is a far more economical way of caring than institutionalisation is, and it brings many bonuses for all concerned. The home care team will usually consist of nurse, doctor, and sometimes also a social worker and chaplain. Their main function will be to support, listen, and advise. They should be readily available by telephone; often the very fact that help can be called upon in this way will diffuse a potentially frightening episode for patient and family alike.

# Day Care

For the patient not ill enough to require a 24-hour program of nursing care, but whose life style is severely handicapped by progressive illness, a visit once or twice a week for care in a day unit run for dying persons can bring great pleasure and quality to life. Often it will be the highlight of what has become a somewhat drab, depressing existence, particularly for the person living alone. Where family members are caring, it will give a day off for them and so relieve their burden. The day should be short, but include plenty of stimulus. Bathing facilities should be available, as well as consultations with physicians, nurses, and physiotherapists. The attendance of hairdresser and beautician will be an added bonus. Simple forms of occupational therapy often fill most of the time, but the greatest benefit will usually be the opportunity to socialise with others. "Ninety per cent of respondents to a questionnaire thought that the support provided was of great importance to both patient and family; and over two-thirds of the patients were said to have benefited from improved control of symptoms" (Wilkes, Crowther, & Greaves, 1978, p. 1053).

# Dying in Hospital

The hospital is seen by many mainly as the place for investigation, treatment, and cure of illness. The training of medical and nursing students is to that end, and very little guidance is given or time spent on teaching the student how to care for the patient dying of progressive disease or how to talk to sick patients and their relatives. The assumption, then, is that death is the result of a failure to cure. Because students are at a loss when faced with a dying patient, they carry out nursing care as quickly as possible and purposely avoid dialogue in case of being asked "an awkward question." Thus, the patient becomes more and more isolated, lonely, and frightened. This can result in withdrawal or a very demanding patient, neither of which are very acceptable states. It is too easy for the dying patient to be an embarrassment in the acute hospital ward. A single room may be allocated— sadly, not to enhance the quality of caring or to allow more family involvement, but so as to avoid the possibility of the death's embarrassing the other patients. It also makes it easier for staff to pass by and avoid significant interaction.

In contrast to all of this, the hospice movement encourages greater involvement with dying persons and their families in order that they may guide caregivers in identifying and satisfying their particular needs. As terminal illness is an experience of the living, these needs will most often be found to have much in common with concerns that we all share. Where such needs are peculiar to the situation of the dying, their proper apprecia- tion most often reveals what might be done for their satisfaction. Skilled professionals will have much to offer, but in the end simple caring, a will- ingness to share one's own humanity, and a commitment to keeping com- pany with the dying are often most helpful.

It may be difficult for overworked, understaffed wards to achieve as much as specialised hospice units. But much can be accomplished when things are seen in their proper perspective. Thus, curing must always be rooted in caring, so that the latter continues even when the former is no longer possible. Likewise, palliative care with its emphasis on control of distressing symptoms must be recognised—as it always has been in the tra- dition of good nursing—to be an active, demanding, and rewarding task. Perhaps the implementation of the nursing process, which helps to restore the prestige and individuality of the patient, will contribute to improve- ments in the lot of the dying person in hospital wards. Also, it should be evident from the above that much of hospice-type care can be carried out in hospital wards, in nursing homes, and in other institutions. This will be- gin with the integration of the hospice philosophy into the basic education of physicians, nurses, and other caregivers. Certainly the experience of the hospice movement continues to demonstrate what can be accomplished. We now, together, face the more difficult challenge of applying these prin- ciples within the mainstream of our health care systems.

## Conclusion

Due consideration must be given to each individual before deciding where the death should take place. But whether in a hospice, in hospital, or at home, good symptom control is essential. Then, the aim should be to allow as much quality as possible to the life that remains, the patient being allowed to live until a quiet, peaceful death intervenes.

## References

Saunders, C., "The Last Stages of Life," Nursing Times, 1965, 61, 1028–1032.

Wilkes, E., "Effects of the Knowledge of Diagnosis in Terminal Illness," Nursing Times, 1977, 73, 1506–1507.

Wilkes, E., Crowther, A. G. O., & Greaves, C. W. K. H., "A Different Kind of Day Hospital—For Patients with Preterminal Cancer and Chronic Disease," British Medical Journal, 1978, 2, 1053–1056. [See also Chapter 23, this volume.]

# 11

# Hospice: A New Horizon for Social Work

*Nina Millett*

## Introduction

The year 1980 marked the 75th anniversary of social work in health care settings. The first organized department of medical social work was developed at Massachusetts General Hospital in Boston, at the request of Richard Cabot, to help meet the psychosocial, environmental, and economic concerns of patients and families.

Since 1905, the basic goals of social work have remained the same, but as the delivery of health care has become more sophisticated and technological, social work skills have become more refined, and social workers have become accepted as an integral part of the health care team in steadily increasing numbers of hospitals and health care settings.

Several factors have contributed to the growth of hospital social work departments during the past 15 to 20 years. There has been increasing recognition that quality health care must include social and environmental factors, in addition to meeting physical needs. In addition, government involvement in the financing of health care in the United States, via Medicare and Medicaid, has led to increasing bureaucratic restrictions limiting the length of stay in acute care settings. At the same time, an increasing proportion of elderly persons in the population has resulted in more persons suffering from chronic, lingering illnesses, many of which need continuing care.

Emotional effects of a progressive, life-threatening illness can be disruptive to the functioning of an entire family. Sometimes these social problems are more difficult to deal with than the patient's physical symptoms are. Social workers focus on the fact that people are total human beings, and that each individual's physical, social, emotional, and spiritual needs are interrelated. From this perspective, a variety of skills—such as individual, family, and group counseling; crisis intervention; casework; and understanding of family dynamics—can be utilized in approaches to problem solving with families under stress or in crisis due to the effects of a life-threatening illness.

## Areas of Involvement

Hospice programs offer the social worker a unique and challenging opportunity to be involved at various levels, including direct service to patients and families, collaboration and consultation, policy and planning, education, research, and legislative involvement (Millett, 1979, 1982).

### Direct Service

Terminally ill persons and their families are constantly assaulted with losses of all types, both real and anticipated. Purtilo (1976) provides a framework for consideration of some of these losses from the perspective of a physical therapist. Each "little death" experienced during the progression of an illness is a reminder of the ultimate loss of death. Her model is easily adaptable to a social work perspective in her discussion of three major areas of loss: privacy, body image, and relationships. Within these major areas, however, an infinite number of "little deaths" occur. For example, one fiercely independent woman who had no children and had lost two husbands prior to her own diagnosis of cancer was faced with the prospect of moving from her second-story apartment to a smaller, ground-level apartment in a different neighborhood, because she could no longer climb stairs. In moving to this smaller apartment, it was necessary for her to dispose of many pieces of furniture and household items that had been in her family for many years. Consider some of the losses she was facing: Two husbands had already died, and she was in the process of losing her own health and physical strength. She was losing her home and many favorite, meaningful possessions. Because of constant medical bills, her financial security was threatened. She was losing her independence due to progression of her disease, control over her present life and future, and her own sense of usefulness to others—all of which were extremely important to her. Relationships with friends were changing, since she was no longer able to participate in many of their (and her) favorite activities. Ultimately, she was facing the loss of her own life.

Situations such as this one are not uncommon among terminally ill persons. Such losses can be overwhelming and devastating, and, frequently, much intervention and support is needed by all team members to help people work through them constructively.

Several years ago, a study conducted by Ronald Koenig (1968) explored the social service needs of a group of 60 persons suffering from a terminal illness. This group reported more than 700 instances of problems they found moderately or severely difficult to manage. These problems included financial difficulties (71 separate financial problems were reported), as well as illness and symptom problems related to fear and anxiety about the course of the disease (i.e., fear of pain, loss of energy, physical limitations, changes in physical appearance and body image, and fear of undergoing possibly painful medical tests). Another set of issues identified by Koenig included social problems such as changes in communication patterns with spouse and other family members, increased demands on others for care, sexual concerns, and feelings of worthlessness due to inability to carry out familiar roles within the family. Patients also expressed concern about the effect on family members and friends of their mood changes and emotions of anxiety, depression, hostility, and irritability.

In addition to the above, terminal illness seldom occurs in a vacuum. Preexisting problems and difficulties are unavoidably aggravated by additional stresses and crises imposed by a chronic, lingering illness. Koenig concluded that patients seldom experience the full benefits of medical and/ or palliative care unless all these factors are taken into account.

The social worker, as part of the hospice interdisciplinary team, can help to insure the inclusion of these factors in patient/family care and can provide assistance in helping people deal with problems arising from their situation.

Direct service with patients and families requires familiarity with and appropriate use of various approaches, including (but not limited to) crisis intervention, short-term casework, advocacy and provision of concrete needs, and longer-term therapy. Good listening skills, as well as knowledge and understanding of family and group dynamics, are essential. As Ruth Abrams has shown (1966), social workers and all other caregivers must take their lead from the dying person himself or herself and from his or her family unit.

CRISIS INTERVENTION
During the terminal phase of an illness, problems frequently occur that require crisis intervention. Jeannette Oppenheimer (1967) suggests that techniques in this situation focus on (1) helping the patient and family to be fully aware of the problem; (2) assessing the total situation; and (3) helping the patient and family to mobilize their existing resources or to develop

new, more effective coping mechanisms for problem resolution. For example, in families already under considerable tension from preexisting problems, the additional stress of a long-term illness eventually ending in death may increase the strain to an intolerable level, precipitating a family crisis. In home care programs, assurance of provision of adequate care for the patient at home during resolution of the crisis frequently compounds the difficulties for all concerned. For example, weekends were an especially critical time for one large family with a long history of quarreling and alcohol abuse. The family (the patient, her husband, eight adult children, and several young grandchildren) agreed on only one factor—the patient was to remain at home as long as possible, and if possible to die there. While this was our goal also, it was necessary to recognize and accept that their wish for this came from negative rather than positive motives—the majority of the family members had an abhorrent fear and mistrust of hospitals.

During the last few weeks of this patient's life, nearly every weekend precipitated a crisis requiring repeated interventions by the staff person on call. Family members would gather in the small home, and the drinking and quarreling began, intensifying as the patient's condition deteriorated. As a result, she experienced greatly increased anxiety and pain, and when the prescribed medication relieved neither, the staff person was called in to act as mediator and to try to get the patient comfortable again.

Teamwork and collaboration were essential in this situation, and resolution involved assessing the two or three most responsible people in the family, discussing the situation in depth with them, and assigning each of them specific tasks regarding the care of the patient. To help them carry out the tasks, a written schedule was made, especially for the administration of pain medications. Use of this method, in addition to a great deal of support, encouragement, and reassurance of staff availability at any time of the day or night, was successful to the mutual goal of caring for their mother at home, where she died peacefully. Unfortunately, it is doubtful that the long-standing, preexisting problems will improve substantially, though contact will be maintained with the family and help provided if desired.

SHORT-TERM CASEWORK

Parks (1963) describes the appropriateness of short-term casework in a medical setting, when used selectively, to work with clients on specific problems. *Short-term casework* is defined by Parks as "from one to five one-hour interviews with the client, including all activity connected with the interviews" (p. 89).

Time and energy are always critical factors when working with a terminally ill person and his or her family. The short-term casework model is easily adaptable to working with hospice families and helping to make decisions regarding specific problems. For example, one frequently encountered problem involves communication difficulties between patient and family members. In an effort to protect the patient from additional worries, he or she may be shielded from some of the problems and stresses that occur daily within families. As a result, the patient becomes increasingly isolated within his or her own family, causing mistrust, increasing anxiety, and loneliness—all of which can lead to an increase in physical symptoms. Usually, within a few sessions, family members can be helped to understand the importance of including the patient in all aspects of life and can learn how to improve overall communication within the family.

CLIENT ADVOCACY

Assisting with provision of concrete needs, as well as acting as a client advocate, are traditional social work functions, and they remain so in hospice care. Awareness of communty resources and knowledge of their appropriate use are both essential for social workers in hospice care, especially in the home setting, where a variety of supplies and equipment may be necessary to insure quality care. Financial problems are common, due to many medical expenses over a long period of time before hospice care is indicated. Client advocacy is frequently necessary, since few hospice patients are physically able to act in their own behalf, and family members are busy caring for the patient, having neither the time nor the energy to work through agency red tape and bureaucracy.

Little more needs to be said about this role, since it is familiar to most social workers and differs little among settings.

LONGER-TERM THERAPY

Some patients and families remain in the hospice program for several months, providing an opportunity for longer involvement in terms of counseling or therapy if this is indicated by individual needs. Bereavement programs, common to all hospice programs, also provide opportunities for additional involvement with family members. Trained volunteers do much of the bereavement follow-up for those experiencing normal grieving patterns, but for those who need additional help to resolve their grief, the social worker is available to help them work through this process. For example, the son of a hospice patient was experiencing great difficulty accepting his father's death. He and his father had been extremely close, but he had had a poor relationship with his mother. Help was needed for him to deal with his anger about his father's death, as well as his guilt feelings in wishing his mother had died instead of his father. During several sessions, it became increasingly obvious that while grief had exacerbated his problems, other long-standing difficulties were at the root of much of his distress. For a time he resisted referral for more intensive therapy, but eventually recognized the need and agreed to seek further help.

Patients and families vary greatly in their need for social work involvement. Some need help primarily with provision of concrete needs, others for supportive care; still others may need counseling to help resolve their specific problems. Whatever the level of involvement, hospice care provides opportunities for a unique blend of social work skills.

## Collaboration and Consultation

Collaboration and consultation include services to or on behalf of patients and families—services that help to interpret and evaluate social, economic, and emotional factors that may affect the patient or family's response to their whole situation, including efforts of the hospice team. Participation with other team members in interdisciplinary conferences insures inclusion of social work input in the planning process for patient and family care.

Ideally, the social worker functions as a full-fledged member of the hospice team and provides direct services to patients and families on a regular basis. In reality, however, organizational structure and financial restrictions in individual programs may limit the extent to which social work is available or utilized, and when one component of the team is limited, collaboration and consultation assume even greater importance as a mechanism to insure input from all disciplines. Regardless of how programs are structured, however, collaboration and consultation remain continuing processes among all team members to insure provision of quality care.

## Policy and Planning

The social work perspective tends to broaden the traditional medical model of investigation, diagnosis, and cure, used by many health care planners. This model, while useful for many individuals who are ill, is usually less effective when applied to program development for groups such as terminally ill persons and their families. Social workers, knowledgeable of the community as a whole, its strengths and weaknesses, its resources (and gaps), and its cultural components, can include this knowledge in discussions of policy issues and program development. Just as teamwork is essential to provide quality care to patients and families, the expertise of several disciplines is necessary for the establishment of a broad, well-balanced program.

## Education

Education is a continuing process, involving self as well as others. Social workers have a responsibility to keep abreast of new developments and knowledge within their own field, as well as to understand the perspectives of other disciplines. Mutual sharing and understanding of various disciplines leads to a broader, more comprehensive program.

Education also includes involvement with patients and families to increase understanding of their own emotions and anxieties resulting from their particular situation. Each patient and family's entire social network is dealing with loss, changes in family roles and relationships, and fluctuating emotions. Increasing awareness and understanding of these issues among family members helps to reduce fear, isolation, loneliness, conflict, and misunderstanding.

Social workers also have a responsibility to participate in community education. Communities need to develop more sensitivity to the issues surrounding death and dying, as well as to the needs of terminally ill persons and families, and the concept of hospice care.

Hospice programs can be valuable practicum settings for both undergraduate and graduate students. The level of social work involvement can give students valuable practical experience as they prepare for their professional careers. Even students planning a career outside the health field can learn much about helping people deal with loss and change, which are universal issues encountered constantly in any area of professional or private life.

## Research

Research in the areas of death and dying, quality of life, the needs of terminally ill persons and families, and control of pain and other symptoms is in its infancy. Only for the last decade has there been recognition of the need for research on the control of chronic pain, for example. Early studies indicate that control of chronic pain is a complex, sophisticated process that combines the art and the science of medicine. In some instances, the use of techniques such as hypnosis and biofeedback have proven useful in helping to control pain to the extent that lower doses of narcotics are necessary. Early evidence also indicates the need for considering environmental and psychological factors, in addition to physiology, in effective control of chronic pain. Much more research is needed in all aspects of hospice care, and social workers can play a vital role in doing research in such areas as program evaluation and consumer satisfaction, prevention of staff burnout, characteristics of persons who work in hospice care, the role of environment in reducing anxiety, and the relationship between anxiety and pain or other symptoms, to name just a few. As more hospice programs develop, and competition for funding sources increases, research will assume even greater importance.

### Legislation

Most health care legislation currently in effect fails to account for the special needs of the terminally ill, as evidenced by the meager financial or social resources available to help families deal with a lingering fatal illness such as cancer. Most legislation (hence the primary emphasis of most existing resources) relates to acute curative care, and/or rehabilitation. The terminally ill seldom fit either of these categories, and as a result, the dying person frequently spends his or her last days being shuffled between a hospital and a nursing home, neither of which is equipped to meet the needs of the individual or family under stress.

Reimbursement by private or public (Medicare, Medicaid) carriers for hospice care, either inpatient or home care, is limited to a few pilot programs that are beginning to assess both quality of care and cost-effectiveness. As results of these studies are analyzed, it may be hoped that reimbursement will become more universal.

Awareness of legislation, both proposed and in effect, must be an integral part of the hospice movement. This is needed to effect change in current laws and requirements in order to benefit patients and families coping with a terminal illness. Educating legislators at local, state, and national levels in the hospice concept of care, as well as being involved in drafting new legislation, is a role appropriate to social work.

## Characteristics Unique to Hospice

The goals and objectives of hospice are different from those in traditional health care settings. Four major characteristics are discussed here: teamwork, role blurring, working under constant stress, and the ability to tolerate uncertainty.

### Teamwork

Teamwork in hospice is more than a concept or an ideal. In order to provide quality care, the interdisciplinary team must function as a cohesive unit, utilizing the expertise and resources of each discipline represented, both professional and nonprofessional. Formal team meetings are held on a weekly basis to review each patient/family situation, to discuss changes in approaches to problems, and to revise care plans as needed. Informal conferences occur almost daily among staff members to keep everyone informed about each situation. Changes can occur rapidly, either in the patient's physical condition or in the emotional condition of the family.

Working closely as a team also provides an important fringe benefit —a mutual support system for staff members, who deal constantly with stressful situations.

## Role Blurring

As a result of close teamwork, there is some inevitable role blurring. In traditional health care settings, professional and nonprofessional roles are well defined, and each discipline understands the limits of its own boundaries. In hospice care, especially in the home setting, roles often overlap. For example, if a family member ventilates concerns about family problems or expresses the need for a community resource during a nursing visit, the nurse deals with it as fully as possible at the time, rather than promising to send the social worker to handle it (although collaboration with the social worker as soon as possible is part of the problem-solving process). Conversely, during a social work visit, the patient may request some form of physical care, such as a back rub or assistance from bed to chair. Calling a nurse to the home to perform such a task would be irresponsible. It is important, then, particularly in home care, that nurses have some basic counseling skills and understanding of family dynamics, and that social workers learn some basic physical care procedures. Most of all, it is crucial that all team members realize and accept that role blurring is inevitable. The primary goal of hospice care is to provide physical and emotional comfort to both patient and family, and this can only be done with the combined roles of all team members, utilizing all available skills and resources.

## Working under Stress

Functioning under constant high stress levels involves everyone, including staff, patient, and family. Families have primary responsibility on a 24-hour-a-day basis for care of the patient, while at the same time they are trying to prepare emotionally for the inevitable loss. The staff experiences stress because of the nature of the work, the level of emotional involvement with patients and families, and the constant need to deal with loss and grief. The combined result of these stresses can lead to staff conflict, which in turn produces more stress. Each hospice program must find mechanisms for dealing with stress, since ultimately the patient and family suffer most from unresolved stress and/or conflict. Some programs have formal time set aside on a scheduled basis with a psychologist or psychiatrist. Others deal with it on a less formal basis. Whatever method is used, it must be effective for the individuals in that particular program.

Pilsecker (1979) gives suggestions that may act as prevention for excessive stress. Before beginning work with terminally ill cancer patients, it is advisable to explore personal reactions to death and dying and working in close proximity to it; to be aware of personal reactions to cancer as a disease and the body disfigurement it sometimes causes; and to examine individual ability to tolerate uncertainty.

### Ability to Tolerate Uncertainty

All three of these factors are important, but perhaps the most crucial is the ability to tolerate uncertainty. The issue of uncertainty has been alluded to earlier within the context of the necessity for frequent staff conferences. Because it is such a constant factor in hospice care, it is addressed here a little more fully.

Uncertainty is always present—in the physical condition of the patient, which can change rapidly, and in the physical and emotional health of the caregiver(s). For example, the wife of a bedfast patient with a tracheostomy and left-sided paralysis called early one morning to inform us that she was to be admitted to the hospital within the hour for a suspected urinary tract infection. From the beginning, she had resented the responsibility of her husband's care, and even though supplemented with volunteers to help with his care and give her some "time off," her resentment had not lessened. The suddenness of her decision, however, precipitated a crisis, since there was no other family member in the area to stay with the patient. Because of his condition, he could not be left at home alone, and his wife made it clear that she was leaving regardless of whether or not someone was found to stay with the patient. In order to prevent his hospitalization, 24-hour-a-day care at home had to be arranged, beginning immediately and continuing until his wife returned from the hospital and was able to resume his care. Fortunately, someone was found (within the range of their financial capability), and he was able to remain at home, as he desired.

These types of situations are not uncommon, and the staff must be flexible enough to handle them as they arise. Schedules frequently must be altered to accommodate emergency situations, and not infrequently, a whole day's schedule must be rearranged after one phone call from a family needing immediate help. For someone unable to handle this type of uncertainty, hospice (especially home) care would be intolerably stressful.

## Difficulties

The hospice movement during the past 5 years has experienced phenomenal growth in the United States, but not without its share of problems and critics. Elisabeth Kübler-Ross's consciousness raising of the American public concerning the needs of terminally ill persons began only slightly more than a decade ago. The modern hospice movement, which began in England, is less than 15 years old. Although much attitudinal change has occurred, the whole topic of death and dying remains difficult for many to deal with, both within the medical profession and in society as a whole.

Within the medical profession, the concept of palliative care rather than aggressive treatment remains difficult for many to accept, despite the fact that palliative care is widely practiced in programs not involving terminal illness. Death still represents failure to our cure-oriented system, and as such, it is usually fought against rather than acquiesced to, even though palliative care may be more appropriate.

Symptom control has been another problem, although the lively debate of a few years ago concerning legalization of heroin for control of severe chronic pain has been essentially resolved, with tests showing that morphine controls pain effectively when given in adequate doses. Giving the right type of medication regularly and in large enough doses, however, remains a problem. Since research is so new in this area, many physicians either are unaware of the findings or are reluctant to prescribe appropriate narcotics on a regular schedule and in large enough doses to keep pain under control. As research continues and new results are reported, it may be hoped that the medical profession as a whole will become more aware of the needs of patients who experience severe chronic pain associated with a terminal illness such as cancer.

Another complex problem area relates to funding and financing of hospice programs in this country, as mentioned earlier. Many programs have had to rely on private donations, grants, or development of all-volunteer programs in order to begin or continue functioning. Evidence of some change in this area is encouraging, as a few private carriers begin to include hospice care in their benefit packages.

Yet another problem related to funding and financing difficulties has been lack of development of a definitive model for care. On the surface, this might be perceived as an asset rather than a liability, allowing considerable latitude in development of individual programs. Without definitive models, however, there are no enforceable standards for care. Lack of such standards disallows formation of licensing or accrediting boards to ensure quality of care. With the rapid growth of the hospice movement, it is virtually inevitable that some programs would provide substandard care. The National Hospice Organization is currently struggling with this issue and is trying to develop standards that all programs must meet. The next step will be the development of an accrediting or licensing board and survey process to insure consumers that quality hospice care is being provided.

## Conclusion

Despite difficulties and problems, the hospice movement appears to be taking root in North America. There are several interrelating reasons why the appeal of hospice is so great at this particular time. One is undoubtedly due to increasing awareness of the needs of terminally ill persons and their families, resulting from Kübler-Ross's influence. Another is related to the steady increase in numbers of persons suffering from chronic, lingering illnesses of the type that need continuing care. Yet another relates to spiraling health care costs over the past 10 to 15 years, with the resultant search for new ways to render services and alternatives to institutionalization that provide cost-effective, quality care. Perhaps the most significant reason is that hospice offers a humanizing alternative to increasing technological coldness found in many acute care settings, as well as to the warehousing effect of the elderly and sick in extended care facilities. Whether care is provided at home or in a homelike, inpatient setting, hospice emphasizes the individuality of each patient/family, allowing a "patient" to remain a "person" even though critically ill. This concept represents one of the most traditional and basic values of the social work profession since its earliest days.

For social workers, hospice offers challenging and rewarding opportunities to utilize a wide variety of skills and knowledge through direct service to patients and families; through indirect service via collaboration and consultation; and, at the administrative level, through policy and planning, education, research, and legislation. In all of these arenas, there are ample opportunities for individual social workers, as well as for the profession as a whole, to influence profoundly the future of a new, humanistic movement on the health care horizon.

## References

Abrams, R., "The Patient with Cancer: His Changing Pattern of Communication," *New England Journal of Medicine*, 1966, *274*, 317–322.

Koenig, R., "Fatal Illness: A Study of Social Services Needs," *Social Work*, 1968, *13*(4), 85–90.

Millett, N., "Hospice: Challenging Society's Approach to Death," *Health and Social Work*, 1979, *4*, 130–150.

Millett, N., "Terminal Illness, Teamwork, and the Quality of Life: Hospice," In T. S. Kerson (Ed.), *Social Work in Health Settings: Practice in Context*. New York: Longman, 1982, pp. 453–468.

Oppenheimer, J. R., "Use of Crisis Intervention in Casework with the Cancer Patient and His Family," *Social Work*, 1967, *12*(2), 44–52.

Parks, A. H., "Short-Term Casework in a Medical Setting," *Social Work*, 1963, *8*(4), 89–94.

Pilsecker, C., "Terminal Cancer: A Challenge for Social Work," *Social Work in Health Care*, 1979, *4*, 369–379.

Purtilo, R. B., "Similarities in Patient Response to Chronic and Terminal Illness," *Physical Therapy*, 1976, *56*, 279–284.

# 12

## The Place of Physiotherapy in Hospice Care

*Patricia A. Downie*

Death has a hundred hands and walks by a thousand ways.
He may come in the sight of all, he may pass unseen, unheard.
Come whispering through the ear, or a sudden shock on the skull.
A man may walk with a lamp at night, and yet be drowned in a ditch.
A man may climb the stair in the day, and slip on a broken step.
A man may sit at meat, and feel the cold in his groin.

—*T. S. Eliot,* Murder in the Cathedral, *Part I**

In these graphic words, T. S. Eliot reminds us vividly that death can come in any form, and that it is not possible to predict how, when, or where. A person may start to cross a road and not reach the other side—that is sudden and unexpected death; a person may develop a progressive muscular disease such as motor neurone disease and watch a daily deterioration over many years ending in total dependence—that is a slow, painful, and inescapable death. Within these two extremes there are many variations, and it is mainly on these that this chapter concentrates its comments. Of necessity much will be philosophical, for a therapist's approach to a progressively ill or dying patient will, to a great extent, be fashioned upon a personal belief.

I do not propose to discuss what is euphemistically known as "terminal care." That would be wholly negative, for it implies only care of the dying, whereas one should be thinking about long-term care of the progressively ill or, as I would prefer to put it, treatment and care for those

*Quoted by permission of Faber & Faber, London, and Harcourt Brace Jovanovich, Inc., New York.

with a vulnerable future. This will include care of the many with neurological conditions such as multiple sclerosis, motor neurone disease, or hemiplegia; respiratory cripples with pneumoconiosis, severe emphysema, or bronchitis; persons with chronic cardiac failure; and those with any form of cancer.

For the patient with a vulnerable future, the word *rehabilitation* means hope and a way to maintain independence. I like to think of rehabilitation as meaning "total care," and for this reason I think it is wrong to limit its use to the active physical requirements following traumatic injury or a medical catastrophe such as a cerebral vascular accident. Rehabilitation means involving oneself with the total care of a patient through all his or her ups and downs until death. Unashamedly I stress this throughout the chapter: If you become involved in any form of hospice care, this total involvement is most important. At the same time the ability to "switch off" is equally important; this is why a positive approach by all concerned is so necessary, and why death should be seen as a natural part of life and *not* a disaster. By our own outward showing of a love of life, we can provide, in most cases, the much-needed stimulus for patients to respond. Watson-Jones (1952, Vol. 2, p. 1021) has defined rehabilitation as "letting the patient understand his disability, regaining confidence and being inspired."

In his book, *True Resurrection*, Father Harry Williams wrote:

> The only suffering of which we can fully or ultimately be aware is our own. It is true that by imaginative sympathy we can, to some extent, understand what others are feeling. . . . All we are generally capable of understanding is an experience of our own, in the past. We feel or live their sufferings by re-feeling or reliving our own. If somebody suffers in a way in which we have never suffered, we may indeed know that they are suffering, but we shall be unable to feel with them because what they are feeling is to us a closed book. (1972, p. 142)

It is often said that once a patient has reached the end of active treatment from the medical standpoint, then there is nothing else that a therapist can offer. This is not true, for if patients have been known and treated over a number of years, or even for only a short time, it is most unkind to forget them at the time of life when they require all the help that can be offered.

In the care of the dying patient, common sense and experience will govern the majority of decisions, and a sure faith and understanding of people will help. If a patient has been in the care of an understanding team whom he or she trusts, this latter stage will fall more naturally into place.

It must be remembered that these patients, while not minding being alone, fear loneliness almost more than anything else. Often they require only someone to sit with them and to listen to their expressions of feelings and thoughts. Whom they choose to do this with is their own concern, but it may well be the therapist, and, time-consuming though it is, this is a task which must be fulfilled willingly.

As death approaches, patients are less able to make adjustments, and this again is why they look for the familiar face. Gradual acceptance of the ultimate will come, but each person must meet this in his or her own way, and no one of us can really imagine how someone else will react.

## The Therapist's Approach

Many therapists (I use the word generically to embrace physical, occupational, music, speech, and art therapists) are reluctant to acknowledge the part that they can play in the overall care of the dying and those with a vulnerable future—except in the acute phases. Therapists are often frightened, not only of the questions which such patients might ask them, but also of their own reactions to what may be (but seldom is) a distressing situation.

What then should be the approach to such individuals? I suggest that basically it must be one of calmness, of reassurance, and of matter-of-factness. There is no place for sentimental slush; but this does *not* mean being hard and unsympathetic. Rather does it mean showing understanding and care, and, above all, being realistic. The Latin word *caritas* (love) covers this meaning so well—not the shallow meaning of physical love, but the deep compassionate understanding of a person's whole being.

For example, the deeply depressed person who has just learned that he or she has multiple sclerosis is not going to appreciate the therapist who arrives all hearty and jolly at the bedside and breezily announces, "Come on now, we're going to the gymnasium to get you walking, and soon you'll be home and everything will be all right." The dying patient will not appreciate this approach either, for everything will not be all right for either person. What they are craving is a sympathetic ear. The slower atmosphere of the hospice will allow for as much time as is needed for that sympathetic ear, but in the busy hurly-burly of a general hospital department, the therapist does not always appreciate that the finest treatment he or she may give is just to sit down and listen.

Therapists will meet with progressively ill patients all through their professional careers, and they need to accept that to effect adequate treatments on and off for many years, a trusting relationship will need to be established. This relationship does not cease until such patients die, and at that stage the therapists may well find themselves continuing to see spouses or other relatives; this is right, for families may have relied upon the therapists to enable these patients to remain independent at home during the last weeks of life rather than becoming bedbound and dependent.

Therapists must also understand that they are as much part of the caring team as if they were attached to a cardiothoracic surgical unit or an orthopedic unit. They will have their own individual skills to offer, but equally they will learn to work with all the team and to realise that this is an area of care where there are no rigid lines of "who does what." The only criteria for care are those of patients' well-being and their desire to remain as independent as possible for as long as possible.

Hospices, continuing care units, and home care programmes are expanding all the time in the United Kingdom and the United States, as well as in other countries throughout the world. They should not be solely for dying patients, nor for those with cancer. They should be available for all with progressive illnesses who require special care. In many cases such patients will be admitted and discharged at varying intervals and followed up by regular visits to the home. In this way an ongoing relationship can be established not only with families and friends, but also with community services and family doctors. Total care can then become a reality, with everyone sharing in it without any feelings of rancour.

Another ingredient in the required approach to these patients is what I will call *intuition*. Graeme (1975), talking about care of the dying, has said that the yardstick should always be "to improve the quality of life remaining, and this could well mean keeping one person drowsy and unaware of pain while allowing another to live more actively and even more dangerously than would normally have been considered." Always, one must remember that the dying remain individuals, even though they may daily become weaker and weaker; all those involved in the care of such patients must beware of imposing their ideas upon them. Aims of treatment need to be realistic, and any goal that is set must always be within a patient's capabilities. With a progressive disease the goals may need to be set in decreasing aspiration, but always they must emphasize independence, however limited that might be. This is particularly true with motor neurone disease.

We must not be tempted to tell such patients that they cannot do something. Let them try and thus allow them to find out for themselves what they can and cannot do. Frequently, therapists can communicate confidence to such patients, so that their achievements may rise above their expectations. Dying and progressively ill patients *must* be allowed to retain their independence to the last moment.

Even more important to remember is that patients are very vulnerable when removed from their own environment. Their feelings and wishes, however far removed from reality, must be respected; all who care for such patients will have their own stories of strange requests. My own relates to the hair-raising request to break and enter a house because the key was mislaid and the dying lady who had just bought it wished to see the alterations!

## Therapy and the Progressively Ill Patient

For any patient with a progressive disease (e.g., motor neurone disease, multiple sclerosis, disseminated malignant disease, and others), the aim must always be to maintain independence for as long as possible. Even when the stage of dependence happens, it should still be possible by judicious help to allow patients to partake in satisfying their bodily needs.

### Aids

The use of aids as a permanency, such as tripods, quadropods, and walking frames, should be stoutly resisted. Their use should be restricted to enabling the patient to become mobile either as the result of extended bed rest or as a progression from crutches and before a walking stick is sufficient. In the latter category, I think of the recovering paraplegic, possibly due to an extradural tumor that has been removed surgically, who will have learned to walk again through using parallel bars, then elbow crutches, then a walking frame, and finally a stick. Tripods, quadropods, and frames, while allowing restricted walking, can be extremely limiting, for they leave patients unable to use their hands for carrying. If walking aids do become absolutely essential, they must be of the correct size for the patient.

As well as walking aids, there are gadgets such as a combined knife and fork for those only able to use one hand. Long-handled combs, toothbrushes, and so on, are helpful for those with restricted shoulder and elbow movements. Difficulty in gripping can be helped by careful padding of the handles of knives, forks, spoons, and so forth—care being taken that the handle is not overpadded so that it becomes totally impossible to hold. Other aids that may be useful include a nonslip mat in the bath, raised lavatory seats, nonslip plates and saucers, plates with a lip to prevent spillage, and elastic shoelaces. The use of Velcro can be a boon as a replacement for hooks, press studs, and buttons. I realise that in some places aids of the sort mentioned in this paragraph are considered to fall outside the province of physiotherapy, but other professionals may not always be available and, in any event, as hospice caregiving is governed by the needs of the patient, we cannot permit narrow professional boundaries to frustrate satisfaction of those needs.

## Breathing Exercises

Normal healthy persons, by reason of their everyday activities, exercise their lungs efficiently and maintain adequate aeration. In sickness, as a patient slows down physically, the lungs are very often the seat of minor infections, which if not treated can become serious. Patients with progressive illness will benefit by being taught simple breathing exercises and encouraged to carry them out regularly. The use of resistance, either by the patient's own hand, a relative's hand, or a wide webbing strap, will help to focus attention on each area of the lungs. Patients who are confined to a wheelchair should also be encouraged to sit up, and those who have weak musculature should be fully supported so that they do not sit in a slumped position with head on chest. Any sputum (phlegm) should be coughed away; sometimes vibrations or shakings of the chest wall will help this. (If vibrations or other motions are necessary, they should be carried out by a qualified physiotherapist or taught by one to either the nursing staff or relatives. This is important, for, unless such techniques are performed correctly, it is possible to produce the opposite effect to the one desired.)

## General Exercises

Almost all patients will benefit from some form of exercise suitably tailored to their ability. The paralysed person requires daily passive movements to maintain joint range of muscle extensibility as well as to aid circulation. Limitation of joint movement can inhibit mobilization and the regaining of independence when voluntary movement is returning. The very weak person, such as one with motor neurone disease, requires assisted movements. These can be achieved with the help of another person, such as the physiotherapist or a relative. It may also be achieved by the use of slings and pulleys, which will support the weight of the limb and allow the patient to use what muscle he or she has. This method can be utilised over a bed to assist feeding, washing, and other activities.

More active patients, including those in wheelchairs, can carry out a programme of active exercises that they should be taught by the therapist. These may need to be adjusted daily according to the condition of the patient, and, as this deteriorates, the accent on any exercises must be that of maintaining some degree of independence.

Ball games of all kinds can be played with the patient in a sitting posi-

tion, either on a chair or in a wheelchair. Such games may vary from simply throwing a lightweight inflated ball back and forth to playing a type of
hockey with sticks and balloons. With a little imagination, much pleasure
can be derived from these simple ideas. Darts and table tennis both offer
excellent exercise and can be played sitting as well as standing.

Such activities can be helpful in assessing a patient's true pain or discomfort. When patients are engaged in such activities, observations of
their ability to move without effort can be of great help to the medical
team. This is not to say that the pain is *not* physical, but it probably indicates that the person is also worried and distressed and that this distress is
being projected as an acute awareness of physical pain. Working together
as a group is both a leveler and an incentive—and can lead the patient to a
realisation that "I am not alone with my disablement."

*Wheelchairs*

Wheelchairs should be regarded as an insurance policy and not always as
an indication that walking is not possible. However, their usefulness cannot be dismissed, and the patient who has been confined for many months
can achieve tremendous pleasure from being wheeled outside for short
periods or from sitting out for a longer period of time on milder days.
Nowadays there are many types and models of wheelchairs, and it is most
important that the right chair is prescribed for a particular patient. It is not
possible to go into detail about this, but in general it is better to have a
slightly smaller chair width than to have one too large; detachable arms
and leg rests make for easier lifting and storage of the chair; desk-type
arms allow for the chair to be wheeled right up to a table, thereby allowing
the user to remain part of a family. All users and handlers of wheelchairs
need to be properly taught how to manoeuvre them and particularly how
to negotiate up and down curbs, cross roads, and enter and leave a lift (ele-
vator).

There are those who would suggest that active physical treatment
harasses the progressively ill patient. This is a shortsighted and often mis-
guided view. No one likes being helpless and dependent on others, and any
active help to maintain even a tiny degree of independence is almost always accepted with alacrity.

## The Therapist and Pain Control

*Pain* can be defined as an unpleasant or distressing sensation due to bodily
injury or disorder. Tolerance to pain is essentially individual, and this is
why there can be no standard prescription for pain control. Chronic pain

of low intensity can be extremely wearing, and while some patients will admit more readily to it, others tend to "grit their teeth" and ignore it.

A therapist treating such a person in the latter category may well be the one who breaks through the patient's defence and suggests that there really is no need to suffer such discomfort. A lot of people do not like taking analgesics, however mild; they have a built-in fear that they will become addicted and incapable of sensible thought. If this fear can be overcome, much help can be offered. While therapists are not able to prescribe, they can certainly help in assessing the degree of pain; having won the confidence of patients, they can then make a useful contribution to working out an acceptable solution.

Apart from the use of analgesia, chronic pain can be eased by correct positioning of the aching limb(s); aching muscles, or muscle spasm as in multiple sclerosis, can often be eased by ice packs or by towels wrung out in iced water placed along the affected areas. (In both methods, the area must first be oiled to prevent ice burns, and the ice pack should not be left in position for more than 3 minutes on the first application. Progression in time must be very slow.) Heat in various forms (e.g., hot packs, infrared lamps, hot water bottles, etc.) can also help to ease discomfort; it must be used with care and, in some cases, is not as effective as ice. Where it is known that the person has a deficit in skin sensation, very great care must be taken.

A firm mattress and well-placed pillows are essential for the long-term patient; for the dying patient, comfort will and must take precedence over everything else. Time spent on making any patient comfortable and relaxed is time well spent. There is nothing worse than for a beautifully tidy patient in bed to be acutely uncomfortable because of his or her neatness. Observation, perceptiveness, and the willingness to take time whenever it is necessary to ensure a patient's comfort might reduce the use of analgesics quite considerably.

In more severe pain, nerve blocking may be undertaken, particularly if the pain involves the sacral and lumbar nerve roots. Intrathecal alcohol or phenol are the agents most usually used. Side effects from such injections can include loss of control of bowel or bladder, numbness and weakness of the legs, and difficulty in walking. Adequate preblocking explanation is essential.

Physiotherapy can be extremely helpful to overcome the walking difficulty that may result from blocking. Usually it is due to the numbness and consequent inability to feel the feet on the floor. Frenkel's exercises are very useful to help reestablish positional sense, and these can be progressed from being done in sitting to carrying them out while walking between parallel bars. (Frenkel's exercises are coordination exercises based on the principle of repeatedly carrying out specific movements in a precise manner. For example, sitting on a stool or chair, a person is asked to lift one foot up and put it down to the side; then to pick it up and bring it back to the starting point. He or she then repeats this with the other foot. This may be repeated a given number of times on several occasions during the day. When that simple movement can be correctly carried out every time, it can be progressed. This may be done by asking the patient to perform the movement without looking at his or her feet, or it may be done by carrying it out in standing. It may also be progressed by making the actual movement more complicated—for example, by asking the patient to lift the foot, circle it, and then put it down.) Some form of walking aid, preferably only a walking stick, is quite justified, if for no other reason than as a boost to morale. I think it is true to say that such patients are so grateful to be rid of their hitherto intractable pain that they accept the annoyance of the numbness as of minor importance. In cervical spine lesions, a collar may help to relieve the tension of the neck extensors and give comfortable support to the head, provided it is correctly fitted.

Physical pain can be intensified by mental anguish; if this latter can be identified and helped, the physical pain may become more tolerable. The therapist who is willing to massage aching limbs and move uncomfortable joints is well placed to help these patients by the mere fact of having time to listen. The "ministry of touch" can be of real value; confidences uttered at such times must be respected, and only if the therapist feels the need of more skilled help should they be revealed. In such circumstances the patient's permission must be sought. Pain makes most people vulnerable, and there are very few who willingly pour out their troubles unless they trust the hearer/recipient. Therapists should be on their guard, remembering that they are primarily listeners, and they must not be overcurious and pry. Having myself been the recipient of such expressions of fear, troubles, doubts, or simple unhappiness, I know that the patient's reaction is invariably "Oh, thank you for listening, I feel better for having got it off my chest," and that both the professional and the personal relationship has been strengthened.

Finally, as I have indicated in the previous section, general classwork and suitable games with other patients can help toward a better acceptance of the pain; so, too, can helping others who are more disabled. Classwork can be very revealing in the assessing of pain and other limitations. Frightened patients can often be helped by others in ways that are not possible for the professional, and the role of volunteer in continuing care homes can be so helpful.

Helping patients with pain problems, be they mild, severe, or chronic, can be a stimulating challenge to the therapist. If, finally, it entails only sitting and allowing the hand to be held, that must be accepted as the challenge to provide the help that is needed at that moment in time.

## Therapy and the Dying Patient

Therapy for dying patients, and physiotherapy in particular, should not be regarded as a waste of a scarce professional's time. Death is neither a disaster nor a failure of medicine, but a natural event that terminates a human being's earthly existence. Physiotherapy that helps such patients to accept their dying and eases their physical discomfort should be prescribed without hesitation. Complicated treatments are not advocated, but with perception and adroitness it should be possible to help many patients to the point of death. There is no doubt that physiotherapy has much to offer patients who are reaching the end of their lives. Active encouragement to continue to live each day will help such a patient to a better adjustment to approaching death, and the mere fact that someone is interested in a dying patient's whim or fancy can be therapeutic. For the paralysed and bedridden patient, passive and active assisted movements of limbs will help the circulation and ease uncomfortable joints. Massage must not be derided as old-fashioned and of no value; it has the dual advantage of giving physical help and, when performed with olive oil, of helping the condition of the skin, and it allows for an opportunity for patients to talk if they so wish. It needs to be reiterated continually that the prerequisite of care for the dying is the ability to give time and to be able to listen and to offer support.

Doctors do not prescribe physiotherapy *because* a patient is dying; but if there is a mutual understanding between a physiotherapist and a medical practitioner, then the doctor may well ask the therapist to treat a dying patient so that the patient may be enabled to die more peacefully. Into this category comes the progressively ill patient who develops pneumonia—"the old man's friend," as Osler described it. Often, simple physiotherapeutic measures such as vibrations (fine shakings) to the chest wall to loosen sputum (phlegm), or simply encouraging a few extra deep breaths, can relieve distress; this is fully justified, but heroics in such cases are to be abhorred.

Relatives also need support and advice. If a dying patient is being nursed at home, the visiting physiotherapist can help by showing the relatives how to give or rather how to offer unobtrusive help, how to move painful limbs, and how to support where necessary as the patient potters round a room. This help with involvement in care will go a long way to alleviate the feelings of inadequacy and despair which are so often encountered in families who are trying to cope and do not know how.

I have raised the question and, I hope, have answered it, as to whether physiotherapy should be prescribed when a patient is dying. Equally, I ask the question, when is a patient dying? I remember a lady, aged 45, with disseminated carcinoma from a primary breast tumour. She developed "pneumonia," and, because the family could not cope, she was admitted to a nursing home for care and comfort. A year later she was still in the nursing home, being kept in bed and comfortable on opiates. It was decided to seek another opinion, and she was reassessed. Following this she was mobilised, weaned off drugs, and returned home, where she was able to remain reasonably active for 18 months before dying—at home.

In addition to helping the patient, the physiotherapist can help the nurse. Frequently the patient may have an advanced malignant disease that particularly affects the bones, and nurses are often afraid of handling such limbs in case of fractures occurring. Nothing transmits itself more readily than fear, and if the nurse is afraid of handling such a limb the patient will soon become aware of this. Firm yet gentle handling is necessary, and often the presence of a physiotherapist who is used to handling injured limbs can give the required confidence to both nurse and patient. Efficient and comfortable ways of lifting can be illustrated, just as principles for preventing joint contractures—which often lead to difficulties in positioning and to pressure sores—may be demonstrated.

## Conclusion

I have made no mention of those psychological reactions to death and bereavement that Kübler-Ross (1970) has laid such stress upon: those stages of denial, anger, bargaining, depression, and acceptance. These so-called stages are by no means peculiar to the dying; they are, in fact, normal reactions to any unpleasant truth. They account for the bloody-mindedness of the poliomyelitis and paraplegia victim, for the withdrawn attitude of the young man who loses a leg in a road traffic accident, or for the acute depression of the newly diagnosed multiple sclerosis sufferer. While therapists should appreciate *why* dying and progressively ill patients react in certain ways, they must also understand that not every patient will go through these stages as defined. Each person will react differently and according to his or her own time scale. It is very dangerous to think in terms of Stage 1, 2, 3, 4, and 5; we must take patients as they come each day, adapt our treatments accordingly, adjust our approach to suit the needs of particular persons, and always remember that we are treating individuals.

I firmly believe that a simple, commonsense approach to the dying and to those with a vulnerable future makes for a more constructive understanding of that person's needs than do all the psychological explanations that are uttered in learned papers and books. No one will escape death, and each of us has to work out our own understanding of it; some deaths will make no impact on us, and that too is natural.

In summary, I say to any therapist who may work within a hospice or outside in hospitals or the community, and who has dealings with dying persons or those with a vulnerable future:

DON'T feel embarrassed or afraid when approaching these patients.

DON'T opt out of your responsibility to them.

DO be realistic in your approach.

DO be prepared to listen.

DO be prepared to use the simple tools of your trade rather than the sophisticated.

DO be prepared to help the families as well as the patients.

DO try to consider the facts of death and dying and so come to your own philosophy of how to face it.

# References

Graeme, P.D., "Support for the Dying Patient and his Family," in R. W. Raven (Ed.), *Marie Curie Memorial Foundation Symposium on Cancer, the Patient, and the Family*. Altrincham, England: Sherratt, 1975.

Kübler-Ross, E., *On Death and Dying*. London: Tavistock, 1970.

Watson-Jones, R. J., *Fractures and Joint Injuries*. Edinbrugh: E. & S. Livingstone, 1952.

Williams, H. A., *True Resurrection*. London: Mitchell Beazley, 1972.

# Bibliography

Downie, P. A., *Cancer Rehabilitation: An Introduction for Physiotherapists and the Allied Professions*. London: Faber & Faber, 1978.

Downie, P. A., & Kennedy, P., *Lifting, Handling, and Helping Patients*. London: Faber & Faber, 1981.

Forsythe, E., *Living with Multiple Sclerosis*. London: Faber & Faber, 1979.

*Handling the Handicapped* (2nd ed.). Cambridge: Faulkner-Woodhead, in association with the Chartered Society of Physiotherapy, London, 1980.

Rogers, M. A., *Paraplegia: A Handbook of Practical Care and Advice*. London: Faber & Faber, 1978.

# 13

# Occupational Therapy in Hospice

*Kent Nelson Tigges*

### Reconstituting Our Goals

Traditional occupational therapy education and practice in the United States and England focus on treatment and rehabilitation with the aim of returning the injured or the disabled to the mainstream of living. Pathology and/or the pathological implications of illness or injury are the springboard in assessment and treatment planning. The majority of patients referred to occupational therapy are those people who have diminished physical and/or emotional function or capacity, of a temporary or permanent nature, which interferes with their ability to function. Although some of my colleagues would adamantly disagree, "quality of life" and "treating the total person" are not of primary or even secondary importance in our customary therapeutic practice. This is true, not because occupational therapists and other health care providers fail to care about their patients or to openly advocate "quality of life" and "treating the total person." Rather, it comes about because no one of the health professions can or does treat the total person. Economics, education, and professional specialization do not permit that. Health professionals treat only that portion of the person as envisioned or described by their limited professional scope of practice. As Eric Wilkes (1980) has said, our greatest liability in dealing with patients is our "professional blinkers." We have been taught, technically, how to preside over what goes wrong physically with patients, but, unfortunately, not how to commune with them when something happens to them. Our emphasis on cure, enthusiastic reassurance, and hope for a long and productive life is often misplaced, but never more sharply than in the case of those with an incurable illness and for whom death is imminent.

Contemporary life in itself is transient and all too frequently empty and purposeless for a large percentage of people. People become lost, confused, and bewildered by a rampant, helter-skelter, and high-speed existence. It is little wonder, then, that when incurable illness occurs, many people panic and become disillusioned with life. Therefore, we should not be surprised that voluntary euthanasia groups are mobilizing and gaining momentum. Life without self-direction, independence, self-esteem, purpose, and the ability to interact constructively with or to influence other people seems to have no value or meaning.

When a person becomes ill and is put into a hospital, a nursing home, or for that matter a hospice bed, independence is always diminished and sometimes completely lost. As soon as a person's normal and familiar environment changes, he or she loses a sense of control and mastery. The problem with inpatient care, as Holland (1980) stresses, is that patients are immediately put into a passive and dependent role, through which they lose their sense of independence. It is little wonder, then that patients have difficulty adjusting from being at home to being institutionalized. Because they prize their autonomy, most people want to stay at home as long as they can. However, despite its advantages, even the home environment can pose similar problems when well-meaning family or friends place the person in a role of passive dependence. And where there are no family or friends, isolation, loneliness, and inactivity can be devastating.

Adult life is executed through prelearned and preconceived sets of values and routines involving both independent and interdependent actions. If health professionals are truly to be about the business of preserving the integrity of a person's life, then they must look beyond the periphery of their "professional blinkers" and examine what services are necessary for the concept of quality living that is being advocated. As the goals of occupational therapy are centered on restoring and/or maintaining role performance skills, one would tend to think that the role of occupational therapy, be it in an acute, long-term, or hospice facility, would remain constant. That is not true. As Doyle (1980a) has said, "[Caregivers are] foolish if they think that the management of people's lives in a terminal care facility is merely a professional side-stepping from one professional role to another."

If occupational therapy is to play its proper part in hospice programs and in serving the needs of dying persons and their families, it must reexamine and reconstitute its goals. Hospice care is centered upon maximizing quality of life in the present moment. Such care cannot be limited to medical or nursing services. Nor can it be construed as rehabilitation, where that is taken to mean restoration of full functioning and return to prior modes of living. Hospice does not abandon rehabilitation of that sort

or the possibility of cure, but for many dying persons the attitude that tomorrow will bring a new chance and an opportunity to learn a new skill or
to maintain an old one is inappropriate and foolhardy. For some people
there will be no tomorrow. What exists, exists now; there is no future or
future planning. The cliches used in acute and long-term care facilities are
out of place here.

> If obsession over "staying alive" by all means supplants the deeper meaning
> of life, man can never experience the transcendence that guides the spiritual
> side of his nature. It is only when we accept the inevitability of death that we
> attain meaning and balance in our lives. In performing miracles on the dying,
> the radical Catholic priest Ivan Illich has said, modern medicine is depriving
> man of a natural vision of death. And it is this vision, he thinks, that adds
> meaning to a life that is more than mere biological existence. (Dempsey,
> 1975, p. 39)

In the context of a hospice program, occupational therapy must serve an
apparently paradoxical set of ends: hope without a future, a future without time.

As the American Occupational Therapy Association has recognized
(1979), humans are active beings whose development, adjustment, and
coping, irrespective of illness, are influenced by the constructive use of
time. Human life is a kaleidoscope of experiences; as such, it demands a
continuous process of adapting. People can adapt, they can cope—but
only when their environment is conducive. Occupational therapy is centered on the realization that a person's integrity, equality, purpose, self-
esteem, mastery, and adaptation rest in the ability to be purposefully engaged in regular and familiar life experiences. In Wilkes's language, "the
way a patient feels about his health depends very much more on his attitude to his work, his family, and his society than to any mere physical or
psychiatric diagnosis" (1976, p. 874). Fear, loneliness, and anxiety encourage and exacerbate pain and symptoms.

Occupational therapy stresses the need for and a balance between
work, self-care, and play/leisure in self determination. Each person and
his or her personal environment must be carefully assessed so as to determine what influences cause them either to react or not to react, and to do
so in a positive or a negative manner. "On the surface, providing opportunities to work and be active is relatively straightforward. But in fact,
sensitivity to the persons' previous and present life style, their physical
and mental stability, and daily fluctuation in their abilities is of constant
concern. The grading of activities to match the fluctuation of continuous
deterioration and remission is critical" (Holland, 1980). This should not be
confused with what some call "diversional therapy":

It is an insult to divert a person's attention from life and that is what diversion implies. Life is a delicate balance between independence, interdependence, and dependence. It is a matter of coping, adapting, being needed, productive, independent, and above all of being of value. Occupational therapy can provide the mechanism in facilitating a person's sense of mastery and competence, and in putting substance into quality of living. (Tigges, 1980, p. 14)

## The Occupational Role Performance Paradigm

The Occupational Role Performance Paradigm focuses on and stresses the human need for mastery—productive use of time, energy, interest, and attention. The occupational role performance assumptions (Tigges & Talty, 1979, p. 18; see Table 13.1) do not focus on the centrality of pathology, but rather emphasize a person's sense of self—what he or she feels is essential to be a competent person. People do not live in isolation, but rather within and involved in the world around them—society, a community, no matter how extensive or narrow it may be. It is this involvement with community or environment that is central to role performance.

Mastery in role performance is expressed in three basic areas: self-

Table 13.1
Occupational Role Performance Assumptions

1. Human beings have vital needs for occupation and mastery of their environment.

2. Individuals possess an innate drive toward mastery/competence.

3. Enduring properties (genetic, demographic, personality) make each individual unique.

4. Quality of life is determined by how humans can influence and be influenced by those in their immediate environment.

5. An individual's total (inclusive) environment affects his or her learning and adaptive behavior.

6. The development of an individual's role performance is both horizontal at any given age and longitudinal over the life span.

7. Psychological, biological, and social trauma can interrupt/disrupt the role performance process.

8. Intervention can produce change in an individual's role performance.

9. Role appropriate activities are a successful means for intervention.

10. Role performance skills are learned in a sequential manner.

11. Mastery of subskills, skills, habits, and performance is necessary for the successful development of satisfactory coping/adaptive behaviors and role performance.

care, work, and play/leisure. As Figure 13.1 (Tigges & Talty, 1979, p. 22) illustrates, these three areas overlap to some extent, but their characteristic concerns are easily distinguished. *Self-care*, or daily personal care, involves such things as grooming and hygiene, feeding and eating, dressing, mobility, and object manipulation. *Work* relates to socially purposeful and productive activities, whether carried out in the home, at school, on the job, or in the community. Thus, it encompasses such components as home management or homemaking, child care or parenting, and employment preparation. *Play/leisure* refers to activities undertaken for the sake of amusement, relaxation, spontaneous enjoyment, or self-expression.

*Role dysfunction* means the inability to perform in one or more of the areas or to perform at the level the person sets as his or her level of expectation in performance. One identifies role dysfunction by assessing the three basic performance areas. Where external intervention is required, one must go further to establish the cause of the role dysfunction. This is accomplished by assessing the social, biological, and psychological/per-

Figure 13.1.    Occupational Role Performance: Performance Components

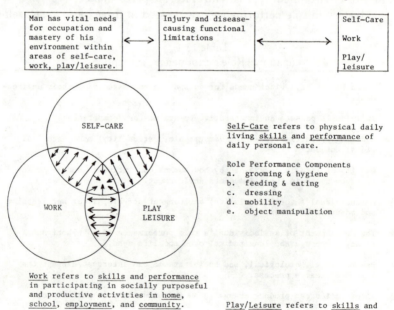

Man has vital needs for occupation and mastery of his environment within areas of self-care, work, play/leisure. ⟷ Injury and disease-causing functional limitations ⟷ Self-Care / Work / Play/leisure

SELF-CARE

WORK

PLAY LEISURE

Self-Care refers to physical daily living skills and performance of daily personal care.

Role Performance Components
a.  grooming & hygiene
b.  feeding & eating
c.  dressing
d.  mobility
e.  object manipulation

Work refers to skills and performance in participating in socially purposeful and productive activities in home, school, employment, and community.

Role Performance Components
a.  home management/homemaking
b.  child care/parenting
c.  employment preparation

Play/Leisure refers to skills and performance in activities for:

Role Performance Components
a.  amusement
b.  relaxation
c.  spontaneous enjoyment
d.  self expression

sonal component areas indicated in Figure 13.2 (Tigges & Talty, 1979, p. 26). Disturbances in any or all of these component areas can result in role dysfunction. Assessment seeks to identify the disturbance in the component area and to match it to its effect on role performance.

The objective of this paradigm is the restoring of role performance. Restoration may involve reduction of the biological, social, and/or psychological factors; it may be maintenance, or the learning of adaptive (manipulative) coping behaviors. In the situation of a person with terminal illness, occupational therapy makes a major diversion from standard practice when it sets out to determine priorities for reducing pathological involvement. For example, in a case where the carcinoma has metastasized to the central nervous system and presents a classic hemiplegia, it is tempting to focus treatment on the reduction of the pathology so as ultimately to enhance performance. But in terminal care all goals are short-term, and therefore, first and foremost is restoration of performance. Reduction is only applicable when it relates to function (i.e., assistive devices, or a splint that would facilitate independent eating). Further, the term *terminal* is relative. Both Twycross (1975) and Wilkes (1980) have stated that, irrespective of pathological indications, the person's mental, social, and personal desire or drive to see the next day or month through is the most highly unpredictable factor in hospice care. "Through occupational therapy, the incentive to be productive, make a contribution, be involved, and have a genuine sense that tomorrow holds a promise and hope, has the greatest influence on how long the term *terminal* means" (Martin, 1980). Thus, the Occupational Role Performance Paradigm, with its focus on role performance rather than on pathology, appears to be the most appropriate occupational therapy approach in terminal care.

## Assessment

Irrespective of how the physical environment is designed or how the style of medical care is altered, in the majority of cases a person's role performance is affected when he or she enters a health care facility. When at home, a person maintains intrinsic and extrinsic control of his or her thoughts, acts, and actions; the individual is the controller of what happens. Personal habits are maintained and carried out in privacy, and the "door" can be closed upon demand to any outside interference. Although admission to an inpatient hospice facility is substantially different from admission to an acute or long-term agency, admission is nonetheless traumatic. Personal independence is diminished, and the individual becomes subject to a routinized environment.

Figure 13.2.   Occupational Role Performance: Performance Elements

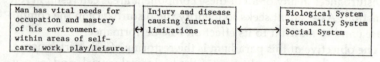

| Man has vital needs for occupation and mastery of his environment within areas of self-care, work, play/leisure. | Injury and disease causing functional limitations | Biological System Personality System Social System |

Biological

Sensorimotor components refers to the <u>skills</u> and <u>performance</u> of patterns of sensory and motor behavior which are prerequisites to self-care, work and play/leisure performance.

Social

Social refers to <u>skills</u> and <u>performance</u> in relating to another person, groups of people in typical and/or atypical social settings and environments.

dyadic interaction, group interaction

neuromuscular (reflex integration, range of motion, gross-fine coordination, strength/endurance) sensory integration (sensory awareness, visual spatial awareness, body integration).

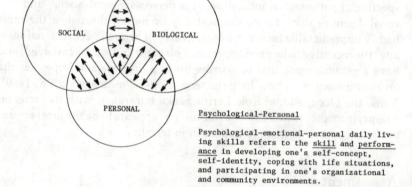

Psychological–Personal

Psychological-emotional-personal daily living skills refers to the <u>skill</u> and <u>performance</u> in developing one's self-concept, self-identity, coping with life situations, and participating in one's organizational and community environments.

self–concept, self–identity, situational coping, cognitive components, psychological components.

## Preadmission Assessment

The purpose of the preadmission assessment is threefold. The first is to become familiar not only with the patient, but also with the family. In this regard, the occupational therapist will be gathering specific information about the patient's life style, likes, dislikes, interests, and in particular regular and routine life experiences.

The second aim is to assess the role performance components (see Figure 13.1) in order to establish in which areas the patient is encountering difficulties and in which areas the patient can function—whether independently or with assistance. Where independence is lacking, it is important to establish which of the areas the individual feels are most important for retaining control. Starmer (1980) stresses that self-care needs are the single most important factor in the maintenance of a person's personal integrity. By the very nature of our upbringing, people avoid and fear vulnerability. A sense of vulnerability can result from being physically exposed, or simply from being shaved, fed, dressed, or taken to the toilet by someone else. The occupational therapist provides an invaluable service to the nursing staff by providing information on how patients feel about their self-care. Occupational therapists can provide that very necessary link—what self-care nursing services are required and which services the patient can do and wishes to do independently. Information obtained at home, within the patient's own territory, consistently is qualitatively different from information obtained after admission. Patients are people and are reluctant to be open or candid. Therefore, they feel obligated to comply with the standard operating procedure. They will not risk not being accepted, being disliked, or being thought of as "difficult." Instead, they will agree and comply. Patients with a terminal illness (cancer or otherwise) cannot afford to risk being alienated. Time is too short and precious to take any chance of offending the medical or nursing staff and of being considered a "troublemaker."

The third purpose of the preadmission assessment is to prepare for being part of the admission of the patient at the hospice. The occupational therapist should be in the position of (1) having made preadmission home visits; and (2) not being considered "medical staff" and therefore not being associated with the physical side of the cancer problem. In hospices, considerable effort is made to receive the patient with personal attention. Just as a nurse is essential to greet the incoming patient, so also is the occupational therapist. It is as important that a nurse is there to immediately attend to and give reassurance to the patient who is in severe pain or having severe symptoms, as it is for the occupational therapist to be there as the "friend" to reassure the patient that all efforts will be made to continue, as much as possible, his or her normal life style.

*Admission Assessment*

In traditional hospitals, the occupational therapist does not see or assess most patients until they are well settled—that is, until the reason for admission is "sorted out" and physical care established. In hospices, physical care and quality independence are not separated. Therefore, the occupational therapist must be involved from the onset of admission. Correct positioning and support at the elbow, for example, may enable a patient to use an electric razor when he would otherwise be dependent on assistance for his shaving needs. Similarly, adaptive equipment and/or functional splints can provide complete or partial independence in eating, grooming, or bathing. For these reasons, the therapist and the nurse can assist each other and must be familiar with each other's admission and assessment procedures. Further, it is essential that the initial care plan is articulated and charted for the next nursing shift.

In the majority of cases, the first 24 hours are the most important in establishing the true sense of hospice care. If all physical care is provided— that is, if the patient is put on bed rest and the primary aim is to control pain and symptoms to the exclusion of any other objective—patients tend to succumb to (1) enjoying being dependent, in which case they may become unnecessarily dependent; (2) believing that in fact they cannot do any of their self-care because others are providing it; (3) giving up hope of ever getting out of bed again; and (4) resisting becoming involved in life activities once the symptoms and pain are well under control.

The most difficult of admission assessments are those of patients who are admitted directly from acute care hospitals where aggressive curative or palliative measures have been the primary goals. In the majority of these cases, patients have become profoundly dependent on their medical care and procedures. Caution must be taken so that the "withdrawal of care" and the encouragement of independence is not interpreted by patients as a withdrawal of concern for them. Nevertheless, it is essential for the occupational therapist to have immediate contact with patients during and on admission and to be involved closely in the first 24 hours of care so that a subtle "weaning" from dependence in self-care can be obtained as soon as possible. If early contact is not made, many patients withdraw from their surroundings and resist any effort to take an active role in "living."

*Day Unit Assessment*

Day unit assessment is substantially different from inpatient assessment in that the physical condition of day unit patients is such that they continue to live relatively independently, even though they may be largely confined to their homes. Day units, which are managed almost exclusively by occupational therapists, provide the following:

1. A very necessary opportunity for patients to escape the confinement of home.
2. The opportunity to be engaged in regular and familiar work and

social activities, thereby encouraging productive living and a genuine sense of self-worth.

3. The opportunity to maintain skills that will foster the ability to continue living at home.
4. Training of adaptive skills.
5. A monitoring of physical ability (i.e., of physical deterioration that may indicate the necessity for inpatient admission) and the quality of pain control.

Twine (1980) stresses that it is only when patients are actually engaged in regular life activities that true pain control can be assessed. An increase in apparent pain cannot automatically be attributed to the illness. Increased isolation at home, the death of another day unit friend, or decreased ability in independence all have a definite effect on pain.

Day unit assessment, like preadmission for inpatient status, begins in the home. This is accomplished by establishing a regular and familiar acquaintance with the patient and other family members who reside in the same household. Assessment is carried out partially by having the cup of tea, the social call, for this is important. However, the essence of the assessment is not only to observe, but also to participate side by side with individuals in their regular routine activities. It is only in this manner that the occupational therapist can adequately gather the necessary information so as to organize day unit programs in a manner that will strengthen and/or maintain consistent patterns of living.

In its practice and philosophy, the day unit concept is based on enhancing and maintaining home living (Wilkes, Crowther, & Greaves, 1978). Assessment in the day unit takes on the form most closely resembling traditional occupational therapy. A planned program of assessing self-care, work, and play/leisure is carried out in a relatively formal manner with the aim of establishing strengths and weaknesses in the patient's role performance. The occupational therapy facility in a day unit program must have available all traditional facilities for assessment. Such facilities are essential not only for assessment and treatment purposes for day unit patients, but for inpatients as well.

## Treatment Planning

Traditional occupational therapy education and practice stress a relatively formal style in the patient-therapist relationship. Objectivity is essential if the therapist is to maintain a professional attitude. To become personally involved, either in the treatment situation or in the patient's personal life, is considered unprofessional. In hospice care, relationships between staff, therapists, and patients are made quickly. They may become intense and deep, although they are usually quite short. It is commonplace in hospices for doctors, therapists, and nurses to sit on patients' beds, hold their hands, and pray aloud if that is what the patients wish (Doyle, 1980b). In hospice care, the occupational therapist must operate first as a solid, mature, and secure person—a person who can easily and comfortably put aside the traditional practice role and commune with the patient as one would do with a guest in one's home. The patient-therapist relationship in a hospice setting is a role reversal from standard practice. As a provider of professional services, however, the therapist must gather data, make evaluation judgments, and construct a plan of treatment.

In terminal care, treatment planning as such focuses not only on the concrete role performance components, but also on the status of the patient's intrinsic security. Long, detailed treatment plans are inappropriate. In most cases, treatment plans are formulated simultaneously with the assessment and are immediately implemented. Treatment plans are as temporary as the patient's needs. Thus they must be discussed collaboratively with the patient as they are being formulated. This does not imply that the occupational therapist does not use persuasive techniques, as many patients need reassurance, encouragement, and assurance that they can live to the fullest until their death. But in all situations, the patient is the leader in finally determining what should be done and when.

The area of persuasion, reassurance, and encouragement presents another role alteration for the occupational therapist. As stated earlier, traditional occupational therapy purports to instill hope and faith in a long and productive future. In the treatment planning of patients with terminal illness, an extremely fine line must be drawn between encouraging the patient to try to achieve and become as independent as possible without raising false hopes that cannot be fulfilled either by the patient or by the therapist. Further, it is essential in a hospice setting to monitor closely the intervention process, as the physical, social, and emotional status of patients can fluctuate rapidly and, with that, also their role performance needs.

Once it has been determined that a patient has role dysfunction requiring external intervention, therapy proceeds in two simultaneous dimensions: (1) to plan implementing self-care, work, and play/leisure treatment toward reducing the dysfunction; and (2) to reobserve, reassess, replan, and treat through self-care, work, and play/leisure activities. This last point reaffirms my emphasis above that occupational therapy intervention does not focus exclusively on just one, but on all three role performance areas.

Aschoff (1965) stresses that humans operate on circadian rhythms—the timing of given life activities to a relationship of performance. This theory coincides with the premises of occupational therapy in that people have certain and specific needs for self-care, work, and play/leisure, and that time relationship directly relates to performance. Thus, a day begins with self-care, is then generally spent in work, and ends with relaxation. When this pattern is maintained, results can be seen in the patients' role restoration.

Occupational therapy in a hospice setting (unlike standard practice) is scheduled according to each patient's individual needs. The treatment process begins as the self-care needs begin each morning. A general standard for occupational therapy services is 7:00 A.M. to 7:00 P.M. The majority of the day must focus on work—productive use of time. To provide a wide variety of fun, leisure, and/or social activities during the waking hours for patients is not only not in compliance with the occupational role performance paradigm, but also not in compliance with standard values of life. Life is not all fun, games, and entertainment. In providing such activities, one deprives individuals of their need to live life as productive persons.

General rules for treatment programming are these:

1. The role performance activity must comply with the appropriate time for doing the activity (e.g., self-care, grooming, and hygiene when the patient is awakened in the morning; feeding at all three meals). Feeding training or assistance at 3:00 P.M., for instance, is totally inappropriate.

2. The activity must meet the immediate needs of the patient.

3. Activities, particularly work activities, should be ones that require few instructions and can be completed in a short period of time. Work activities that can be completed in 1 to 3 hours are highly desirable. Activities that cannot be put down and picked up easily, those that have complex instructions or processes, or that have a high risk of poor completion results are to be avoided. "It must be stressed that by the time a patient requires inpatient or day unit care, the illness generally is well advanced. As a result, many patients are physically weak. Their physical and emotional endurance is short" (Holland, 1980).

4. A wide variety of work activities must be provided to match age, interest, and gender needs.

5. Play/leisure activities—individual as well as group—are selected according to the needs of individual patients. The programming of play/leisure activities should, as mentioned earlier, represent

the smallest time allocation in a given day. Programming should include passive as well as active involvement. It is not uncommon that by midafternoon many patients are growing tired. It is not inappropriate at this time, on a daily basis, to offer a wide variety of leisure activities. It is at this time that the occupational therapy department becomes the "family room" in a hospice for inpatients, day patients, and their friends or family members. Many patients look forward to playing a game of bingo, chess, or cards, watching television, or reading a book or magazine—all activities going on simultaneously. Patients should be made to feel free to move from one activity to another as their mood so determines, or to return to their room or ward as they wish.

The mid- or late-afternoon leisure program, although informal in nature, must be managed with a keen eye by the occupational therapist. Quality of life does not necessarily mean quantity. Patients have special needs in a leisure situation as they do in the other areas of role performance. Putting a group of people in a room and providing a circus of activities can be as devastating to a person as total neglect or isolation can be.

Although the five general rules for treatment programming are applicable, special attention must be given to the patient confined to bed. The bed confinement may be due to further metastasis, insufficient pain or symptom control, or general deterioration. Some may be mentally alert, others confused or disoriented. Particularly for those patients who are alert, every effort must be made to keep them active and involved in the mainstream of daily living. When possible, their beds should be moved to the occupational therapy department where they can either actively or passively participate with other inpatients and day unit patients alike. For those patients for whom it is inadvisable to leave their rooms or wards, efforts must be made so that their confinement and isolation does not result in withdrawal, depression, increased anxiety, or fear—thus significantly affecting their quality of living. These principles can be illustrated in the following case history.

Mrs. R., age 44, weighing 82 pounds, married, with three children, confined herself to bed because she was so emaciated and did not want anyone to see her, and because she feared that any physical activity would aggravate her "severe" respiratory condition. She demanded a private room next to the nurses' station, as she was fearful that if she could not see a nurse about she would have another "breathing attack." She was in a constant state of anxiety, fear, and agitation, and demanded almost constant nursing attention. A week following admission her medication had to be doubled to control her pain, which was attributed to her self-imposed isolation and distress.

The occupational therapist talked with Mrs. R. daily to gain her confidence and to encourage her to leave the confinement of her room. Assurance was given that she would be taken from her room and the hospice without having to see anyone, visitors or patients. Ultimately, wrapped in a blanket and in a wheelchair, she was taken to the park adjoining the hospice. After 3 days of walks in the park, her mental status markedly improved. Once outside the hospice she became eager and willing to talk about her fear, anxiety, and guilt about not letting her husband or children visit her. Mrs. R. eventually expressed an interest in seeing her family and was eager to make gifts for her children. Although she was confined to bed the majority of the day, her room became a beehive of activity. With an over-the-bed table and a variety of adaptations, she was capable of involvement in a wide variety of work activities.

During this period of time, there was a significant decrease in demand for nursing attention and a 40% decrease in pain medication. In the last few days before she died, Mrs. R. was relatively happy and contented. Meetings with her family were happy, and much of their conversation focused on the craft activities of which she was so very proud. Although her last 3 weeks were spent in relative confinement, her life was quite rich and meaningful.

Often, following pain and symptom control, patients are allowed to return home, provided that they and their families can cope. For these patients, the occupational therapist can provide that link between hospice and home, just as for patients who remain at home throughout their illness and who may never be admitted to a hospice. For the person who will live alone or with a spouse who is working during the day, retraining in homemaking (adaptations and/or work simplification) and meal preparation, with adaptive self-help equipment for bathing and dressing, can change being at home from a life of isolation and dependence to a life where the patient can remain a productive and contributing person.

Considerable assistance can also be provided to family members who will be primary caregivers. Instruction on transferring (i.e., from bed to commode, bathtub, or toilet) and in the use of adaptive equipment provides family members with skills and confidence in caring for their ill relative. Special guidance also prevents family members from inadvertently rendering the patient totally dependent.

It must be remembered that a patient's home is his or her territory and, as such, must be respected. Although many patients are keen to have physical alterations made in their bathrooms, bedrooms, and kitchens, there are people who do not want their homes looking like "handicapped houses." This must be respected; the alternative is the learning of adaptive skills. Unlike a hospice setting where many activities and a variety of environments can be "brought to the patient," in the patient's home this is not possible. Although being at home is most desirable for most people under any circumstance, being ill at home presents problems for the patient that can challenge the occupational therapist. The incentive to get up and face each day as a housebound person, with friends making token visits, demands initiative on the part of the occupational therapist to make daily living convenient, productive, and meaningful.

## The Occupational Therapy Process

The occupational therapy process, as discussed in assessment and treatment planning, provides guidelines for formulating occupational therapy services. If accurate and adequate care is to be provided in hospice programs, we cannot permit traditional lockstep "roles." Unlike traditional settings, the occupational therapist cannot operate solely from a geographic department. The occupational therapy process must be patient-centered. Quality care cannot be fragmented. All staff members not only must know everything that is happening with a patient, but must be prepared for and capable of providing almost any care at any time, under any circumstances. In a hospice setting, one cannot say, "I'll call the nurse," "You had better talk to the doctor about that," or "When the minister comes you can ask him to pray with you." Similarly, if a patient is about to die, one cannot rush out of the room, ward, or home. Occupational therapists must be as competent and comfortable changing a colostomy bag, sitting with a patient for as long as an hour without saying a word, or laying out a body, as they are in providing therapy. When a patient says, "What do you feel about death?", "Do you believe in God?", or "I'm going to die soon, aren't I?", an immediate, sincere, and trust-provoking response must be given, and the time needed by the patient must be provided.

There are times when an occupational therapist will be working with a patient in the occupational therapy department in a somewhat scheduled manner. There will also be times when the occupational therapist will be functioning as a member of the unit staff, alongside the nurse or doctor. Apart from the regular medical ward rounds, the occupational therapist should make daily ward rounds and see each and every patient. In a hospice setting, the occupational therapist cannot just pop in every third day and spout out platitudes like, "Is everything all right?", or "Do you need any more materials?" In some instances, the occupational therapist may make as many as three or four visits to a given patient in one day. It all depends on how one defines "quality of life" services.

Similarly, the nursing staff must be more than just casually acquainted with what occupational therapists provide. Should patients on the evening or night shift be distressed, be upset, or have an urgency to complete a project that has special meaning to them, the nurse must feel comfortable and confident in providing the necessary assistance. It is not a matter of "This is my role and you stick to yours." It is a matter of cooperation in delivery of skills and abilities. If true cooperation between the occupational therapist and the nurse is to exist, then they must work together, share responsibilities, and know—irrespective of their former traditional roles—when it is important to relinquish their roles in the true spirit of giving their best to people whose earthly lives are about to be fulfilled.

## Looking to the Future

In order to prepare occupational therapists to assume these new roles, innovative educational and training programs must be developed. Such programs must emphasize distinctive theoretical and practical components for working with dying persons and their families. And it is most important for the practical component that therapists be affiliated with a fully operational hospice service in the immediate locality of the training program. As Wilkes has pointed out, one of the greatest missions of a hospice is to provide training programs where medical and therapeutic disciplines would receive academic and practical experience. The emphasis in this is not to train personnel to work in hospices, but rather to expose them to changes that are so urgently needed in standard practice. "One cannot justify the proliferation of hospices merely to provide care for the terminally ill person. Economically, it is unrealistic" (Wilkes, 1980).

As we develop these new educational programs, caution must be exercised to prevent the concept of "specialization" from creeping in with its associated implications of narrowness and limitation. There is not one segment of health care where the concept of a "specialty" has not become a perpetuation of the professional specialty—a certain select few, a fraternity, all of whom become preoccupied with their own preeminence. So many specialists lose sight of the conceptual intent of their mission because their mission is to be different.

What is different, and what must be different in the hospice philosophy, is that each patient is treated as a person: The patient tells you what he or she needs, wants, and cares about—not the doctor, nurse, or therapist. What is special about the education of people who wish to enter this field is teaching, or reteaching, people how to care about other human beings. We must teach people who live in a complex, high-speed society of instant disposability that human beings can and do care, and that life can be fulfilling. Quick and shallow rewards are not what bring people together into communion with each other. What brings people together is more than education can provide. People come together in life and at the end of life, because they truly care about others, and sincerely believe that they are their brother's keeper.

# References

American Occupational Therapy Association, *Occupational Therapy Newsletter*, 1979, *33*(1), 6.

Aschoff, J., "Circadian Rhythms in Man," *Science*, 1965, *148*, 1427–1432.

Dempsey, D., *The Way We Die*. New York: Macmillan, 1975.

Doyle, D. Conversation with the author at St. Columba's Hospice, Edinburgh, July 10, 1980. (a)

Doyle, D., *Education for Health Professionals*. Paper presented to the United Kingdom National Society for Cancer Relief, Abingdon, England, December 1980. (b)

Holland, A. Conversations with the author at St. Luke's Nursing Home, Sheffield, August–November 1980.

Martin, A. Conversations with the author at St. Luke's Nursing Home, Sheffield, September 1980.

Starmer, E. Conversations with the author at Cynthia Spencer House, Northampton, October, 1980.

Tigges, K. N., *Independence Through Occupational Role Performance*. Paper presented to the United Kingdom National Society for Cancer Relief, Abingdon, England, December 1980.

Tigges, K. N., & Talty, P., *The Occupational Role Performance Handbook, No. 1*. Unpublished manuscript, State University of New York at Buffalo, 1979.

Twine, J. Conversations with the author at St. Luke's Nursing Home, Sheffield, July 1980.

Twycross, R., "Relief of Terminal Pain," *British Medical Journal*, 1975, *4*, 212–214.

Wilkes, E., "The Trouble with Patients," *Journal of the Royal College of General Practitioners*, 1976, *26*, 874.

Wilkes, E. Conversations with the author at St. Luke's Nursing Home, Sheffield, July–September 1980.

Wilkes, E., Crowther, A. G. O., & Greaves, C. W. K. H., "A Different Kind of Day Hospital—For Patients with Preterminal Cancer and Chronic Disease," *British Medical Journal*, 1978, *2*, 1053–1056. [See also Chapter 23, this volume.]

# 14

# Hospice Chaplaincy in the Caregiving Team

*Trevor Hoy*

## Spiritual Concerns for the Dying: The Hospice Experience

> Yea though I walk through the valley of the shadow of death, I will fear no evil; FOR thou art with me; thy rod and thy staff comfort me.
>
> —*Psalm 23:4**

The little preposition "for," tucked unobtrusively in a psalm that is recited at almost every funeral service, lies at the heart of any spiritual or religious support of the dying. It is my assumption that this chapter is addressed primarily to those of the Judaeo-Christian tradition, who know a God who has been revealed in the shadows of history, in the suffering and joys of our own lives, in the story of the People of God preserved in Scripture, and supremely, for Christians, in the life and death and resurrection of Jesus Christ. We have much to learn in this age of religious pluralism from Eastern religions, or even from some of the emerging "new" religions. But no minister can be all things to all people, and his or her commitment need not be compromised to serve those who many not share it. What distinguishes the chaplain from other members of a caregiving team is the representative and symbolic nature of the role, which transcends physical and emotional support and points to God's action and presence: "FOR thou art with me; thy rod and thy staff comfort me."

*All quotations from the Bible in this chapter are from the New English Bible version. Copyright 1981 by Trevor Hoy.

The chaplain is more than another counselor on a hospice care team, though pastoral counseling and emotional support are important services. The chaplain represents God and the religious community that has nurtured a patient's pilgrimage of faith. Indeed, one of the insights derived from my 5 years of experience delivering hospice care has been to recognize that few dying patients need counseling—in the therapeutic meaning of that term. Family members and caregivers do require such support from professional staff. But it is not uncommon for dying patients to minister quite intentionally to their family and to their chaplain. Thus the spiritual dimensions of hospice work are manifold, and hospice programs—both as modern efforts and as medieval programs of care for the dying—have properly been firmly grounded in religious values (Stoddard, 1978).

Hospice chaplaincy, then, is practiced in the midst of inherent tension between work with those whose faith is secure and the need in our secular society to serve those who entertain a variety of humanistic beliefs that see "spiritual support" as virtually identical with "morale building." The Appendix to this chapter contains a statement that defines in detail the corporate nature of chaplaincy that is shared by professional staff or volunteers on a hospice interdisciplinary team. The adjective *interdisciplinary* means that *disciplines* are represented by persons having training, experience, and recognition in that particular field. It should not seem strange, therefore, that the caregiving team should include a *disciple,* or designated ordained minister, to provide the supervision of spiritual/religious support and to assure its credibility in the community where it is offered. It is as inappropriate for a chaplain to intrude his or her advice into the analysis of physical symptoms or pain and their management, as it is for a nurse to assess and attempt to meet effectively the spiritual/religious needs of a patient or family. Each discipline needs to respect the special competence and experience of the other. There is a growing danger, as third-party reimbursement becomes normative, that hospice care may revert to a traditional medical model, being at best multidisciplinary instead of interdisciplinary.

Most hospice programs will depend heavily on members of the clergy volunteering themselves on a part-time basis. Nevertheless, commitment to their services should be reflected in a significant line item in the budget to cover their expenses and training. Some hospital-based or inpatient facilities may have a full-time chaplain. It can well be argued that it is often better for clergy to fill more than one function on a staff. Some of their responsibilities could be in administration, coordination of volunteers, counseling, bereavement work, or (as in my case) coordinating a national professional training program. A particular chaplain cannot and should not be involved with every patient or family admitted to the hospice program of care. In numerous instances the services of a chaplain are neither requested nor appropriate, and I say more of this matter later. But the risks of burnout can be severe if any staff member is personally involved with a large number of patients. It is because of such limitations that every hospice program must seek the support of clergy and congregations in its community. Just as a hospice makes it clear to a physician that he or she remains responsible as the patient's primary or attending physician for the care of his or her patient, so spiritual/religious support must remain the prerogative of a patient's pastor, rabbi, church, or synagogue. One of the major duties of a hospice chaplain is to identify and encourage such ministry and to serve as a backup when needed. Among the most promising developments of my chaplaincy has been the creation of a strong "clergy support group," which includes three Protestant clergy (one a woman), a Catholic priest, and a rabbi. It is the authenticity and resourcefulness of this group that undergirds the religious credibility of hospice care. Through regular ecumenical training workshops that the group sponsors several times each year, clergy throughout the county have become better informed about how they may care for the sick or admit members of their congregation to a hospice. In addition, they have had opportunities to share with one another many of the skills and sensitivities they require in their ministry to the dying.

As indicated in the principles and standards developed by the National Hospice Organization (1979), hospice care emphasizes supporting a patient to live fully during a time of decline, so that this may permit a quality of life that includes opportunity for extraordinary personal or religious growth. Focusing on the needs of the dying is like watching the ripples from a pebble cast into a lake; their effect touches caregivers, family members, friends, and professionals, and can reach the furthest limits of our culture. It has been said that a civilization can be measured by how it regards and takes care of the dying. By such a standard we have fallen far short of our humanitarian ideals, not to mention the implications of our faith. Confronting our own death or being confronted by the dying challenges the basic belief systems and values of our society. In his excellent guide to counseling the depressed, Roy Fairchild (1980) of the San Francisco Theological Seminary reflects the essence of hospice philosophy when he says,

> The enlargement of hope is even possible in the situation of the fatally ill person, but we must ask, "Hope for what?" For long-range survival, no. For an end to agony, perhaps. For a richer life now, yes. For a life after death? Chris-

tians are confident of that. Hope, even in terminal illness, can be enlarged. Despite the medical prognosis, the pastor's task is to help the person *live fully and creatively whatever time he has left.* (pp. 121–122)

For some people, the shock of impending death does its own work, and they reevaluate their values as in a conversion. Humanistic psychologist Abraham Maslow spoke of his "post-mortem life" after a heart attack:

> One very important aspect of the post-mortem life is that everything gets doubly precious, gets piercingly important. You get stabbed by things, by flowers and by babies and by beautiful things—just the very act of living, of walking and breathing and eating and having friends chatting. . . . I am living an end-life where everything ought to be an end in itself, where I shouldn't waste any time preparing for the future. (quoted in Fairchild, 1980, p. 122)

The National Hospice Organization, in its statement of standards (1979), sums up this approach well:

> Hospice affirms life. Hospice exists to provide support and care for persons in the last phases of incurable disease so that they might live as fully and comfortably as possible. Hospice recognizes dying as a normal process whether or not resulting from disease. Hospice neither hastens nor postpones death. Hospice exists in the hope and belief that, through appropriate care and the promotion of a caring community sensitive to their needs, patients and families may be free to attain a degree of mental and spiritual preparation for death that is satisfactory to them. (p. 3)

Then, under Principle 7 and Standard 7, it affirms: "Personal philosophic, moral, or religious belief systems are important to patients and families who are facing death," and "Hospice care is respectful of all patient and family belief systems" (p. 7).

It is in this context that hospice care is interdisciplinary and interactive in yet another way. As Robert Twycross has said (1980), control of chronic pain has as much to do with social, psychological, and spiritual support of the patient as it has to do with the chemicals ingested. Thus, just as nurses can provide needed emotional and spiritual comfort, so a minister may be in a position to contribute to the patient's physical welfare. Often the patient will speak of a symptom to the chaplain rather than "bother the doctor." Similarly, the nurse may be the first to whom patients will confide their fears that they are dying rather than "bother their priest." Team members share perceptions, identify family dynamics and resources, and agree on the proper intervention, for it is a central axiom of hospice care that no one person can undertake the total care of the dying. Clergy, who are not always well noted for their reputation as "team players," must be prepared to submit themselves to the requirements of this approach and perhaps even to the judgment of the team as to the appropriateness of their visits. It is for this reason that attendance at weekly patient care conferences is mandatory for all hospice staff members—whether salaried or nonsalaried.

I would like to conclude this section by quoting what William Lamers (former medical director of Hospice of Marin and now with the Tom Baker Cancer Centre, Calgary, Alberta, Canada) has written recently (1981), interpreting from the perspective of another discipline the value of religion in the care of the dying:

> Religion gives me a great deal of support. Belief in an afterlife and the potential for eventual reunion is comforting. Prayer and ceremony not only help to close a relationship that has ended with death, but provide a sense of satisfaction from knowing that important traditions have been fulfilled. All the talk of death in recent years has taken away some of the mystery about the scientific aspects of death . . . and opened up for wonder the larger questions of life and death, time and eternity. Our search for knowledge has brought us back to fundamental questions that cannot be resolved by science and medicine. Religion offers a promise, a comfort, and a hope. (p. 146)

## Meeting People Where They Are

> There is a special Providence in the fall of a sparrow . . .
> If it be not now, yet it [will] come—the readiness is all.
>
> —*William Shakespeare*, Hamlet, *Act V, Scene ii, ll. 219–222*

Hamlet, just before his fatal duel with Laertes, beautifully summarizes the goal of hospice care for patient and family—to insure that their "readiness is all." Every member of the caregiving team, including volunteers, contributes to that readiness. However, if there is one insight that I would hope might spare other chaplains some grief, it would be this: Do not be unduly concerned if you appear to be underutilized, whether regarding the number of patients you may be called upon to serve, or the limited number of visits you may enjoy with them. It is one of the criteria of successful hospice care that the patient and family be so "ready," so able to cope, that only the very minimum number of visits or telephone calls by professionals are really needed.

One of the characteristics of an effective pastor is the continuity of care for people through a wide span of their life and a spectrum of life experiences ranging from birth to death, from joy to sorrow. In contemporary nomadic industrial societies, few parishioners or clergy remain pastorally connected for more than 10 years. But at times a chaplain may have to enter the life of a patient and family for at best months or only for days. Sometimes the hospice chaplain may be called upon to conduct the funeral of a patient whom he or she has never met. It is well for such a chaplain to be clear that it is *need*, not membership in a congregation, that undergirds this sort of care. A century ago, the Church focused her energies on carrying the Gospel to those who had never known Christ in distant lands. Today's mission can be to the churched, the unchurched, or even the antichurched close to home in our own communities, who are our brothers and sisters in need: the sick, the poor, the oppressed, the lonely, the refugees, the aged, the minorities—yes, and the dying. Hospice challenges our congregations to look again at their care of the dying and to make this a contemporary frontier of their mission of love and service.

Hospice care of the dying raises discomforting questions when those who have seemed indifferent, or who have scarcely darkened a church door for years, suddenly want all of the rites, sacraments, and privileges of the informed and dedicated believer. It is here that the metaphor of the "magician" seems to typify the expectations that a family may have of the chaplain or pastor. I confess to finding such last-minute demands distasteful and will do everything I can to seek earlier referral in order to provide an authentic basis for ministry. Nevertheless, Jesus spoke of rewarding the laborer who was hired at the last hour of the day as much as the one who had worked throughout its heat. We can be clear with people that we will not offer cheap or magical answers to the mystery of life and death. And we can discover, if we will be open to this possibility, that more often than not God works a miracle of healing grace in the "desert" of faith and theological literacy—a term that describes the barren spiritual/religious pilgrimage of some of those we are called upon to serve. Often patients regress to earlier moments in their lives where religious values and practices were vital. We recently had a patient and her husband request baptism, since they could not find records in the small congregations they came from in the Midwest. In another instance, a Protestant patient who had been divorced from his wife a year previously sought through our chaplaincy the opportunity to be reunited with his family the week he died. During that period we were able to locate the Catholic priest who had performed their marriage ceremony 12 years earlier, and he agreed to "remarry" them 2 days before the patient's death. In this case there was time for important, unfinished business (religious, emotional, and financial) to be undertaken. Funeral arrangements were completed, and I have seen few families that shared greater love and compassion during those closing days together climaxing years of painful alienation. The contribution to the grieving process for this widow and her young children was immeasurable. God worked redemptively through the seeming ambiguities and confusions of that family's story to make this final chapter of the father's life a victorious one.

It was, in fact, reflection on this family that suggested to me a metaphor for ministry unlike that of the "magician" (which I fiercely resist)—a metaphor that defines the essence of the function of chaplaincy. It is that of "story hearer" and "story teller." For the dying wish to tell their story and find in it new meaning and new evidence of God's loving care, which still sustains them. And the chaplain can help connect that individual story to the larger tale of the People of God, of whom all are a part in this world and in the life to come when we walk through that "valley of the shadow of death."

A diagram that has proven helpful to me in describing the context of ministry to the dying and its story-telling theme has been adapted here in Figure 14.1. I first encountered this in a seminar presented in 1977 by John Scherer, a Lutheran pastor who now serves as a member of the faculty of the Graduate Center for Applied Studies, Whitworth College, Spokane, Washington. It is reproduced here with his permission and ties in well with the fine article by E. Michael Brady (1979). The dotted line running horizontally across the center of the page represents the patient's life, with the present moment in the middle, the past to the left, and the decreasing future to the right. The vertical axis on the left depicts the tension between

Figure 14.1. The Context of Ministry to the Dying

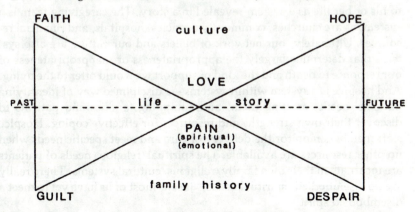

*Adapted from:* John Scherer's schema. Reproduced by permission of John Scherer.

faith (trust) in God's goodness in history or in our life and the negative feelings of guilt or regret that surround our own limited efforts to live up to our ideals or His standards. Similarly, the vertical axis on the right, defining the future, reflects the tension between hope and despair, between being a victor or a victim. It is in the present, the "now," that we experience both love and hurt (or spiritual/emotional pain). The "now" approaches the boundary of transition marked by death and finally merges in those swings of mood—from hope to despair—that mark patient and family alike. Few patients pass through life or their decline focusing exclusively on either the upper or lower dimensions of their life story. More often, there appears to be a movement of the patient's concerns from agendas of the past (the injustice of being stricken by a terminal disease), to the confusions of the present (selecting appropriate treatment and support), to consideration of options for the future. Often a patient appears to regress to some happy period of childhood or marriage where events or persons are more sharply perceived than even the present circumstances are. There seems to be a cycling of focus from past to present to future, leading to a blurring of memories and hopes. As Cantor (1978) suggests, our task as chaplains and caregivers is to assist patients and families to take charge of the "writing" of this last chapter of an earthly story. Generally, we can expect persons to face death much as they have lived, revealing familiar strengths and weaknesses. Yet in those final days we are often privileged to observe rare nobility and courage of the human spirit. The quality of faith, hope, and love may never be more transparent or strong as in those final moments of transition we call death.

These remarks point to the fact that spiritual/religious care, however personal and private it may eventually become, requires a "systems orientation." It requires orientation to the patient's family as a system, and to his or her life as a system revealed in a story. The caregiving team is a system, as are churches, community agencies, hospitals, and financial resources. Ultimately, our network of beliefs and our culture are also systems that determine largely the appropriateness or inappropriateness of our response to death and the kind of support we would offer to the dying. And hospice is a system within systems—a disciplined way of identifying patients' needs, meeting them, and equipping families and patients to discover their own strengths and resources for effective coping. Hospice staff members monitor the delivery of care and meet specific needs when no other resources are available. The spiritual/religious needs of patients are incarnate in their own family/religious/cultural systems. There really are no disembodied "spiritual needs," just as most of us have yet to meet a disembodied spirit.

The Christian faith is articulate about this truth, for we affirm that "the Word became flesh, he came to dwell among us" (John 1:14). We believe that God had to reveal Himself in human form in Jesus Christ, a historic person who endured the depths of human suffering. We believe that the Church, with all of its limitations and failings, remains nothing less than the Body of Christ. It remains possible for us to know and receive God's presence in mundane physical signs: water, oil, bread, wine used in the sacraments. The transactions of ministry begin with the simple presence of one who is quiet, who listens, who holds a hand and shares a tear. Patient and priest may pray together. One patient I visited for a year never let me leave without praying for our hospice, for me, and for my family. In the Episcopal tradition, as in that of the Roman Catholic Church, the anointing of the sick becomes another visible sign of the larger fellowship of faith and of healing. It has taken the place in Catholic practice of "last rites," which have become increasingly limited. Should the patient desire it, those having special gifts of healing or prayer may be called upon. A few words, supplemented by ritual acts, go far at a bedside. But no matter what may be the faith or affiliation of patients or families, the theme of "story hearer" and "story teller" runs through the pastoral relationship. Dying patients are dealing with grief as they have to surrender much that is valued and as options become fewer and fewer for the future. Dreams go unfulfilled, mobility and alertness may be reduced, and past memories and relationships become more and more precious. A number of patients have reported that they are communicating with a deceased spouse or parents, anticipating a reunion with them.

It is the goal of hospice chaplaincy to meet people where they are, and any member of the team may have to assess what are the appropriate spiritual/religious needs of patients that they are visiting or admitting to the hospice program. Because individuals have no current active affiliation with a congregation, this by no means indicates that they may not wish contact with a pastor or priest of their preference. It is also unlikely that many have had direct experience with the ministry of a chaplain, unless they have been hospitalized or have served in the armed forces. But while we try to respect the wishes of each patient, we should not forget that the chaplain is representative of a God whom we believe reaches out to us when we are in the valley of the shadow of our denial or rejection of Him. The interdisciplinary team, including the chaplain, represents the ever-available grace of God to those who face death, loneliness, and loss. The needs of those who profess no formal religious roots are no less real than those who do. In his useful summary of such needs, John Pumphrey (1977) reminds us to be sensitive to how different individuals may wish to meet their needs or to whom they may wish to turn for spiritual/religious support. Those of us who are ordained also need to be comfortable emotionally and theologically with the prospect that many will not request our spiritual/religious support.

## Identifying the Spiritual/Religious Needs of the Patient

> No wonder we do not lose heart! Though our outward humanity is in decay yet day by day we are inwardly renewed. Our troubles are slight and short-lived; and their outcome an eternal glory which outweighs them far. Meanwhile our eyes are fixed, not on the things that are seen, but on things that are unseen; for what is seen passes away; what is unseen is eternal.
>
> —*St. Paul, II Corinthians 4:17, 18*

We turn now to another model that I have developed to assist in determining the variety of spirtual/religious needs that exist for the patient and his or her family. This "taxonomy" can suggest what the appropriate style of ministry or resources might be. None of us likes to be placed in a category, yet this simple analysis can clarify the minimal religious predispositions of the patient/family system. The unit of care in hospice work is the patient/family—the patient in a living context. Yet it is precisely here that we encounter difficulty when providing religious support. For it is rare today for many family units to remain intact throughout a lifetime, let alone have cohesive spiritual/religious beliefs. Those assessing a patient's needs at admission will find that persons who have a profound faith and strong religious support will probably have little hesitation in acknowledging this. Those who have limited faith or who are indifferent or hostile to formal religion will probably not long conceal their feelings. In some families there is compatibility of religious preference; in others there may be open conflict. Figure 14.2 portrays four quadrants that correspond to the differing needs of patients and their families and the options available for meaningful spiritual support. I would invite anyone involved in hospice chaplaincy to identify for themselves what the needs and appropriate resources for ministry are in each category. For the sake of brevity, I here summarize just a few of the distinctions as they affect the immediate role of a chaplain or pastor.

> *Quadrant A (upper left).* Committed personal faith/strong religious support. Most such patients/families will have their own clergy, as well as active support from their local congregations. The primary function of the hospice chaplain in such circumstances is to be sure

Figure 14.2. Religious Support/Personal Faith: Differing Needs of Patients and Their Families

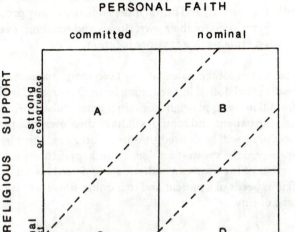

**PERSONAL FAITH**

that such clergy are informed, available, and supported by the chaplain in their ministry. At times, the chaplain may be invited to fill in when the primary clergy are unavailable.

*Quadrant B (upper right).* Nominal personal faith/strong religious support. The chaplain attempts to provide support for such a family while minimizing stress to the patient. Here the family may take the initiative in planning for the impending death, anticipating grief, or setting the funeral arrangements. Because the family's own pastor is probably not suitable, the chaplain may be called upon or can in turn make an appropriate referral to someone else.

*Quadrant C (lower left).* Committed personal faith/minimal religious support. The patient's commitment is strong, with little encouragement from family or others. Often this patient has been "transplanted" from a distant home and is living with relatives who have no church. This person may take the initiative in preparing for death, seeking the chaplain or other ministry, and leaving specific instructions for a funeral.

*Quadrant D (lower right).* Nominal personal faith/minimal religious support. Neither patient nor family professes any active faith or religious preference. Often there is a clear rejection of "organized religion" and all that it stands for. The family may face issues of death, the funeral, and burial independently of any professional services. Some prepare their own rituals and readings, even scattering cremated remains in a favorite location.

There is one other value of the taxonomy diagrammed in Figure 14.2. The diagonal dotted lines running from Quadrant C in the lower left to Quadrant B in the upper right contain segments also of A and D. Above these lines, the patient and family will have their own spiritual resources; below them none will be desired. It is in the area contained by the parallel lines that there is the greatest ambiguity and opportunity for chaplaincy. Every member of the team can collect data to determine the depth of spiritual/religious needs of a patient and to monitor how this may change with the passage of time.

## Three Kinds of Hope—Three Functions of Ministry

> There are three things that last forever; faith, hope, and love; but the greatest of them all is love.
>
> —St. Paul, I Corinthians 13:13

We have explored the "context" of ministry and a means of clarifying the spiritual/religious needs of those whom we serve. I would like now to consider three functions of one who has established a sound relationship as pastor, priest, or chaplain with a patient facing the remaining days or months of his or her life. These address physical, emotional, and spiritual needs, and correspond to the prophetic, pastoral, and priestly dimensions of ministry. They also represent three kinds of hope for which the patient is searching. I define these as the hope for

1. Physical healing and the remission of the disease; a prophetic hope.
2. Healthy and loving personal relationships, where alienation and sin are forgiven or remitted; a pastoral hope.
3. Meaning in the face of the ultimate mystery of death; a priestly hope.

Table 14.1 describes spiritual support in terms of these three dimensions. In the first case, there is the need for a patient or family to cope with fear and uncertainty arising from the physical realities of disease, the complex systems that come to entangle them, and medical options for treatment. Here the chaplain can be an informed mediator and an effective advocate for the patient, fulfilling an ancient prophetic function to proclaim justice and truth in the midst of confusion. Secondly, support focuses on personal and interpersonal relationships, and on pastoral counsel that can enable people to cope with disappointment, termination of significant relationships, and loss of control. In these two related efforts, religion seeks to "re-collect" or "bind together" the fabric of the life that is ending so that

Table 14.1
Spiritual Support

Providing hope during phase of:

| | |
|---|---|
| 1. REMISSION-I:<br><br>COPING WITH FEAR<br>AND WITH UNCERTAINTY<br><br>Focus on the physical;<br>chaplain in "prophetic"<br>role. Dealing with<br>reality of disease and<br>systems. | *Clergy as confidant at time of trauma<br>for patient, spouse, family as they<br>seek to make a sound choice of physic-<br>ian and treatment.<br>*Chaplain as an informed advocate/<br>mediator of conflict.<br>*Knowledge of community resources;<br>professional and volunteer.<br>*Prayer; Healing; Meditation; Scripture.<br>*Facing financial anxieties with family. |
| 2. REMISSION-II:<br><br>COPING WITH DISAPPOINTMENT,<br>LOSS OF CONTROL AND RE-<br>LATIONSHIPS<br><br>Focus on the personal;<br>chaplain in pastoral and<br>counseling role. Dealing<br>with personal and inter-<br>personal relationships. | *Getting affairs in order; personal,<br>financial, legal.<br>*Dealing with unfinished business, re-<br>grets, alienations.<br>*Facilitating family communication.<br>*Clarifying arrangements. Saying "Goodbye".<br>*Recollection and thanksgiving for life<br>story.<br>*Dealing with anger with God. The re-<br>ality of forgiveness. Sacrament of<br>penance.<br>*Living fully, coping with risks of<br>attachment in the anticipation of loss.<br>*Taking charge of these days. Giving<br>of patient to others. |
| 3. REMISSION-III:<br><br>COPING WITH ULTIMATE<br>MEANING BEYOND ACCEPTANCE<br>OF DEATH<br><br>Focus on the spiritual;<br>chaplain in "priestly" and<br>symbolic role. Dealing with<br>ultimate meaning. | *Open discussion of death with patient<br>and family.<br>*Planning the funeral and the grieving.<br>*Reconsidering suffering and injustice.<br>*Accepting dependencies, the community<br>of caring.<br>*Sacraments, prayer, ritualization of<br>waiting.<br>*Letting go--by patient, family, care-<br>givers.<br>*Discovering peace--continuing the "fight".<br><br>*CELEBRATING THE TRANSITION AT THE TIME<br>OF DEATH<br><br>*CONTINUING THE COMMUNITY OF CARE FOR<br>THE FAMILY. |

it can complete its story. And thirdly, the priestly and symbolic role of the chaplain may come to take precedence as the patient copes with ultimate meaning beyond the acceptance of death. None of us is very comfortable speaking of the dying as "patients," yet there can be no disputing that among the great virtues of those we serve in hospice, beyond their faith and courage, is their patience as they wait (sometimes with eagerness) upon the experience of these mysteries. It is here that open discussion of death can occur and ritualization of waiting begins, with the appropriate offering of prayer, sacraments, and family visitations, with the aim of achieving new meaning and hope through redirection or "re-mission." When there has been continuity of spiritual support through these three phases of need, the patient and the family will be "ready" for that final transition at the moment of death, and the groundwork will be well laid for the continuing care of the surviving family members during the period of their bereavement. But, as with other "stages of dying" that have been proposed, these phases of hope should not be taken too literally or "imposed" on others. None in fact is ever completed; each can "recycle" or reappear as live issues at any moment. They do, however, suggest useful underlying themes to set priorities and focus for appropriate roles, rituals, and ministry.


## At the Time of Death and Afterward

> How blest are the sorrowful; they shall find consolation.
>
> —*Matthew 5:4*


It is easier for the chaplain to make an appropriate intervention when there has been an opportunity for the establishment of that level of relationship referred to earlier as "re-mission" prior to the time of death itself. If so, it will be possible to clarify the expectations of patients and family members regarding the physical, emotional, and spiritual realities they will face. The ritualization of waiting requires simple liturgical and devotional actions, translated into a minimum of words and a maximum of feelings. That is why, for the religiously literate, and even for some who have not shared such commitment, ancient prayers and rites or sacraments bring solace. Christians may wish to be anointed by the chrism, not so much as a "last rite" but as a sign of that final healing bond with God and community of faith. The Eucharist may well be the last physical and spiritual meal received by the dying. We have much to learn about the level of consciousness of a person who may appear to be in a coma. It seems likely, however, that hearing may be the last of the senses to fade, and family and friends at bedside need to avoid inappropriate comments, weighing words that may convey their last good-bye. It is also possible that there may be a final "brightening" that allows for lucid conversation to resume a short time after a period when a patient was comatose.

If the family is "ready," they will have decided whom they wish to call at the time of death. They will have discussed arrangements with the funeral director or burial society, and they will consider whether they wish certain members of the family, friends, or clergy to be called. They may wish their physician to be notified and invited to pronounce the death. When hospice staff have been involved, the nurse on call is usually alerted, and sometimes the chaplain is requested to lead the family in prayers. It has been our experience that it is important for the body to be lovingly prepared and dressed, and for those closest to have a reverent time of quiet before their loved one is taken from the room or home. Also, we recommend that the head remain uncovered as the person is taken to the hearse. Those last glimpses leave indelible memories.

Staff attending the dying need to be well informed about the special religious or cultural traditions that must be considered. Mormons and Jews are among those who follow strict customs continuing through the burial and often for weeks or months of bereavement for the surviving family members (e.g., Lamm, 1969). One of the important relationships that a hospice program needs to cultivate professionally is that with the funeral directors in the community. We have found them to be collaborative and helpful. They are willing to learn and also willing to teach our staff about their work. A number of funeral directors nationally have initiated the development of their local hospices. The National Funeral Directors' Association, and other similar groups, have prepared valuable educational materials supportive of the hospice concept.

Chaplains and clergy officiating at funerals have a major responsibility to prepare a service that is appropriate for the family and in keeping with the wishes of their loved one. Sometimes a conflict occurs between the bereaved and instructions left by the person who has died. Usually there are ways of compromising, but the chances for avoiding such difficulties are greatly increased if there has been a proper discussion of the issues prior to the death. While the desires of patients for disposition of their bodies, perhaps for cremation, must be honored, the special spiritual needs of the family commonly have priority regarding funeral arrangements. For it is this service of worship that permits them to pay their respects and to say their "good-byes"—a word we sometimes forget is derived from the phrase "God be with ye." During the funeral, a basic support group that will be available to the bereaved during the difficult months ahead emerges. Hospice programs always offer an extensive bereavement service, with counseling offered by a marriage/family counselor, social worker, chaplain, or other staff member. In addition, gatherings are scheduled where the survivors provide significant support for one another.

When there has been little contact with the deceased, it is difficult to personalize a service. The Episcopal Church wisely guards against sentimental or trivial eulogies by recommending that the person who has died be appropriately referred to in prayers or in the context of a homily to be preached. Often clues can be discovered in a patient's home—from photos, paintings, or favorite books or poems—and these can be incorporated into a liturgy. In more informal settings, members of the family may wish to read a favorite selection or say what is in their hearts. The important thing is that there be a spirit of hope and thanksgiving—one that yet allows for the pain and tears accompanying loss. Those in the congregation are themselves confronted with their own mortality as they support the family in its grief.

Often there should be an opportunity for friends, relatives, or even children to view the person who has died in the funeral home, if they wish to do so (Grollman, 1977). This may help those involved to deal with the reality of death and permit the casket to be closed during the service itself. It is increasingly common for the body to be interred or cremated prior to a memorial service.

## Ethical Concerns

> How blest are those who hunger and thirst to see right prevail; they shall be satisfied.
>
> —*Matthew 5:6*

Hospice chaplaincy must pay particular attention to those ethical concerns that arise in caring for dying persons and their families. In the first place, these relate to the work of the chaplain as a member of the caregiving team. For example, clergy need to be very clear with patients, family members, or other members of the hospice team when strict confidentiality is expected, or when others may be privy to information disclosed. There are still proper moments of confession "under the seal" that no priest can violate. Nevertheless, patients and families must appreciate that effective care can only be promptly delivered if there is a frank exchange of critical data among the staff involved.

More broadly, hospice chaplaincy should offer guidance and witness to the ethical and religious principles that undergird this sort of work. Thus, the chaplain, along with others, should be an effective advocate for community responsibility to respect the individual worth of those for whom we care and their legitimate spheres of autonomy in such matters as truth telling and decision making (Vanderpool, 1978). Finally, as indicated in the hospice philosophy quoted earlier in this chapter, hospice care "neither hastens nor postpones death." It is important to articulate the implications of that perspective in anticipation of questions (which are sometimes quite insistent, even though they may not be spoken aloud) about euthanasia. In practical terms, patients may sign a "living will" (which, under stipulated circumstances, can now have legal force in certain states); request that "heroic treatment" be withheld; or refuse further surgery, radiation, or chemotherapy. Very occasionally, someone may threaten suicide, but those who are then offered good pain and symptom control, together with a caring environment, usually discover emotional and spiritual support that discourages such plans. Generally, it is wise to separate hospice care from the debate about euthanasia, which can best be continued in contexts and organizations that have long ago been founded to explore the frontiers of medical ethics (Oden, 1976). Still, it is important for the chaplain to be a member of the professional advisory committee of a hospice, for it is in this group that the ethical issues bearing on the hospice program are clarified and appropriate policies developed.

## Conclusion

It is not uncommon for a hospice chaplain to be asked: "Don't you find this work depressing?" My answer is that I rarely do, though there need be no illusion that death is pleasant or always peaceful. But the knowledge of the tragic alternatives currently available for the dying and their families is infinitely more depressing. The generous gratitude of those we serve, the privilege of associating with many wonderful families demonstrating the rarest kind of human courage and self-giving love, is reward enough for this demanding ministry. When we are really honest, I suspect there is a legitimate element of self-interest in our hope that the day may come when our death or that of someone close to us will be eased by others who have grasped, and been grasped by, the hospice philosophy and practice. We prefer to face death boldly as a normal climax to living, acknowledging that we may need to become as dependent on others as we were when we entered this world at birth.

Most of us prefer to avoid euphemisms for death and dying, which are popular ways of denying death in our society: "Mary has passed on," "John is no longer with us." St. Paul long ago used a term in the closing verses of his second letter to Timothy that seems to me to be realistic while capturing that special quality of his full life as it entered that final transition in martyrdom for which he was prayerfully preparing. He wrote:

> As for me, already my life is being poured out on the altar and the hour for my departure is upon me. I have run the great race, I have finished the course, I have kept the faith. And now the prize awaits me; . . . and it is not for me alone, but for all who have set their hearts on his coming appearance. (II Timothy 4:6–8)

The original Greek word for *departure* (*analousis*) reflects so well not only the life journey of St. Paul, but the values of hospice care that are the goals of our spiritual/religious support of the dying and their families. For it draws on three metaphors marking the end of life's earthly journey and the beginning of a new one. St. Paul was a tent maker; how fitting that one meaning of *analousis* is the striking of a tent, the pulling up of tent pegs before departure. St. Paul, as must have all people in Biblical times, understood the burden of animals that plowed the rocky soil. *Analousis* is also the release of an animal from the yoke to which it has been harnessed. Death brings us release from the burdens of this earthly pilgrimage. Finally, St. Paul traveled far throughout the ancient world on ships. *Analousis* means the casting off of a ship from the dock as it departs on its voyage into unknown, uncharted waters.

I trust that this analysis (a word so close to *analousis*) has offered its readers some understanding and resources to minister with new love, sensitivity, and power to those whose "hour of departure" and of death is upon them, as it will inevitably some day be upon us all.

## Appendix: Hospice Chaplaincy

Chaplaincy is a specialized, interfaith, institutional ministry to persons confronted by clearly defined physical, emotional, and spiritual needs. Hospice chaplaincy is ministry to those who are dying and to those who are experiencing the loss of a loved one.

As used here, *hospice chaplaincy* is a collective term denoting a variety of resources and persons engaged in meeting the spiritual/religious needs of families facing terminal illness. While it includes the traditional prophetic, pastoral, and priestly dimensions of ministry, it is not restricted to the hospice chaplain, but brings in all who share in providing spiritual support—other members of the interdisciplinary hospice care team and the religious leadership and resources of the community.

It is a role that must be negotiated with each patient/family unit to take into account their history, belief system, any differences in beliefs within the family, affiliation with a particular faith/church, and available resources when referral is appropriate. Hospice chaplaincy is limited by time, by the information available about the family, and by little prospect of extended follow-up. It is a specific service provided within a particular framework.

Chaplaincy is a listening role. It can help the patient to recollect what is past, to deal with regrets and unfinished business that may be causing pain, and to rejoice and give thanks for what has brought love and meaning to life. It can help the patient to see his or her life in a new perspective and increase awareness and readiness for what lies ahead.

In a hospice program, it is the responsibility of the chaplain to make sure that patients and families are offered spiritual support in keeping with their belief systems. Specifically, the chaplain will ascertain whether a family is affiliated with a particular faith or church. If so, the chaplain will offer to contact clergy of that faith on the family's behalf, to serve as liaison for that support, and to support the family's pastor in his or her ministry.

If the family has no affiliation but desires spiritual/religious support, during the illness the chaplain will provide direct spiritual support or delegate care to one of a resource group of clergy of various faiths in the community. Such support can help the patient to recognize God's presence and love in the midst of uncertainty, suffering, and death, and can encourage the patient or family members to "let go" by offering appropriate prayer, scripture, sacraments, or rites during the patient's decline.

At the time of death, the chaplain will prepare and conduct a funeral service for nonaffiliated families who desire a religious service. Such a service can provide continuity of care to surviving family members and can help, along with the work of other hospice team members, to initiate a wholesome grieving process.

# References

Brady, E. M., "Telling the Story: Ethics and Dying," *Hospital Progress*, 1979, *60*, 57–62.

Cantor, R., *And a Time to Live: Toward Emotional Well-Being During the Crisis of Cancer*. New York: Harper & Row, 1978.

Fairchild, R., *Finding Hope Again: A Pastor's Guide to Counseling the Depressed*. New York: Harper & Row, 1980.

Grollman, E., *Living When a Loved One Has Died*. Boston: Beacon Press, 1977.

Lamers, W. M., Jr., "How Doctors Feel When A Patient Dies: Grief Is the Price for Love," in E. Grollman (Ed.), *What Helped Me When My Loved One Died*. Boston: Beacon Press, 1981, pp. 142–147.

Lamm, M., *The Jewish Way in Death and Mourning.* New York: Jonathan David, 1969.

National Hospice Organization, *Standards of a Hospice Program of Care* (6th revision). Unpublished booklet, 1979.

Oden, T. C., *Should Treatment Be Terminated?* New York: Harper & Row, 1976.

Pumphrey, J., "Recognizing Your Patient's Spiritual Needs," *Nursing '77,* 1977, *9,* 64–70.

Stoddard, S., *The Hospice Movement.* New York: Stein & Day, 1978.

Twycross, R. G., personal communication to Dr. William Lamers, St. Christopher's Hospice, London, England, June 1980.

Vanderpool, H. Y., "The Ethics of Terminal Care," *Journal of the American Medical Association,* 1978, *239,* 850–852.

## Bibliography

Bailey, L. R., Sr., *Biblical Perspectives on Death.* Philadelphia: Fortress, 1979.

Bane, J. D. et al., *Death and Ministry.* New York: Seabury, 1975.

Becker, E., *Escape From Evil.* New York: Free Press, 1975.

Freese, A., *Grief: Living Through It and Growing with It.* New York: Harper & Row, 1977.

Jackson, E. N., *You and Your Grief.* New York: Hawthorn, 1962.

Kübler-Ross, E., *Death: The Final Stage of Growth.* Englewood Cliffs, NJ: Prentice-Hall, 1975.

# 15

# Psychotherapy of the Dying Patient

*Averil Stedeford*

The role of the psychiatrist in a terminal care unit was described in general terms . . . by Stedeford and Bloch (1979). This paper focuses on the clinical experience gained while offering psychotherapy to the patients who were referred, and attempts to highlight the psychodynamics which they showed and the psychotherapeutic interventions which were used. [Colin] Murray Parkes (1978) has reported that much of the physical pain in terminal illness goes unrelieved. Cartwright et al. (1973), in their retrospective study of the symptoms suffered by patients in the last 12 months of their life, reported an incidence of 36 per cent for both depression and mental confusion. Our preceding paper [1979] confirms this in the cases referred to the psychiatrist, and in addition shows that family problems related to the terminal illness are even more common. Much of this suffering can be alleviated when the psychology of dying is understood and appropriate psychotherapy is provided.

## The Therapist's Approach

When considering the psychology of dying patients, Kübler-Ross (1969) inevitably comes to mind. She described the stages through which they may pass during the course of their illness. Her work provides valuable guidelines for the therapist, but he must avoid interpreting it too rigidly, or he may lose sight of the wide variety of ways in which terminally ill pa-

*From:* Averil Stedeford "Psychotherapy of the Dying Patient," *British Journal of Psychiatry*, 1979, *135*, 7–14. Reprinted by permission.

tients cope. There is obviously not one way which is ideal, and the therapist should approach patients with an open mind, recognising that they are often more aware of their strength and limitations than is the therapist, and use coping mechanisms which they have learned to depend on during previous crises. Some have retained the flexibility that enables them to try new ways, and for them the experience of dying can be even one of growth. Others are frightened into withdrawal from the therapeutic relationship by anything other than support for their familiar pattern, coupled with the gentlest attempts to modify those aspects that are especially maladaptive. As the therapist explores with the patient the problems confronting him at that moment, he should ask himself about each one, "How is this patient coping with this? If his reaction is adaptive, can it be reinforced? If maladaptive, how much attempt at change will he tolerate?" The more secure a person feels, the greater is his capacity for change. The relief of physical symptoms, the warmth of the therapeutic milieu, and a growing rapport with the therapist may combine to transform a patient who is initially frightened and rigid to an open, more flexibile person who will respond to a programme of psychotherapy. Then quite brief but precisely aimed intervention may bring about marked improvement, as case illustrations in this paper will show.

The dying patient should never be considered in isolation, because his interaction with those around him profoundly affects his own well-being and theirs. Therefore an *adaptive reaction* is here defined as one which brings most relief or causes least suffering to the patient himself and also to his family and those patients and staff with whom he is in close contact. It is sometimes assumed that however difficult or destructive a patient's behavior may be toward others, it should be accepted just because he is dying. It is always appropriate to support those who are coping with the patient, giving them opportunities to ventilate their pain or frustration. But it may also be necessary to confront the patient himself with what he is doing and to explore with him the reasons for his behaviour. For example, hostility in dying patients is usually a mask for inner distress or fear, and where the psychotherapist can help the patient to cope with these, the resulting improvement is rewarding for everyone. Even if the patient does not change, discussion with relatives and staff about the causes of the behaviour enables them to tolerate it more easily.

## Establishing Communication

The dying person experiences many fears and often feels isolated because there is no one with whom they can be shared. The basic aim in therapy is therefore to establish good rapport so that the patient feels free to talk and thus to discover the relief that comes from being understood and accepted. This interchange often leads the therapist to explore with the patient whether he wishes to share what has passed between them with a relative, friend, or priest. Often he does, but is reluctant to begin. The therapist can offer to meet the other person and prepare the way, or suggest that a joint discussion take place. Where the relationship was previously close, a single bridging interview may suffice. As soon as the patient begins to receive the emotional support he needs from his family and the regular staff, the therapist can withdraw. The main focus of attention will be on those patients who for one reason or another lack supports or are not able to use them.

## Defences

One obstacle to close relationships during the patient's illness may be his use of certain defences. Relatives do not know what to say, for instance, to a patient who is talking unrealistically about his future. They either collude or retreat from him by visiting infrequently or communicating at a superficial level, leaving him feeling lonely and isolated. But defences are an essential aspect of coping, and the therapist needs to know which are being used and whether they are maladaptive, before he plans his intervention. Some patients go through an initial crisis of adjustment, experiencing shock, anger, depression, and then acceptance, followed by a period of relative calm. Then the various defences operate to enable him to cope with each new sign of the progress of the disease without re-evoking the fear of death. Few people can tolerate facing death for any length of time, and the therapist should be content simply to monitor the situation, intervening only if there is a resurgence of persistent anxiety and suffering. Forceful disclosure of the truth when a patient does not need to hear can be as harmful as evasion when he does.

The commonest defence is probably denial, and this will be discussed in detail to illustrate how it may be dealt with in various circumstances. The use of other defence mechanisms, such as displacement, projection, and regression, will be mentioned more briefly.

### Denial

Pattison (1977) has contributed to our understanding of denial by differentiating three forms: existential, psychological, and nonattention denial. *Existential denial* refers to the universal capacity to suppress awareness of the hazards inherent in everyday life. It is necessary for a continuing sense of security that we should be able most of the time to ignore such threats as nuclear warfare or sudden accidental death. Persistent awareness of these possibilities would cause overwhelming anxiety and paralyse the individual's ability to respond selectively to those immediate threats that jeopardize his well-being, and to which an effective response is possible.

*Psychological denial* is a defence against the anxiety evoked by danger or the threat of it. The dying patient who initially seems to accept the truth about his illness but behaves as if he has never been told is using this defence. He shows anxiety at the nonverbal and physiological levels, but denies it if questioned. He may repeatedly ask about his condition and respond to the answers he is given as if no such conversation had ever taken place before. This behaviour may indicate that he believes at an intellectual level that an honest approach is best, but at a deeper level is not prepared to know. If this is the case, he will continue to "ask round" the staff until someone gives him a reassuring answer to which he can cling. More often this pattern gives the patient time to assimilate gradually information which would overwhelm him if he appreciated its full import at once. Over the passage of time he makes less use of denial, and his behaviour indicates that he is making adjustments in his appraisal of his situation. No intervention other than sensitive support is necessary here.

I agree with Mansell Pattison's observation that psychological denial is a problem only when it is the sole or prominent defence. It then blocks communication with family and friends and prevents the patient from making suitable plans for the future. It is often accompanied by severe anxiety, distressing dreams, and either attention-seeking behaviour or withdrawal. The case of a farmer's wife with breast cancer illustrates this clearly. Her relatives reported that she had always been "nervous and difficult to get on with" and that her habitual method of coping with stress had been a refusal to speak about it and an attempt to live as if nothing amiss had occurred. On admission she reacted angrily when she overheard a doctor talking with another patient about death. "No one must ever talk to me like that," she declared. This request was respected until she reported a dream in which she had been trapped in a corner of an enclosure by a large herd of her husband's pigs. She had cried out for help, but although her husband could see her, there was no way he could rescue her. Her readiness to talk about this dream seemed to indicate a change in attitude, and it led to her acknowledgement that she felt "cornered" by her illness and afraid because there was no escape. Later she was able to talk with staff about the death of other patients she had come to know, and through this came to accept that she too was dying. She lost most of her fear and achieved a peace which was remarkable for a woman whose life style had always been one of anxiety and denial.

Three patients who persisted in using denial as a defence were found to have suppressed their grief over the death of close relatives in the past.

One who was referred because of vomiting which was thought to be psychogenic could not recall experiencing grief when either of her parents died, and appeared unconcerned over her own malignant disease. The other two were referred for chronic anxiety and depression and had never mourned the death of a husband and a daughter, [respectively]. It seems likely that successful grief work in the past prepares people to approach their own death with more equanimity. Conversely, a history of previously unexpressed grief should alert the therapist to the problems he may encounter when he treats such patients.

*Nonattention denial* differs from psychological denial in that it is at least partly conscious and not usually accompanied by undue anxiety. It occurs in those patients who, having accepted that they are terminally ill and made necessary practical arrangements, pretend to themselves and others that they will recover. The purpose of this form of denial is not to escape the truth, but to prevent the pain of it from spoiling the quality of life in the present. It enables patients to live as normally as possible for as long as possible, and is adaptive unless it reaches a level where they deny the severity of the illness to such an extent that they refuse further treatment and endure unnecessary pain.

## Displacement

Patients use the defence of displacement as a means of coping with powerful emotions which would be most appropriately felt about themselves or their predicament. By directing their feelings onto others, they remain relatively calm except when thinking about those who have become the focus. This defence may be adaptive in some respects for the patient, but causes suffering to the person who has become the target. A man who showed considerable nonverbal anxiety denied that he was at all worried about himself. He declared that he had witnessed death in the Army Medical Corps and had learned to accept it. Now his sole concern was for his wife. He remained calm for most of the day with a detached attitude to this illness, but became increasingly apprehensive as visiting time approached and quite agitated if his wife was a few minutes late. When she did arrive, his reproachful attitude and his anxious questioning about her activities distressed her so much that she curtailed her visits and consequently felt guilty. Psychotherapy aimed at allowing him to experience appropriate anxiety about himself corrected this displacement. Temporarily he was more disturbed as he worked this through, but his relationship with his wife improved so much that she was able to sit for hours by his bedside, knitting and keeping him company as she would have done at home.

Anger about the terminal illness is often displaced onto doctors, who are blamed inappropriately for making the diagnosis too late or giving wrong or ineffective treatment. Relatives are sometimes blamed for not showing sufficient concern, and nurses may become the butt of innumerable petty complaints. A patient who displaces anger in this way can disrupt relationships with those on whom he depends for his care, and psychotherapy which allows him to express the anger and frustration he feels because he is dying often changes the situation for the better.

## Projection

Paranoid states in terminally ill patients can often be understood in terms of projection. The unconscious recognition that a man is soon to die is turned into a belief that someone is trying to kill him, and may result in frightened or aggressive behaviour in apparent self-defence. I have described elsewhere (Stedeford, 1978) how this happens most often in acute confusional states in which impaired consciousness can result in disinhibition and the release of florid psychotic material. Guilt about events in the patient's past may appear as ideas of persecution and accusatory auditory hallucinations. Although it may be necessary to control the resulting disturbed behaviour with major tranquilizers, it is also worth attempting psychotherapy with these patients. They usually retain some capacity to relate to a sympathetic person and may—during or after the acute episode —be able to perceive the relationship between their psychotic experience and their real guilt or fears. When this occurs, the abnormal experiences usually cease.

## Counterdependency, Dependency, and Regression

There is an appropriate level of dependency for each stage of the illness, and the psychiatrist may be able to help his patient to achieve this. In the terminal phase, a patient's heroic attempts to maintain his independence can cause suffering both to himself and to his relatives. The person who is determined to walk unaided despite frequent falls often needs help to recognise that it is not shameful to "give in" at this stage and accept assistance. The man or woman who "has always been a fighter" needs permission to stop struggling and, having received it, often experiences great relief when able to let go.

On the other hand, the regression which accompanies dependency may be maladaptive in terminal illness, as it deprives the patient of independence which he could still enjoy and makes him expect more attention from others than he needs. A patient who became breathless on walking a few yards claimed that he was too ill to walk at all, and thus denied himself the freedom to move about the unit at will. During psychotherapy he revealed that while he was taken everywhere in a chair, he could sit and imagine he was still able to walk well if he chose. The last attempt he had made had forced him to recognise how ill he was, and he would rather stay put than be made aware, day by day, that his strength was waning. When he understood why he had taken to his wheelchair prematurely and had accepted that he would gradually be able to do less, he resumed walking and was pleasantly surprised at how much he could still do.

Later in the illness regression is appropriate, and allows the patient to accept without loss of dignity the personal help and attention which he needs. The closeness that results from the giving and receiving of tender care can be one of the compensations for the suffering of terminal illness, for both patient and family, and for nursing staff too. Adaptive regression can be an enriching experience, as a dying psychoanalyst discovered. She asked for psychotherapeutic help to ensure that her defences did not deprive her of full awareness of what she was experiencing. When she gave up her vigorous attempts to be independent, she became almost childlike in her attachment to the therapist, and the new intimacy that followed gave her intense joy. This emotional regression in no way impaired her ability to ponder about the philosophical and spiritual aspects of her dying, which led to deep and stimulating conversations almost to the end.

## Hope

This discussion of defences and their management leads on to the subject of hope, particularly because some clinicians maintain that it is cruel to remove defences and confront patients with the truth about their illness, as this will inevitably undermine some of their hope. The idea that truth destroys hope is often used as a justification for keeping patients in ignorance. Some doctors with such a view may well have seen patients in a stage of shock, anger, or despair after news has been awkwardly imparted, and [may] not be aware that their emotional state can change considerably over a few days. Dying patients have a great facility for holding two incompatible ideas without feeling that they are incongruous. They make appropriate preparations for imminent death, and at the same time can plan for a splendid holiday a year hence. As death approaches, it is not that hope gets lost, but that its object changes. At first a patient hopes that the doctors are wrong and that he will recover. Later he accepts limits, and sets his sights on an event such as a wedding, which he hopes to attend before he dies. Later still, he speaks of his aspirations for members of his family who will survive (as if he envisages himself living on in them) and for himself he asks only for a peaceful death. If he is religious, his hopes turn to eternal life, and perhaps to reunion with beloved relatives who have already died. Only the patient who knows he is dying can make these natural adjustments. To withhold information about prognosis when a patient is seeking it is therefore to deny him something which is essential if he is to do the work of rounding off his life in a fulfilling way.

## Depression

As the preceding paper [1979] indicates, depression is common in dying patients who have many losses to mourn. Some staff and relatives find it hard to accept that depression is appropriate and inevitable, and their well-meaning attempts to cheer a patient may jar and make him feel that he is not understood. There may be pressure on the psychiatrist to prescribe antidepressant drugs, motivated by the need to feel that something is being done for the patient. It should be recognised that giving support and understanding, together with the facilitation of the expression of anger where necessary, is in itself active treatment. Patients who have always had a positive attitude to life emerge from this kind of depression with a new appreciation of the good things that are left. Once they accept that their time is limited, they begin to make the most of every opportunity that presents itself, and outsiders are often surprised by their capacity to experience so much happiness. Other patients who are naturally of a gloomy disposition do not change much. But even they may respond to the staff's friendly individual attention, and this, together with freedom from customary responsibilities, may bring about improvement in mood.

The only patient in this series with completely intractable depression believed that an intrathecal block done for the relief of severe pain had caused her paraplegia. When seen by the psychiatrist, she began to reveal her feelings, and it soon became clear that she had suppressed a considerable amount of resentment. The display of any negative feelings was taboo for her, and she refused to discuss the matter further or to see the psychiatrist again. She remained most unhappy until her death.

Some patients whose pain is disproportionately severe and unresponsive to analgesics are suffering from *atypical depression*. One such woman with severe facial pain had a personality disorder, characterized among other features by a belief that the only acceptable way to respond to trouble was to treat it as a joke. Her attempts to laugh her way through her illness did not evoke the sympathy and support she needed, and the only way she could obtain concerned attention was through pain. Psychotherapy enabled her to begin to express her distress more directly, especially to her husband, who in his turn learned to support her. Her depression lessened, and although her pain never left her, it receded into the background so much that she could return to her home and her role as housewife, and her requirement for analgesics diminished.

## Anxiety

Anxiety too is common in the dying, and the defences discussed above are used in an attempt to cope with it. When a patient expresses anxiety directly about himself and his condition, it is often helpful to explore it by breaking it down into its various components. Existential anxiety, the fear of nonbeing, was seldom in evidence in our patients. More common were fears about the suffering which the process of dying might entail: pain, loss of control, dependency, and abandonment. Some fears were groundless, and disappeared when they had been spoken about. Others were realistic, and here patients responded to reassurance that their fears were understood and were not shameful. They needed to know that their symptoms would continue to be treated as they arose, and that they would never be left alone to cope. We have noted that the presence of a familiar person does much to allay anxiety, and relatives sitting quietly by the bedside contribute greatly to a peaceful death. Anxiolytics are a valuable adjunct to psychotherapy, but no substitute for care and support.

## Organic Brain Disease

The following case history illustrates the management of a variety of problems which one patient presented, and in particular shows how the distress of organic brain disease can be ameliorated.

Mrs. G., a 52-year-old widow whose husband had failed to return from the war, had lived with and cared for her 86-year-old mother until she became too disabled by her illness. At the time of admission she had a severe hemiplegia and some dysphasia, the result of a cerebral tumour. The first problem arose when she convinced her relatives that the nurses had strapped her in her chair all day and prevented her from walking. Her use of this mechanism of projection enabled her to avoid the distress of accepting the full extent of her disability, and to blame the staff instead. Attempts to help Mrs. G. withdraw this pattern of projection were not successful at this stage, but explanation of it to the nurses helped them to cope with her allegations and handle the relatives' complaints with understanding.

She also presented with depression, provoked in part by the loss of her role as head of the household. On her admission to hospital, relatives had abruptly stopped consulting her about the future care of her mother in the belief that she had enough to worry about. When it was explained to them that she was still very much concerned, and that all she had left to offer was her interest and advice, they readily agreed to involve her in their deliberations. Her depression then diminished.

Later, the patient experienced temporal and spatial disorientation and thought that she was in Germany searching for her husband. This was associated with great distress. Staff were instructed on how to talk her back to reality and to separate past and present; their efforts usually brought temporary relief. On one occasion when Mrs. G. was disoriented in time, she angrily blamed her watch for being wrong; it became apparent that she believed "they" had decimalized time. With reassurance that this was not the case, she reflected for a long interval and then said, "It is only a matter of time." This led to conversation about her impending death and her difficulty in tolerating the uncertainty of how much time she had left.

In spite of her confusion, she did have lucid periods. In one of these, she complained that some nurses thought she was mad, and discussion with them led to greater understanding on their part. Through talking about her condition with the psychiatrist, she lost her fear of insanity and slipped in and out of confusion without being distressed. She learned to separate "myself" from "my illness" and summed up her acceptance by saying on one occasion, "I think it is perfectly logical that I should be confused."

## Psychotherapy with the Family

The patient's admission to a terminal care unit confronts the family with the seriousness of his illness. Practical decisions about who shall be told, who shall visit, and how dependent members should be cared for, immediately arise. In this crisis the united family shows its strength, but the problems of a divided family are painfully exposed. In the latter case, the patient is often distressed at visiting time, and family feuds may erupt in a way that disturbs others in the unit. In almost half the cases in this series, the dying patient was so affected by family problems that psychotherapy was indicated in an attempt to alleviate them. Relatives were usually invited to see the therapist alone at first. This often led to conjoint or family interviews.

In one such family, the patient was an elderly man who had always been independent. He had expected to care for his invalid sister until her death, and refused to accept that he would die before her. He obstructed any arrangements that were suggested for her management, and consequently the family were forced to attempt to decide amongst themselves what should be done. The patient then complained that "things were going on behind his back" and became increasingly angry. In this crisis, several interviews were held with the patient, his sister, and various family members, over three days. These resulted in an acknowledgement by the patient that he was dying, and the recognition that his anger and frustration about his illness had become displaced on to his family. A partial reconciliation was effected, sufficient for them to agree on plans for the care of his sister. The patient was also anxious that, because his sister had not made a will, her vulnerable situation after his death might be exploited by various family members who wanted to gain access to the money he planned to leave her. Delicate negotiations continued until the will was made, and she was placed in a nursing home. The old man then became less irascible, both with his family and with nursing staff, and he died peacefully a few weeks later.

Terminal illness puts a strain on any marriage, particularly on one in which there are underlying problems. In eight instances in the series, an important focus of intervention was the couple; the following vignette illustrates the kind of therapeutic approach used. A man of 53 was admitted primarily because he had become so morose and irritable at home that his wife could no longer cope. Theirs was a marriage in which she was dominant, while he could only assert his masculinity sexually and as a skilled labourer. When prostatic carcinoma made him weak and partially impotent, he lost all self-esteem and suffered from depression punctuated by angry outbursts against his wife and sons. Psychotherapy with the couple helped the wife to understand her husband's difficult behaviour and to respond more appropriately to his emotional and sexual needs. He found a new role, taking increased interest in his adolescent boys, whose care and discipline he had previously left almost entirely to his wife. Communication between the couple improved, serious quarrels ceased, and both saw the last months of their relationship as the most intimate of any period of their marriage.

In terminal care there is a tendency to underestimate the ability of the dying patient to give. Relatives may feel that a dying person should not be troubled about other problems arising in the family, and may try to conceal them. This often depresses the patient, who senses that something is amiss and feels deprived of his role as parent or spouse. It is appropriate for the therapist to point out to the family that the sick person still wants to give, and that he can continue to offer his concern and advice. They soon appreciate that he is likely to feel more alive if involved in family affairs, even when they are an additional source of anxiety.

Although the spouse of a dying patient may be painfully aware of the lack of communication between them, he is often reluctant to talk about the impending separation. This may be because he is trying to avoid facing the situation himself, and pointing [this] out to him gently may be helpful. If the spouse accepts this insight, he may still be unwilling to talk, fearing that he might break down in the course of the conversation and further upset the patient. A knowledge of the marital history is important here. If the dying partner has been a source of strength and encouragement to the spouse in previous crises, he is likely to want to do so again, and he can only act in this role when the couple are facing the separation together. Discussion about the future and planning how the surviving spouse will cope helps the patient to work through guilt he or she feels about abandoning a loved partner. In the days and weeks that follow death, there is comfort for the newly widowed in the knowledge that they are carrying out those things which the couple planned together.

## Conclusion

The psychiatrist who provides psychotherapy for the terminally ill needs to be something of a jack-of-all-trades, and the prospect might seem daunting. However, sophisticated psychotherapy is not as necessary as are sensitivity, a willingness to follow the patient rather than lead him, some knowledge of the psychology of dying, and the ability to accept the inevitability of death. In the relief of pain physicians have moved from the era of aspirin and morphine to a wide variety of analgesics, each with its specific indications. To use them well, the causes of pain must be accurately diagnosed and the drugs given in the optimum way. The relief of the emotional pain of dying has traditionally been achieved with tender loving care, and spiritual measures for those patients who are religious. Both still play an essential part, but the experience described [here] suggests that a better understanding of the causes of emotional pain and the use of psychotherapeutic strategies aimed at specific areas of distress may be more effective than devoted care alone.

## References

Cartwright, A., Hockey, L., & Anderson, J. L., *Life Before Death*. London: Routledge & Kegan Paul, 1973.

Kübler-Ross, E., *On Death and Dying*. London: Tavistock, 1969.

Parkes, C. M., "Dying at Home," *Journal of the Royal College of General Practitioners*, 1978, *28*, 19–30.

Pattison, E. M., *The Experience of Dying*. London: Prentice-Hall, 1977.

Stedeford, A., "Understanding Confusional States," *British Journal of Hospital Medicine*, 1978, *20*, 694–704.

Stedeford, A., & Bloch, S., "The Psychiatrist in the Terminal Care Unit," *British Journal of Psychiatry*, 1979, *135*, 1–6.

# 16

# Volunteers in Hospice

*Eve Kavanagh*

Certain qualities seem to be common to individuals who are successful in working as volunteers in hospice programs. First of all, they affirm life and enjoy living. Secondly, they like people and do not consider helping others or giving themselves to be something extraordinary—instead, they usually think of this as a privilege (although many would not use that term). And thirdly, they have the ability to bear the joys and sorrows and all the tensions inherent in life, especially as it nears its fullness in death. What seems to be central here is the attitude of prospective hospice volunteers toward life, their fellow human beings, and themselves.

It is the purpose of this chapter to discuss the role of volunteers in hospice work. In order to do that, some humility and candor are a prerequisite. For example, one must immediately admit that good volunteers are not easy to come by. Thus, we must consider questions of recruitment and selection, and of training, before we can speak of the work of volunteers. Further, it is important to note that, when all is said and done, successful hospice programs do not select their volunteers—even though they often speak as if they did. Rather, prospective volunteers select hospice out of all the many volunteer opportunities offered by any community. One must also recognize that hospice training programs can never give to their enrollees those qualities that will make such people good hospice volunteers. It would be fatal to pretend that this is possible. At best, the hospice can only identify and nurture those qualities offered to it by prospective volunteers. This demands a respect for volunteers and a willingness to search out their individual strengths. Thus, the foundation of a good hospice volunteer program is the attitude of the organization toward the volunteers who supplement, carry out, or even make possible its very program.

## Attitudes toward Volunteers

In large part, the modern hospice movement is the work of voluntary (or volunteer) initiative. Most give credit for its beginnings to Dame Cicely Saunders and her work at St. Joseph's Hospice in northeast London during the early 1960s, and before her to the Irish Sisters of Charity who founded St. Joseph's and other similar institutions to care for the poor, the destitute, and those who are often least appreciated by society, the dying (Lamerton, 1975). As members of a religious order, the Sisters of Charity (like many others, both religious and lay) brought faith, hope, and charity along with skilled care to those whom they served on a voluntary basis. Similarly, first as a nurse, then as a social worker, and finally as a physician, Dame Cicely perceived unmet needs among the dying and trained herself at her own initiative to learn how to respond more effectively. Further, she conceived the idea, initiated the planning, raised the money, and saw to the establishment of St. Christopher's Hospice in southeast London in 1967. In this, as she has often said, there was aid at an early moment from a patient who donated funds and said, "I want what is in your mind and in your heart" (Saunders, 1978, p. 201).

Subsequently, many other individuals across Great Britain, Canada, the United States, and many other parts of the world gave—and continue to give—of their time, talents, and energies to found hospice units and programs of care, or simply to implement some principles for improving care of dying persons and their families in settings that might never seek the label "hospice." Like Dame Cicely, these people had come to realize that the care being provided by existing institutions and programs in relation to terminal illness was all too often inadequate. They did not think of themselves as better than other caregivers. Rather, they viewed themselves as different by virtue of viewpoint, goals, and lack of encumberances or hindrances. The earliest hospice volunteers did not demean the value of acute curative treatment or long-term custodial care. But they grasped the problems of a small group of people who fitted well in neither of these settings and whose needs, as a result, often were not satisfactorily served. This initiative became the first step in what is now a widespread grassroots movement, which has already begun to try to discover how it can strengthen and integrate its affiliation with the larger health care system.

Though neither grand nor especially prominent, our experience in Des Moines is perhaps typical of the way in which many hospice programs have risen from and remain dependent upon their local community. Hospice of Central Iowa could not exist without its volunteers. When we first began providing care in June 1978, we had a volunteer medical director and about 20 trained volunteers. Two and one-half years later, we have about 130 volunteers. Approximately 80 of these are presently active in caregiving teams, while others are inactive for programmatic or personal reasons. We have a part-time patient coordinator, a part-time volunteer coordinator, a part-time social worker, and a part-time office manager. Each of the last four is salaried. They are paid for 10 to 16 hours per week. The rest of their time is donated. Everyone else is a volunteer. Ages range from the 20s to the late 60s and a few early 70s. Both men and women volunteer, and we have six husband-and-wife volunteers who always work on a team together (this arrangement is enormously beneficial to patients and their families). Except for those persons who are retired, all our volunteers work (in their homes and/or elsewhere), and many have growing families as well. Their time is very valuable, and we try to remain constantly aware of this. To date, we have suffered no volunteer "burnout," and we hope to maintain this good record. We believe that our record in this area is good because we value our volunteers so highly. They are not cheap labor. They are an invaluable resource, and the talents and dedication they bring to their work cannot be bought. Therefore, we are as careful of our volunteers as we are of our patients. Our premise is that one does not have to be terminally ill to be important!

*Respect* is a word commonly used. *Reverence* or *awe* might well be a more fitting term to describe the attitude one should have toward the men and women who so generously and simply dedicate their spare time, and all their talents of mind and heart, to the service of the dying and their families, and ask for no reward other than the chance to serve. This attitude has to be spontaneous and genuine—one cannot pretend to have it. It is a difficult attitude to maintain because it is so demanding in itself. It demands that we know our volunteers individually, since knowledge is fundamental to reverence. Knowing them, we can treat them with the confidence (*con-fides*=with faith) that allows them to do the work of hospice with freedom, intelligence, and creativity (all this, of course, without violating the professional norms that are essential for patients' well-being). And, finally, we do not exploit volunteers. It goes without saying that a man or a woman who has a job and a family, and is also a hospice volunteer, needs time to re-create his or her own forces at specific occasions. The moments that always most concern us are those that follow after a death. We insist that all volunteers take time off after "their" patient dies so that they are fresh for each successive patient and do not try to serve one while grieving for another. This time of bereavement or re-creation is different for each volunteer. No two people are alike. We take this difference for granted.

Like most hospice programs, we ask volunteers for 1 year's commitment. However, the time given by each volunteer within a day, a week, or a month is left to the individual, and we do not encourage comparisons. Hospice hours cannot be compared. One hour spent with a frightened patient cannot be compared with 10 hours spent with a peaceful patient. There are many other things that make a volunteer program successful. However, we are convinced that the three things mentioned here—respect, knowledge, and confidence—are basic. Such a program is open, full of loose ends, untidy. It defies description. It requires incredible teamwork, trust, courage, and humor to keep it going. It could quite easily be captured, regulated, tidied up—and destroyed!

## Recruitment and Selection

As mentioned above, our volunteers select us. Recruitment is primarily a matter of making known to promising audiences the needs that are being served by the hospice program and describing accurately the dimensions of its work. Active recruitment will usually only be required before a hospice program begins to offer services, when it alters or expands its services, or when a specific skill is required. One can advertise or publicize the existence of a hospice program through many community, professional, religious, and lay channels; give presentations to schools and organizations; capitalize on visiting speakers or local events; or foster word-of-mouth communication by current members of an enthusiastic program. News releases to radio, television, and newspaper services are often helpful, though stories of successful service to individuals may be most effective. The forms that these efforts take will depend upon the means available in the area being served and the imagination and energies of the hospice staff. There are only two essential points: Do not romanticize the work or mislead prospective volunteers as to its nature; and do emphasize that talents of all sorts are welcome. It is often more difficult to find people to do the necessary but unglamorous clerical chores required by a hospice program than it is to attract those interested in direct service to patients and families. Not everyone needs or wants to be a leader; those who diligently cultivate a modest corner of the hospice vineyard are equally essential.

In order to aid prospective volunteers in deciding that they have chosen the right work and the best program for themselves, we let them know the qualifications that we have learned from experience to be necessary for a hospice volunteer. These qualifications will be recognized by hospice personnel everywhere. They include basic communications skills; ease with sick people and bodily functions; willingness to learn; ability to grow in self-knowledge; respect for religious beliefs other than one's own; ability to be nonjudgmental of others' life styles; ability to define personal time limits and commitments; respect for the confidences of patients, family members, and team members; ability to bear strong emotions within oneself and others; ability to be honest with oneself and others; and ability to work with others in a team situation. Very few individuals look at this list and feel confident that they have the ability to be hospice volunteers! However, most people soon learn that they have more talents than they realize (especially when their attention is on the patient/family unit rather than on themselves), and where one is weak, some other member of the team is strong. Therefore, although all the qualifications are necessary, the last three are perhaps most important for the new volunteer. With time and practice, all skills improve.

Each new volunteer is interviewed. The interview consists of a conversation designed to collect practical information such as skills, professional qualifications if any, education and experience, areas of interest, and so forth. The interviewers also try to isolate persons who might not be suitable hospice volunteers. Needless to say, this is difficult to do, and we usually give the person the benefit of the doubt. However, we do not accept people who have recently suffered an important loss or a death in the family; people who are already dealing with a serious illness within their own family (although we do let them participate in the training program if they think it will benefit them); or people who have ulterior motives, such as a desire to confirm their own belief systems by proselytizing. On the whole, our first important screening process is the training program. People who do not screen themselves out during the training program usually do it when they are asked to be members of a hospice team.

We know of no process of selection that ensures success. People who impress no one during an interview or during the training period turn out to be superb volunteers. Others who seem to be full of promise never get as far as a patient's home. Experience has made us aware of two things. First, the real testing ground is the hospice team. Secondly, when everyone (staff and volunteers) expresses doubt about the competence of a volunteer, the communal sense usually can be trusted, and soon enough the volunteer in question resigns. We have found that it is not wise to be quick to judge. The volunteer who is unsuitable for one patient will be excellent for another. And in the last analysis, it is our patients and their families who tell us who our good volunteers are and why they are good. Many hospices insist on a probationary period for new staff and volunteers, during which the individual can experience actual work within the program and can have time to demonstrate his or her suitability for continued participation.

## Training of Volunteers

Several hospices have published outlines of the training programs that they have used for their volunteers and staff or manuals for the training of volunteers (Baldwin et al., 1980; Cox, 1978; Mount, 1976; see also Chapter 17, this volume). It should not be surprising that these different schemata for training have a good deal in common with each other. Our training program in Des Moines is 10 weeks long and consists of two 2-hour sessions each week. It is required for all volunteers, professional and lay, who will be involved in patient care, and it is open to anyone else who might benefit from it. This program is not geared to produce "finished products" and does not really end until a volunteer has served on a hospice team. From that point on, the emphasis is on continuing education and the uniqueness of each patient/family. We try hard to guard against the illusion that any one of us will ever become an "expert" in death and dying. At the same time, we do everything we reasonably can to imbue each volunteer with the confidence that he or she can do a good job.

There is not a great deal in the program about death and dying. Each person is asked to keep a journal to use in any way he or she sees fit in order to keep in touch with emotions and feelings about death—"my death," "a patient's death," "my mother's death," and so on. Certain readings are required, others recommended. But for the most part the training program is very practical. It stresses such topics as speaking with cancer patients (we concentrate our limited resources on patients with terminal cancer); learning about religions other than one's own; discovering the resources that are available to patients and volunteers within the community (this is quite an eye-opener for most volunteers); investigating what cancer is and what it is not; understanding what medications will be used commonly and what to expect if they are used correctly or incorrectly; grasping the principles of basic home nursing; knowing what to do if death occurs in the home (state laws) when a volunteer is there; grieving and how to help; sensitivity exercises; stories of hospice teams and families; confidentiality; record keeping; and so forth. The program is simple. It is hard work. It is only appreciated in the light of experience.

Usually some volunteers are called on immediately after completion of the basic training program. However, we do not call on volunteers unless they really feel "ready to go." We are convinced that no volunteer should be required to go into the highly charged atmosphere of a hospice family without this feeling of readiness. But we warn everyone (on the basis of the experience of many people) that if they wait to feel totally comfortable and unafraid, then they will never go. And we make a practice of assigning new volunteers to work with experienced partners, especially at the outset. The feeling of readiness can be summed up in a simple sentence: "I think I can do it and I'm willing to try." Each volunteer reaches this stage at a different time. The mystery and constant surprise is that patient needs and volunteer readiness always somehow coincide.

Education continues at weekly team meetings, monthly volunteer meetings, and above all in the home of the patient/family. We have a small library and a volunteer newsletter where books and articles are recommended. After serving on three or four hospice teams, each volunteer has learned the fundamental education philosophy of Hospice of Central Iowa—we are always learning, and each patient/family unit is our teacher. We do not deal with abstract, unchanging universals. We live with people who are dying and with their families and friends. We cannot answer most of the questions that they ask us. However, we can say, "We will be with you." And being "with you" is good for all of us. We go to give a helping hand, and we find that we are filled. We go when we are tired, and we leave renewed. We go in spite of our inadequacy, and we leave immeasurably enriched. Every now and then we go and nothing we do seems to work, nor does our presence appear to make any difference. Then we learn from each other what "support" really means and what "team" really means. We learn that our work cannot be measured by apparent successes or failures. Hospice is a community of love and service. It includes patients and families, friends, volunteers, and staff. It can be partly seen. It cannot be measured.

## Roles for Volunteers

I have already indicated above that volunteers must be integrated and respected as full partners in hospice work, as an integral part of the interdisciplinary caregiving team. The consequences of this for the work assignments of volunteers are as follows: "Volunteers do not replace paid positions; they provide additional services which enhance the care of families and augment the work of paid staff in all departments" (Cox, 1979, p. 3). Each aspect of this statement is essential. First, volunteers ought not to be regarded as cheap labor who can make up for an inadequate number of paid staff members or a budget that is not sufficient to sustain the program. Each hospice needs a core of full- or part-time (depending on scope) paid personnel who unify the program and guarantee its continuity. Nevertheless, the second point is that volunteers are not second-class citizens in hospice work. They are essential to the goal of improving care for dying persons and their families, both because they bring a wealth of talents to this work and because they give it a human face.

Volunteers augment hospice work by lending it their extra resources, which could not be hired. Whether they are professionals or lay persons or bearers of some specialized skills, volunteers flesh out a hospice program and help it to go beyond minimalism. Especially because their very presence is a gift and they usually lack "status" in an organization hierarchy, volunteers have a particular opportunity to offer simple human companionship to all who are involved in or are being served by the hospice program. Also because most volunteers work on a part-time basis, their main life is outside hospice, and they are likely to be fresh in outlook and refreshed in spirit when they come to their volunteer assignments. Of course, paid and full-time staff are also human, but unpaid volunteers represent a kind of neighborliness that is essential to the caring community. It should be noted that volunteers are not uncompensated; service in a hospice program has its own intangible, rich rewards. But because volunteers are not paid, they do not need to depend upon the hospice for monetary support or for their primary vocational identity. Where they do not have a paid career, volunteers sometimes see the hospice as a means of maintaining contact with their profession in a limited and manageable way.

Exactly what volunteers actually do for the hospice program will depend partly on its situation and needs, and partly on the skills and imagination of the individuals involved (e.g., Ajemian & Mount, 1980). In the broadest sense, volunteers develop and strengthen the links from the surrounding community to the hospice and from the hospice to those whom it serves. This may occur in the context of an inpatient hospice unit (whether free-standing or somehow affiliated with a larger health care complex), a consultation team, a home care program, or a day unit service. As appropriate to each of these settings, volunteers might engage in direct service to dying persons and their families, in bereavement follow-up programs, in general administrative and logistical functions, and in such areas as public relations, education, or fund raising. For example, within the limits of legal and professional restrictions—and such limitations should be incorporated into the hospice's volunteer policy and communicated clearly to each volunteer—volunteers can assist with meals, help to make beds, do chores in the home to relieve others, simply sit with a patient to provide companionship or time off for a primary caregiver, visit bereaved families, or help to run support groups for survivors. No list of these possibilities or of all the specialized talents that might be donated to hospice could ever be complete. Roles for volunteers can be expected to change with the evolution of a program, with the arrival of new people, and with the growth of each individual. As always, the task is to explore carefully the real needs of those who are being served and of the program itself, and to respond to them in an imaginative way. Successful volunteer programs permit volunteers themselves to have a hand in defining their roles, and they remain aware of the value of insuring that volunteers are challenged and satisfied by their duties—however limited or simple they may be.

Instead of attempting the impossible task of describing every conceivable role for volunteers in hospice, it may help to look at one program in detail. In so doing, I remind the reader that (apart from a small number of legal and professional restrictions) the involvement of volunteers in this work is limited only by the needs of patients and families, and by the creativity of each hospice unit. For a home care program like Hospice of Central Iowa that is largely staffed by volunteers, direct service to patients and families is the primary task. After the patient care coordinator has visited with the family to discuss their needs and available resources, the patient has expressed a desire for hospice services and signed our consent form, and the primary physician has consented and agreed to cooperate, the foundation is laid and the hospice team goes to work. Usually our teams consist of four people including a nurse, unless this is clearly unnecessary. However, we have had as few as two people on a team at the express wish of a family, and we have had as many as 10 people on a team because of special needs. We designate a team leader. Our team leaders are not "in charge" of a team. Their role is to coordinate and act as the center of communication. The ideal team leader is someone who has the gift of leadership without taking over and telling others what to do. He or she also has a good intuition about the importance of details and has the ability to be sensitive to the whole family. Volunteers are encouraged to act responsibly and creatively within the sphere of their competence and qualifications.

The chief role of our nurse volunteers is educational. When skilled nursing is required, public health nurses are available. We do not replace them. However, our nurses spend a great deal of time teaching the family and the patient how to use medications correctly, what to look for and report to us or to their doctor, how to give good primary care to the family member who is ill, and how to care for themselves as well. When the patient can no longer be responsible for self-medication (or can never have that responsibility, as in the case of young children), the family is relieved by a nurse—for recreation time, church attendance, a good night's sleep, and so on. Hospice nurses are on call for the family every day and every hour. We do not find that families call them unnecessarily. Some nurses must limit their time in such a way that, on the whole, they do confine themselves to the physical care of the patient. When this is so, the situation is explained clearly to the family. However, many nurses fulfill the roles of friend, home help, chaplain, or babysitter, to name a few, according to patient and family needs.

Lay volunteers never act as professional nurses. Apart from this limitation, they do just about everything else. Frequently, the first two things a family needs are rest and equipment of one kind or another. Volunteers go to the Cancer Society and "raid" their marvelous loan closet. Walkers, wheelchairs, comfort items, toilet seat raisers, sheepskins, and even hospital beds may be needed immediately. Families sometimes do not realize the need, they frequently cannot afford to buy or even rent, and hardly anyone knows that they can get these things free, as a loan, for as long as they need them. One of the most satisfying things we know is to inform families of this resource in the community and to share their joy as the necessary items arrive one by one when they are so badly needed. Sometimes the relief in a family eliminates the felt need for immediate rest. However, we do not count on that and try to schedule something regular, whether it be time away from the house or help during the night.

Sometimes the next order of business is to involve other members of the family in the care of the patient. Too often we find a woman caring for her husband all by herself when she has a son and/or daughter living within a short distance. They may be fearful and have young children—a good excuse to keep them at a safe distance. The mother may feel guilty about asking them for help. We do not. We work to get every family member involved to the degree that is suitable for them. We do this not only for the sake of the primary care person, but for the sake of the family members themselves. If someone lives close to a dying parent and does nothing to help, the result may be a lifelong burden of guilt. We suspect this might be especially true when hospice (i.e., a group of strangers!) is involved.

Every now and then, a family welcomes us with open arms from the first visit. On the whole though, the first few weeks are somewhat awkward for the family and the hospice team. It is not easy for family members to welcome a group of strangers into their home at a time when they feel so very vulnerable. We encourage volunteers to keep visiting frequently at this time, in spite of the fact that they feel tolerated at best. We also advise them to bring some handwork, letters to write, or a book to read. We do this so that once the practical chores that may be required are done, the volunteer has something to do if the patient seems tired or just shy. Patients appear to develop ease with an "occupied" volunteer much more quickly, since they learn from the outset that this person does not have to be entertained. Also, a comfortable rapport develops quite rapidly when two people sit together in silence. Usually a family trusts someone that the patient trusts. Practical chores include such things as helping with patient care (a bath, for example) or helping with the housework, the laundry, the grocery shopping, and the cooking. As often as not, we have to wait until a family feels comfortable with us before helping around the house. This comfortable feeling may take a week or two; sometimes it never really comes. We try to be sensitive to the feelings of the family and to do what they want us to do rather than doing things just for the sake of doing. Some primary care persons want to remain with the patient, and the hospice volunteer will free them to do so by attending to ordinary daily chores. Other primary care persons need more time away from the patient, so the volunteer will stay with the patient (not necessarily in the same room, but at hand) while the family member cleans the house, goes for a walk, plays a game of golf, visits with friends, or does whatever will be relaxing. Once, a patient who still lived alone wanted to visit his son in California. He was still strong enough to do so and needed no nursing care. His only problem was his horses. So a volunteer "horse-sat" for 2 weeks! Every talent is useful in hospice.

Volunteers help to alter clothes. Some fix hair. Some make wheelchair ramps. Some just sit and talk, and some just sit. Most spend hours listening—to patients, family members, friends. We find that *listening* is our most valuable skill. In order to develop this skill, we sometimes ask new volunteers not to take notes during a class but to listen and then go home and summarize what they have heard. This is a very good way to practice, since one can hardly go to a hospice family with a notebook and pencil in hand.

We do not require that our volunteers can cook. But we have noticed that people who volunteer for hospice are, with a few exceptions, excellent cooks. The prepared meal is an invaluable help for the tired primary care person. At first families may be reluctant—they object to "charity"—but soon enough they realize that if it is "charity" it is that charity that one human being always owes to another, and if they have any reservations they can always contribute the ingredients and we will simply put them together. Then the exchange of recipes becomes a moment of light relief and a bond of ordinary, normal friendship. The challenge of producing a meal that is tempting to the poor appetite of the cancer patient, and the joy of seeing him or her really enjoy food, breaks through barriers of shyness very quickly.

Once symptom control has been established and a patient regains some strength, outings may be important. Cabin fever can be a very distressing symptom. It deserves the same attention as any other symptom. The help of a few friends may be sufficient. If other arrangements have to be made, our attitude is this: Try! A drive through town or in the country may be all that a patient needs. What may be ordinary to the healthy person is often a joy and a wonder to the terminally ill person. With the help of a patient's friends, we have packed medications, enema equipment, and an oxygen tank into a large car and taken off for a few days in the Ozarks. The patient had been confined to her apartment for 8 months prior to this trip. She suffered no ill effects, and her apartment no longer seems so confining to her.

Sometimes a primary care person who is alone with the patient will merely need companionship at night. A volunteer can stay overnight without losing sleep. This is important for volunteers who work during the day. We must realize that some people adjust to being disturbed once or twice a night and can return to sleep without trouble. It is not lack of sleep that bothers them, but the loneliness of the night. We can relieve this loneliness by simply sleeping over. Nobody loses anything this way—except some fear and loneliness. This simple solution to a common experience of primary care persons also eliminates any reluctance a family may have in asking for help during the night later on when they really need it, especially during the last few days and nights of the patient's life.

The role of the volunteer is endless. Anything that can be done by a human being needs to be done some time or other in hospice. Yet it is not the things to be done that make the difference in the last analysis. Time after time patients and families tell us that it is our *presence* that makes the difference. After talking this over we find that what patients and families appreciate so much is the volunteers as people. They come to look on us as friends and even family. Once two volunteers were sitting with the wife of a patient chatting over a cup of coffee. Her son came running through the kitchen on his way to school. His mother suggested that he say "good morning" to the volunteers. He looked quite surprised and said, "Mom, they're just family, and I don't have to bother with 'good mornings' for the family." When this kind of relationship develops, it is quite natural to attend funerals, to provide support to the surviving family, and to maintain the friendship after death.

## Coordination and Supervision

In our program, the efforts of volunteers working within a caregiving team are coordinated and monitored by the team leader. Assignment of volunteers to team or to other duties and their overall supervision is accomplished by the volunteer coordinator. Different hospice programs will achieve these ends in different ways, but there will always be a need for some system of coordination and supervision of volunteers. That need grows as the number of volunteers in the hospice program increases, and as their skills diversify and they take on a greater variety of duties. As a general rule, the involvement of volunteers in hospice work usually requires some one person to serve as their coordinator. This person represents the hospice to the volunteers and the volunteers to the hospice.

Duties of a director or coordinator of volunteers in hospice are manifold. A typical spectrum might include the following: recruiting, interviewing, and selecting volunteers; insuring proper training at the outset and ongoing continuing education thereafter; maintaining a current file of volunteers that notes availability and special skills; determining needs for volunteer workers; assigning volunteers to specific duties and scheduling working times; insuring that volunteers are properly utilized; monitoring and evaluating their performance (especially in the probationary period); and conducting exit interviews with those who are leaving the program. Volunteer directors usually play an important role in conducting orientation and training sessions, in developing hospice policies, and in formulating a procedure manual for volunteers. A good example of what might emerge from this is the *Hospice Assistant Handbook* (n.d.) prepared by the Hospital Home Health Care Agency of California. Volunteer directors also maintain records bearing on volunteers and on their work. And they normally serve as an important source of informal support for individual volunteers. The position of director or coordinator of volunteers is obviously crucial to the smooth operation and success of the whole hospice program.

## Conclusion

I shall let a patient speak the last word for hospice and its volunteers. We do lots of "jobs" for this patient, but the "jobs" are not mentioned, although we know that she is grateful for them.

> I have had the privilege to have the care, friendship, and support of a hospice team since the middle of December. Without their care and friendship I would be unable to remain in my home since I have no family living in close proximity. They have made the difference of my being in my own home and being "I don't know where."
>
> My experience has shown me that each team member is unique. In addition to their genuine interest in my well-being, my team is easy-mannered and easy to converse with. I have developed a special rapport with one member because we have common interests dating back to the forties; with another because of her interests in reading and art; with a third because of her unhurried and genuine air of helpfulness and kindness. Another member impresses me because she is so kind and considerate. She is usually available only in the evening time after her day's work and I am often not feeling too well then and do not have the energy for visiting. Her patience and consideration are a great comfort. I frequently fall asleep while she is here but I never have to apologize.
>
> Finally, I am blessed with a very kind and unique primary care person. She is also a hospice volunteer who, being single like me, offered out of

friendship to live with me when I could no longer care for myself. Her expert care over the past six months has not only prolonged my life, but has contributed to its quality to the extent that I believe that in me the goal of hospice is fulfilled—I know that I can "live until I die."

Apart from the uniqueness of each personality, there are the constant day-to-day surprises that make life such ordinary, wonderful fun—a bunch of flowers, a mystery novel, a cheese cake, etc. Each of these things is not only a gift of love but a constant reassurance that I am still a real part of the world today in all its many facets. I think too, that some of my friends visit me because of the reassuring presence of the hospice team.

Insofar as we know, my cancer is still terminal, although good care makes me feel so well. In spite of the tensions of living with the reality of dying, it is good to be alive now, and it is a very real privilege to know each of these people and to be blessed with their friendship.

# References

Ajemian, I., & Mount, B. M. (Eds.), *The R. V. H. Manual on Palliative/Hospice Care: A Resource Book*. New York: Arno Press, 1980.

Baldwin, M. V., et al., *Hospice Volunteers: A Guide for Training*. Piscataway, NJ: Office of Consumer Health Education, CMDNJ—Rutgers Medical School, and Riverside Hospice, 1980.

Cox, M. S., *The Connecticut Hospice, Inc., Volunteer Program*. New Haven: Hospice Institute for Education, Training, and Research, 1979.

Cox, M. S., "Volunteer Program," in S. A. Lack & R. W. Buckingham (Eds.), *First American Hospice: Three Years of Home Care*. New Haven: Hospice, Inc., 1978, 47–73.

*Hospice Assistant Handbook*. Unpublished booklet, n.d., (Available from Hospital Home Health Care Agency of California, 23228 Hawthorne Boulevard, Torrance, CA 90505.)

Lamerton, R. C., "The Need for Hospices," *Nursing Times*, 1975, *71*, 151–153.

Mount, B. M., *Palliative Care Service: October 1976 Report*. Montreal: Royal Victoria Hospital/McGill University, 1976.

Saunders, C. M., (Ed.), *The Management of Terminal Disease*. London: Edward Arnold, 1978.

# 17

# Learning and Caring: Education and Training Concerns

*Marcia E. Lattanzi*

In the rapid emergence of hospice care services, education and training programs have been developed as the vehicles that are intended to make the unique caring of hospice possible. Most hospices seek out available information and resources as they struggle to translate the ideals of hospice into tangible caregiving realities. There has been, however, little consistency or standardization of efforts. The training programs for hospices range from limited individual orientations to courses spanning several months of weekly sessions. Training may include all members of the interdisciplinary team, or only volunteers.

The area of education and training raises numerous questions: What are the goals of hospice education and training programs? Who should deliver these training programs? Who should attend? What content areas need to be included? And finally, can we teach people the type of caring necessary for hospice workers?

It is a generally held principle that hospice staff need to be carefully selected, trained, and supported in their work with dying persons and their families (Koff, 1980). In contrast to many death education efforts, the intent of hospice education and training is not to change attitudes of the participants. Rather, hospice training programs seek to encourage an increased awareness of the needs of others, as well as an increased self-knowledge.

In hospices, the education and training programs are designed to prepare individuals to function as effectively and comfortably as possible in their roles. Pine (1977) points out that large amounts of technical material or sophisticated training programs are not a substitute for clear thinking or compassion. Rather, my major interest in exploring education and training concerns centers around encouraging a thoughtful definition of purposes, needs, and approaches. Perhaps the principle of education and training as a foundation for working within a hospice needs to be considered. Why is there a need for education or learning that is greater than the orientation programs offered in most other related settings? Does hospice care involve special needs and problems that are addressed in training programs? Is there a new type of expertise demanded of hospice workers? Does the interdisciplinary team approach influence the type of training needed by hospice workers? Is training more extensive for hospices because of the involvement of many lay volunteers? Or, are we seeking to reorient or expand the past and existing viewpoints of hospice workers? It is my belief, based upon my work at Boulder County Hospice and as a consultant and trainer for numerous other hospice programs, that the reason for hospice training and education programs is not to teach the participants specific skills. Nor is it to change the attitudes of potential hospice workers. Rather, training programs exist to sensitize participants and to encourage them to examine their experiences and beliefs. Efforts are aimed at the outlook, view, or personal vision of the participants. While some hospice training programs may have grown out of an initial need to legitimize services, another reason for their emergence and development is most likely related to the individual and collective concerns and discomforts of hospice caregivers. In acknowledging and addressing the discomfort and the concerns, we are responsibly encouraging excellence in the delivery of care and services.

## Goals for Training Programs

Hospice training programs need to present and clarify the knowledge and values that will enable hospice workers to care for dying persons and their families with quality and excellence. The knowledge and skills necessary to the provision of hospice care are the foundations of a training program. In addition, many health professionals need to learn the care orientation of hospice, which involves an approach of advocacy and participation uncommon in professional experiences. Not only should training programs present this new philosophy and approach, but, also, they should increase the participants' understanding of the needs of dying persons and their families. Understanding is increased by activities that allow participants to explore their personal experiences and feelings toward death and loss. By increasing one's awareness of one's experiences and related responses, there is less likelihood of these experiences negatively affecting caregiving activities or decisions (Simpson, 1979).

Since hospice care is very personalized care, it may be hoped that training efforts can encourage openness and sensitivity of hospice workers. In a very real sense, hospice caregivers enter into the world of the dying person and family. One of the major goals of hospice education and training is to encourage the development of awareness and openness among hospice workers. There is a significant opportunity for hospice workers to enhance the experience for the dying person and family members. Hospice workers also have the unique potential of learning from others' experience (Jourard, 1964). The greatest challenge of hospice training efforts lies in providing a model for caregivers in the management of the "stress" associated with hospice work. Training programs need to present a philosophical orientation that acknowledges the difficulties inherent in caring for dying persons and their families. More importantly, the training program should encourage and promote involvement that recognizes the positive potential of working with dying and grieving persons. Individuals desiring involvement or work in a hospice program are individuals deeply concerned with the importance and meaning of human relationships. They are individuals seeking a deeper personal understanding of human relationships (Brantner, 1977). This need to passionately understand ourselves and others, and thereby to improve human relationships, must be acknowledged in the formation and development of a hospice training and education program.

The training program (and staff involvement in it) is not only the presentation of the philosophical orientation of hospice, but also the communication of the tone set by the leadership of the hospice. The modeling and behavior of the trainers and hospice leaders need to communicate the level of caring necessary for the delivery of services. Treatment of staff and volunteers is reflected in treatment of patients and their families. Hospice training programs need to communicate a policy of valuing staff and volunteers. They also need to contain elements that will encourage caregivers to maintain and develop activities, outlets, and involvements that will increase the quality and enjoyment of their own life experience.

## Training Rationale

Some health care professionals already possess the knowledge and skills that will be utilized in hospice work. Certain lay persons have an innate understanding of human needs and helpful responses. While individual backgrounds and relevant experiences are valued, a training program can present more than the technical information related to hospice care. Educational exploration into the topic of death and grief has the possibility of making life more meaningful (Worden & Proctor, 1976). Personal learning about death and grief also has the potential to stimulate hospice workers to develop their individual life priorities. In addition, learning about death can stimulate people to communicate their esteem and love to those dear to them before they die (Brantner, 1977). There is value in preparing hospice workers for situations they will encounter in their hospice work. Caregivers can learn ways of dealing with traumatic events they will be involved in while working with dying persons and their families. For example, a team case presentation review by hospice workers of a difficult care experience can be very helpful. Often situations of family conflict arise in hospice caregiving. A case presentation can describe preexisting family patterns, situational difficulties, and caregiver definition of goals, as well as the framework and limitations for their involvement and intervention. A retrospective care presentation has the benefit of offering an example of caregiver roles and responsibilities. A concrete statement is presented that difficulties and conflict arise in caring that are sometimes unable to be resolved or easily managed. In addition, caregivers can review the personal and professional lessons learned from involvement with a given family. Because death remains unknowable, training programs need to present a broad view of the many ways individuals can think and feel about death and death-related experiences.

Most importantly, hospice training programs have the great potential for building a sense of community within a hospice. This shared experience, where philosophy and information are presented against the backdrop of personal exploration, can be the important element in the creation of the hospice community. An effective hospice training program will be both cognitive and experiential, with participants learning from one another.

## Trainers

Trainers are those individuals selected by a hospice to translate education and training goals into tangible presentations. If the hospice training program is seen as the presentation of the philosophical and practical approach of hospice care, the trainers need to be individuals with appropriate experiences and expertise. Hospice groups often turn to individuals who have had a positive experience in an existing, established hospice program. A guest speaker, presenter, or trainer can kindle sparks of enthusiasm in a group. It is crucial, however, that each hospice group define its own specific training needs. Local hospice leaders need to be active in the training program to promote the cohesiveness and bonding of the group. Resource persons are generally available in the local community (e.g., members of the clergy to speak to spiritual care concerns, physicians to present current cancer treatments, mental health experts to discuss loss and grief, etc.). By utilizing an interdisciplinary group of local resource persons, the hospice also encourages community involvement and ownership. Suggestions for the selection of competent death educators (Leviton, 1977) can be applied to potential hospice trainers in the following manner:

1. Trainers need to know thoroughly the subject matter they will present.
2. Trainers need to have had some personal or professional experience in the areas of death, grief, terminal care, or hospice.
3. The trainer must have examined his or her own feelings and responses to death and grief.
4. The trainer must support the hospice philosophy and approach to terminal care.
5. The trainer must exhibit the qualities of warmth, openness, effective listening, and communication skills, and the ability to express genuine caring in relation to the concerns of service recipients and coworkers.
6. The trainer must serve as a model for other hospice workers.
7. Recognizing human discomfort with death and grief, the trainer seeks to promote greater personal understanding of human needs and responses to death and grief.

It is essential that the hospice training program be delivered by a group of individuals representing the disciplines involved in the hospice team. A team of trainers exhibits the functional principle involved in the delivery of hospice care. The blending of perspectives in the training process ensures the broad view that training participants will come to see as the hospice vision.

There are a number of well-established hospice programs that have made a commitment to education and training concerns. Most notable among these are the Connecticut Hospice and the Hospice Institute for Training and Research in New Haven, Connecticut; the Hospice of Marin in San Rafael, California; and the Royal Victoria Hospital Palliative Care Service in Montreal, Quebec, Canada. Hospices in England also offer a limited number of resident learning experiences. Other hospice programs have built upon the pioneering efforts by making a commitment to the dissemination of information. The National Hospice Organization lists resource films and manuals, as well as indicates those hospices which offer site visits or speakers. Courses, conferences, and on-site consultations are available nationally. It is wise to consider the experience and motives of the group offering the educational program. In general, educational offerings related to hospice ideally involve or develop with the input of hospice-related personnel.

Finally, hospice programs, however diverse their models, have a responsibility to engage in dialogue and communication with one another. By sharing experiences, questioning assumptions, challenging approaches, and collaborating on efforts at standardization and evaluation, hospice training programs can continue to evolve and improve.

## Selection of Caregivers

Careful selection of caregivers is the essential first step in a hospice training program. Prior to an individual's attending the training program, an application and an interview can be helpful in determining the appropriateness of an individual's participation in hospice. People from diverse backgrounds, age groups, and experiences can be effective hospice workers. The major question is why the person wants to work with or be involved with hospice. The applicant needs to begin considering the reason for desired involvement. If an individual has experienced the loss of a loved one, it is important that the loss has been dealt with and that an appropriate time has since gone by (e.g., 1 to 2 years for the loss of an immediate family member).

People who want to work or volunteer in a hospice program need to bring to this work some successful life experience and/or work experience. Hospice workers need to have a sense of what strengths, skills, and personal gifts they will be using in working with dying persons and their families. Hospice workers should ideally have their glasses half full, not half empty. Hospice is not a religion, or a god, for individuals seeking fulfillment in that sense (Good, 1979). Rather, hospice involvement provides an opportunity for an individual to explore further the meaning of life.

In the selection of individuals for staff or volunteer positions, the following are considered important application or interview questions:

1. What are your reasons for wanting to be involved with hospice?
2. What personal or professional experiences have you had with death or grief?
3. What kinds of support do you have from family or friends?
4. What do you do to have fun (hobbies, activities, etc.)?

The training program itself is also a selection process, eliminating individuals who are unable or unwilling to commit themselves to the time involved. In addition, individuals often realize at the completion of the training program that they are not ready for hospice involvement—a self-selection process. People who are not considered able to work effectively with dying or grieving persons can perform administrative or support service functions. Noncaregiving activities, while often viewed as less glamorous, are essential and are highly valued in the functioning of hospice programs.

Enhancing the quality of life for dying persons and their families is the essence of hospice care. Individuals who do not have the ability to find enjoyment in their own lives have no place working in a hospice program.

If the hospice training accomplishes the goals of increasing personal awareness and understanding of the needs and responses of dying and grieving people, hospices need to consider allowing interested community persons to attend their training programs. Boulder County Hospice has included nurses, school teachers and counselors, ministers, and lay persons from the community in its team training sessions. Also, special training sessions or programs for these populations can increase community awareness and support for dying and grieving persons. Hospice education and training efforts must not exist in isolation from the community. Hospice philosophy and principles have broad application to other medical settings, as well as to the community at large. Hospice principles, in reality, are not new. They are basic truths that need to be learned, relearned, and constantly practiced in a great range of life situations.

## Training and Education Methods

Hospice training programs, like hospices themselves, must be individually designed to address the needs of specific groups and locations. There is no predetermined model for training that can be universally applied. Individual hospices must assess, plan, and design their training programs based upon their own needs and experience.

Planning for a training program goes beyond contacting speakers and arranging for the training environment. Hospice training programs will be consistent and of higher quality if the following factors are incorporated:

1. Qualified trainers/presenters. Training programs are best when delivered by an interdisciplinary group of trainers or presenters. Trainers/presenters need to be persons with relevant experience and expertise who are supportive of the hospice approach.

2. Behavioral or measurable objectives. These objectives allow for a determination of the specific learning it is hoped that participants will achieve. For example, at the completion of the program/ training, the participant should be able to

   a. identify the philosophical framework of hospice care and services;
   b. review the dying and grieving processes;
   c. understand approaches to the physical, emotional, psychological, spiritual, and social needs of dying and grieving people.

   Measurable objectives are ideally designed for the entire training program, as well as for individual sessions or content areas.

3. Outlined content areas. It is suggested that each presenter outline the material to be covered under a given topic or content area. These outlines should be kept on file at the hospice. Outlines are helpful in evaluation, standardization and/or expansion of material, and transitions among trainers/presenters.

4. Diversified learning experiences. Inherent in the goals of a hospice training program is the need for a wide range of teaching/ learning approaches, such as the following:

   a. Didactic presentation. Certain content areas are almost by necessity delivered in lecture format (e.g., pain and symptom control, current cancer treatments).
   b. Discussion/interaction. Participants are actively encouraged to contribute responses to questions, film presentations, and so on. Discussion and interaction can take place both in the larger group and in smaller groups of varying sizes.
   c. Personalizations or experiential exercises. Since one of the main objectives of training involves the examination of personal experience and concerns, opportunities to explore these areas safely are included in the training. Simulated experience exercises are powerful tools for increasing understanding and sensitivity. These exercises should be presented by individuals with appropriate professional experience.
   d. Reading and homework assignments. Learning can be extended by asking participants to explore questions individually prior to or after training sessions. Reading and homework assignments can be chosen to reinforce important elements covered in a session. For example, participants can be asked to answer the question, "What are the major ways in which you personally cope with difficulties?" At the start of each training session, participants can discuss their responses in small-group interactions.
   e. Journal keeping. Many individuals involved in hospice work

have commented on the need to spend time personally reflecting upon one's work and experiences and their meaning. Journal writing can be used during the training program experience to sort through and further clarify responses. This approach offers a significant opportunity for further self-exploration and understanding for those individuals interested in pursuing it.

5. Evaluation by participants and presenters. Written feedback by training participants and presenters as to the program's quality and completeness is essential. Individual content areas should be rated so that weak presentations can be identified. Also, participants should be asked to identify and outline major personal learnings. Recommendations for future trainings and additional learning needs should also be requested.

In the effort to present a range of training experiences, audiovisual materials can play an important role. Recently, a number of hospice caregiver training audiovisuals have become available. (See appended Audiovisual Resource List.) Audiovisuals should be evaluated for use on the basis of their ability to represent with sensitivity and accuracy human experiences, responses, and needs in relation to death and grief. Also, the behavior of caregivers exhibited in audiovisuals should serve as a learning model. Negative or insensitive representations can serve as a stimulus for clarifying the value of various types of responses. Audiovisuals can have emotional impact upon training participants and need to be used responsibly by trainers. Beyond eliciting emotional responses, an audiovisual and the discussion and processing following it should serve to enhance awareness and understanding.

Role playing, team presentations, sociodrama, and small-group exercises all have been used effectively in training programs and can offer means for skill building and greater personal learning. Perhaps the most important element of the training program is the creation of a diverse and meaningful opportunity for practical and personal learning. Training participants must be active and interact with other participants. This element improves the quality of the learning and also provides support to participants.

## Training Program Content Areas

It seems logical that content areas in hospice training programs relate specifically to the needs of dying persons and their families. Schulz (1978) has identified three major needs of dying persons:

1. The need to control pain.
2. The need to retain dignity or feelings of self-worth.
3. The need for love and affection.

It is clear that these needs are the needs of all human beings. In addressing these needs in the hospice context, the following training content areas emerge:

1. Hospice philosophy and approach. Includes content related to the characteristics and principles that define hospice care.
2. Pain and symptom control. Includes presentation of principles related to the understanding of pain and holistic approaches to treatment.
3. Family-centered care. Includes material related to viewing care from the perspective of the individual as part of a family unit. The contrasts among stresses, available resources, and coping styles are appropriate content.
4. Understanding the process of dying. Includes presentation of responses, concerns, and needs of dying persons and their family members.
5. Current cancer treatments and care. Includes presentation of the influence of cancer upon the individual, available treatments, and major physical concerns related to cancer care.
6. Interdisciplinary teamwork and roles. Includes presentation of the functions of various team members, role overlap and role blurring, stress, and support.
7. Personalization/experiential exercises. Includes integration of personal experiences, feelings, and responses through the use of simulation exercises.
8. Funeral practices/mortuary tour. Includes tangible presentation related to practical concerns and consumer information.
9. Helping and communication skills. Includes practice in listening and responding skills. Focus is upon the ability to be present with another.
10. Grief and bereavement. Includes content concerning the grief process and the experiences of grief. Follow-up care for family members is discussed.
11. Caregiving approaches and concerns. Includes assessment of personal strengths and skills, defining one's involvement and limitations, stress management, and the personal costs and benefits of hospice work.
12. Spiritual, psychological/emotional, and social dimensions of

care. Presents hospice care from differing dimensions and focuses on the blending of perspectives. Needs and concerns of aging persons are presented.

Hospice programs may add to this list or emphasize certain topics. Hospice training programs are generally in the 20- to 30-hour range. The team training at Boulder County Hospice includes two all-day (weekend) sessions and three to five evening sessions. All-day sessions serve to intensify the group interaction and personal involvement. Sharing of lunches and extended time together serve to encourage the development of relationships within the group. Involvement and continuity of several of the trainers also contribute to the closeness and level of interaction of the participants. The philosophies of advocacy, facilitation, and enabling care, which are so inherent in hospice, need to be strongly presented and practiced at the training sessions.

## Evaluation

Most hospices receive participant evaluations of their training programs. At Boulder County Hospice, these evaluations have indicated that the training is a meaningful and personal learning experience for the large majority of participants. The true effects of a hospice training program are difficult to measure. However a training program is structured, it should attempt to integrate head and heart. The Socratic method, where the individual transfers and links his or her experiences with the knowledge presented, is a powerful learning process to employ in hospice training. Consistent and objective evaluation of training programs is our responsibility.

Training programs can be evaluated by assessing the following:

1. Participant satisfaction.
2. Degree to which behavioral or measurable objectives are met.
3. Trainer review and assessment.
4. Ability of new team members to function with effectiveness and comfort following training.

Since ongoing education, training, and evaluation of hospice services are standards of the National Hospice Organization, national-level communication and collaboration, especially in the area of evaluation, will be necessary.

On a subjective level, perhaps the best test of our learning lies in our ability to act not just as advocates for the dying and the bereaved, but as advocates for life—advocates for the improvement of the human condition of all.

## Continuing Education

The process of learning never stops. Hospice training programs are the beginning, the foundation upon which further learning will rest. Hospices need to commit themselves to ongoing staff/volunteer education programs. Monthly in-service sessions are considered a staff benefit, an element in the management of stress, a guarantee against stagnation, a factor in the ongoing development of the hospice community, and a consideration related to job satisfaction. By continuing to learn together, questioning past approaches and considering potential new ones, hospice workers enhance their experience.

Hospice principles should not exist in isolation from the existing health care delivery system. Rather, the integration of these principles into the practices of caregivers is part of the potential of the hospice approach.

## Support Systems

Some of the great lessons involved in care of the dying are related to giving and receiving, coming together and letting go. By training and education efforts, we are establishing a value system for care of the dying (Harper, 1977). Significant values include the following:

1. A present orientation.
2. Acknowledgment of an individual's right to participate in and make decisions relative to his or her care and medical treatment.
3. Efforts to enhance the quality of an individual's life.
4. Caregiving that allows an individual to retain a sense of control, dignity, and self-worth.
5. Caregiving that actively involves family members.
6. Provision of options and choices for people.
7. Provision of the highest quality of care, whether or not cure is possible.

These values must not only be applied to dying persons and their families. If we are to be effective caregivers, these beliefs and values have to be applied to ourselves. In the attempt to provide supportive services for dying persons and their families, we must seek support for ourselves and our efforts. Care of dying and grieving persons is not work to be done in isolation from others. Training programs need to emphasize the necessity of receiving support from within the hospice network, as well as from family or friends outside hospice. By learning to give and receive support, we expand not only our professional competence, but also our empathy, compassion, and sensitivity to others. Individuals unable to work in or utilize a support community will not function well in a hospice program.

Training and education deserve major emphasis in hospice programs. In the process of preparing caregivers, hospices are involved in determining their present functioning and future viability. To be effective in improving care for dying persons and their families, hospices must extend their learning to other caregivers and to members of the community at large. There are no fixed or final answers to the human concerns and questions involved with death and grief. In the same context, my perspective on education and training is intended to offer some ideas and elements that may be of use to others in developing or refining their approach. My presentation is based upon the belief that the dying and grieving are our teachers. The task of hospice training and education efforts is to encourage our greater responsiveness and humanity as we are challenged by the complexities and richness that can transform us.

# Appendix: Audiovisual Resource List

*Audiovisuals for Hospice Training*

GENERAL INTRODUCTION TO HOSPICE CARE
*Day by Day*—16 mm film, color, 20 minutes. Available from Hospital Home Health Care Agency of California, 23228 Hawthorne Boulevard, Torrence, CA 90505; 213/373-6373.

*Hospice*—16 mm film, color, 13 minutes. Hillhaven Hospice, Tucson, AZ. Available from Carousel Films, Inc., 1501 Broadway, New York, NY 10036; 212/354-0315.

*Hospice: An Alternative Way to Care for the Dying*—16 mm film, color, 26 minutes. National Hospice Organization. Available from Billy Budd Films, 235 East 57th Street, New York, NY 10022; 212/755-3968.

*Hospice Care: An Alternative*—synchronized slides and audio cassette, color, 26 minutes. Available from Boulder County Hospice, Inc., 2118 14th Street, Boulder, CO 80302; 303/499-7740.

CAREGIVER CONCERNS
*As Long as There is Life*—16 mm film, color, 40 minutes. Available from The Connecticut Hospice, 61 Burban Drive, Branford, CT 06405; 203/481-6231.

*Last Days of Living*—16 mm film, color, 58 minutes. Palliative Care Service, Royal Victoria Hospital, Montreal, Canada. Available from National Film Board of Canada, 1251 Avenue of the Americas, New York, NY 10020; 212/586-5131.

*Terminal Cancer: The Hospice Approach to Pain Control*—videotape, color, 19 minutes; *Terminal Cancer: The Hospice Approach to the Family*—videotape, color, 19 minutes. Both available only to hospitals and medical schools that are members of the National Council for Medical Education; available from Network for Continuing Medical Education, 15 Columbus Circle, New York, NY 10023; 212/541-8088.

### Resource Books

Baldwin, M. V. et al., *Hospice Volunteers: A Guide for Training*. Piscataway, NJ: Office of Consumer Health Education, CMDNJ—Rutgers Medical School, and Riverside Hospice, 1980.

Stewart, K., & Hancock, P. *Care of the Dying Patient and His Relatives: A Resource List of Audio-Visual Teaching Materials*. Unpublished manuscript, 1981. (Available from the NHS Learning Resources Unit, The Centre for Developments in Nurse Education, 55 Broomgrove Road, Sheffield S10 2NA, England.)

Wass, H. et al., *Death Education: An Annotated Resource Guide*. New York: McGraw-Hill/Hemisphere, 1980.

## References

Brantner, J., "Positive Approaches to Dying," *Death Education*, 1977, *1*, 293–304.

Good, J., *Approaches to Staff Support*. Speech delivered at the National Hospice Organization Region IV Conference, Boulder, CO, 1979.

Harper, B. C., *Death: The Coping Mechanism of the Health Professional*. Greenville, SC: Southeastern University Press, 1977.

Jourard, S. M., *The Transparent Self*. Princeton, NJ: Van Nostrand, 1964.

Koff, T. H., *Hospice: A Caring Community*. Cambridge, MA: Winthrop, 1980.

Leviton, D., "Death Education," in H. Feifel (Ed.), *New Meanings of Death*. New York: McGraw-Hill, 1977, 253–272.

Pine, V. R., "A Socio-Historical Portrait of Death Education," *Death Education*, 1977, *1*, 57–84.

Schulz, R., *The Psychology of Death, Dying and Bereavement*. Reading, MA: Addison-Wesley, 1978.

Simpson, M. A., "Death Education—Where Is Thy Sting?", *Death Education*, 1979, *3*, 165–173.

Worden, J. W., & Proctor, W., *Personal Death Awareness*. Englewood Cliffs, NJ: Prentice-Hall, 1976.

# 18

# Staff Stress in Care of the Terminally Ill

*Mary L. S. Vachon*

Increased sensitivity to the needs of dying patients has begun to change the philosophy of treatment for the terminally ill; that is, greater emphasis is now being placed on palliative care. Rather than focusing on extending the lifespan of patients dying of a lingering illness, such as cancer, good palliative care is designed to improve the quality of life remaining for such patients by alleviating the physical, psychosocial, and spiritual concerns of the patient and his or her family (International Work Group, 1979). The emerging hospice movement emphasizes providing this type of care for the terminally ill, not only in separate hospices, but also in palliative care units within general hospitals and through improved home health care programs.

As new services for dying patients have multiplied, the emotional demands made on patient care staff by intimate and prolonged contact with these patients have increased. Those who work with the dying frequently experience considerable stress, and ways of helping them cope need to be developed (Artiss & Levine, 1973; Beszterczey, 1977; Vachon, 1978; Vachon et al., 1976, 1978).

## The Nature of Stress

Stress has been defined as an "organism's response to stressful conditions or stressors, consisting of a pattern of physiological and psychological reactions, both immediate and delayed" (Rabkin & Struening, 1976). One of

*From:* Mary L. S. Vachon, "Staff Stress in Care of the Terminally Ill," *Quality Review Bulletin,* May 1979, pp. 13–17. Reprinted by permission of Mary L. S. Vachon and the Joint Commission on Accreditation of Hospitals.

the basic concepts in current stress theory is that the individual has a finite amount of energy for adapting to stressful situations, and unless this energy is replenished regularly, the supply becomes exhausted. Selye warns, for example, that constant expenditure of energy will result in that energy being "eventually exhausted if we only spend and never earn" (Selye, 1956). This concept is the key to management of stress in all areas of life. Those who work with the dying are particularly at risk of depleting the energy they have to give, because of the tremendous emotional investment such work entails. This fact presents one of the major problems in caring for the terminally ill: if patient care staff only give of themselves without in some way being replenished, they will ultimately have nothing left to give.

## Staff Stress in Acute Care Hospitals and in Hospices

The comparative merits of the hospice versus the acute care hospital for treatment of the dying patient will not be debated here; instead, each setting will be discussed separately. The focus will be on staff who care for patients with terminal cancer, although much of what is said may apply equally well to those who care for patients with other terminal diseases.

### The Acute Care Setting

The acute care hospital is generally oriented toward providing aggressive treatment aimed at curing or controlling disease. The patient care staff in the hospital often presents a fairly optimistic outlook to the newly diagnosed patient, hoping to encourage the patient to initiate and persevere with indicated therapy. In an acute care setting, the staff usually shares the patient's trauma at the initial diagnosis, empathizes with the difficulties of decision making regarding treatment, helps the patient cope with the side effects of treatment, rejoices with the patient and his family over a remission or shares with their despair at a recurrence, and worries with them about maintaining the quality of life in the face of advancing disease and inevitable death.

SOURCES OF STRESS IN THE ACUTE CARE SETTING
Staff who care for terminally ill patients in an acute care setting are exposed to a number of situational factors that can cause stress:

> Staff who care for an individual throughout the course of an illness may come to know both the patient and family well. Watching the patient decline then becomes increasingly difficult for staff to bear.

Hoping for a cure, staff may also give the patient the impression that if prescribed treatment is followed, a cure or at least a good remission can be expected. This increases the staff's emotional investment in the patient's welfare and their frustration when a cure is not achieved.

If treatment does not work, and the patient is clearly dying, staff members may feel responsible, guilty, angry, depressed, or helpless.

Staff members may begin to wonder whether treatment is worthwhile and whether they should encourage a patient to persevere with treatment, especially if he is having trouble with side effects.

Members of the patient care team may disagree about the efficacy of treatment and the value and ethics of research.

Staff members may find personality changes or resentment in the patient caused by the illness difficult to bear and may tire of the patient and his family.

With increasing exposure to the patient and his family, the staff may become more aware of social problems the family faces and feel helpless to deal with them.

The patient and his family may have unrealistically high expectations of the staff, and the staff may experience guilt and anger when they fail to meet these expectations.

If they are unable to control symptoms (e.g., nausea, pain, constipation, bowel obstruction), staff members may feel impotent when dealing with a dying patient.

Staff members who have cared for a patient over a long period of time may feel resentment when active treatment is no longer appropriate and the patient is transferred from their unit.

MANIFESTATIONS OF STRESS IN THE ACUTE CARE SETTING

Anxiety generated by the stressful conditions to which staff are exposed in an acute care setting is frequently translated into staff conflict (Vachon et al., 1978). Individual members of the staff often express the opinion that "If only the doctors (or nurses, social workers, clergy, psychiatrists) were different, things would be a lot better around here." As anxiety increases and team members approach a state of exhaustion, they may try—in subtle and not so subtle ways—to thwart each other's efforts. Certain individuals may be singled out for hostile criticism; hostility generated by the discrepancy between the desired and the probable outcomes in a patient's disease may be displaced, for example, onto staff oncologists or onto anyone in a position of authority who can somehow be held responsible. Patients and their families are also not immune from displaced hostility, and real problems can occur when patients, families, and staff displace their hostility toward the disease onto one another. Family members may blame each other for the patient's disease or blame the physician if there is a recurrence.

To decrease the stress they are experiencing, some staff members in acute care settings may withdraw from patients, especially from those who are unresponsive to treatment or obviously dying. Staff members may even suggest transferring these patients to "more appropriate" chronic care units. Other staff members may become very involved with patients who are dying, but ignore the newly diagnosed. These staff members will describe themselves as summoning up their last reserves to care for patients to whom they have already made a commitment; however, they are also consciously avoiding involvement with anyone new who "will probably just die anyway." One nurse in such a situation said, "I knew it was time to move on when I realized that I was avoiding meeting new patients. I figured that they were all going to die anyway no matter what we did, and I had the feeling that I knew a terrible secret that the new patient and family didn't yet know. I could no longer be optimistic when I talked about treatment, and I knew I had to leave."

Staff members may also find that their jobs begin to interfere with their personal lives. As another nurse said, "I look at other people, and they seem happy and carefree; of course, they have their problems but basically they're happy. They aren't weighted down by the constant exposure to the reality of suffering and death that we live with every day. I'm not really complaining, but I wonder what it does to us." These staff members have probably reached a state of exhaustion (Shubin, 1978).

Once nurses, social workers, and other staff members become aware of their exhaustion, they can take steps to relieve it, even if it means changing jobs. A more difficult problem, however, may confront oncologists who have spent many years training for their specialty without realizing that their role is potentially a very stressful one. The oncologist's role encompasses a commitment to research, ultimate responsibility for the patient's welfare, and a duty to be supportive of the patient; yet often the oncologist is also aware of the importance of the quality of life and may question the ultimate value of what he is doing for the patient. Some current treatment modalities, for example, cause patients extreme discomfort but at best only increase life expectancy and do not promise cure. The sensitive and caring oncologist may come to question the value of putting a patient through so much suffering. The oncologist may find himself working longer and longer hours while he tries to meet the needs of patients and achieve some sense of satisfaction. This can be increasingly frustrating if more time spent with patients means a greater awareness of the needs of the patient and his family and increased guilt at not being able to meet all these needs. To avoid this conflict, many oncologists retain or revert to the medical model of treating only the disease, leaving the patient and family to cope with their personal problems.

## The Hospice Setting

The term *hospice* is used to mean many things and to encompass a wide variety of settings, ranging from separate hospice buildings to palliative care units or teams within acute care hospitals to home care programs. Many of the problems faced by hospice staff in these settings are similar to those encountered by staff in the acute care setting, yet each setting has its own unique stresses that vary with the circumstances. The basic difference is that, unlike the acute care setting where both staff and patient initially hope for a cure and together face the realization that the patient's disease is terminal, in the hospice the focus of the relationship between staff and patient is always on the process of dying.

### Sources of stress in the hospice setting

Stress factors that may affect patient care staff in the hospice setting include the following:

Difficulty accepting the fact that the patients' physical and psychosocial problems cannot always be controlled;

Frustration at being involved with a patient's family only after their emotional resources have been drained by the illness;

Disappointment if expectations for patients to die a "good death"—however this may be defined—are not met;

Frustration at having invested large amounts of energy in caring for people who then die, taking this investment with them;

Anger at being subjected to higher-than-standard performance expectations in prototypal facilities exposed to considerable scrutiny and publicity;

Difficulty deciding where to draw limits on involvement with patients and their families, particularly during off-duty hours; and

Difficulty establishing a sense of realistic limitations on what the hospice service, which is expected to be all-encompassing, can actually provide.

MANIFESTATIONS OF STRESS IN THE HOSPICE SETTING

Staff members in hospice units sometimes come to think of themselves as special people, capable of incredible feats. Although the concept of staff stress may be acknowledged, manifestations of stress in individual staff members may be regarded as a weakness and as a threat to staff image. Open recognition of the fact that a staff member is under considerable stress may lead to decreased tolerance of its expression. Stress may then be expressed in behavior different from that observed in the acute care setting.

Staff stress may be expressed in terms of staff conflict, particularly in hostility toward the leader of the unit, who may be a charismatic figure. If the leader is absent from the unit, hostility is often displaced onto those given authority in his absence. Unexpressed conflict, on the other hand, may lead to deterioration in the expected high level of patient care on the unit.

Staff stress may also be expressed as depression caused by constant exposure to death. Or staff may experience grief reactions due to unresolved sorrow over the constant and often unacknowledged loss of many significant others. Grief, in the form of chronic, unacknowledged depression, may be manifested in fatigue and lack of interest in life. The individual feels drained and cannot concentrate on the patient and his needs. Other staff members may find themselves unable to step out of the patient care situation and may make themselves available to patients and families 24 hours a day, seven days a week. Staff members may develop marital and family problems because of overinvolvement with patients and the belief that the needs of dying patients should come before the more mundane needs of their own families. Staff members may also exhibit various forms of "acting-out" behavior, such as excessive social activity or overuse of alcohol, to affirm life and well-being (Vachon, 1978).

## Suggestions for Decreasing Staff Stress

Suggestions for dealing with staff stress are predicated on the idea that an individual's response to stressful situations is determined by "those characteristics of the stressful event, of the individual, and of his social support system that influence his perception of, or sensitivity to stressors" (Rabkin & Struening, 1976). The suggestions are organized into four categories: staff selection, staff training and orientation, social supports, and working conditions.

## Staff Selection

Preemployment interviews with prospective patient care staff should elicit information about an individual's previous exposure to death, both personally and professionally. Particular attention should be paid to the coping mechanisms the individual employs; evidence of denial of grief or flight into overactivity may be indicative of unresolved grief, which could lead to later difficulty in the care of the dying. Caution should also be exercised in hiring someone who has experienced a major bereavement within the previous year. Unresolved grief reactions could increase such an individual's sensitivity to the stress of constant exposure to grief.

A prospective staff member's social support system should also be carefully assessed. An individual without supportive relationships may be unable to obtain the personal support necessary to offset the emotionally draining nature of hospice work. Many people who want to work with the dying have a sense of calling, an almost missionary zeal. Such people often wish to devote their entire lives to the care of the dying. When unaccompanied by a good support system, this can prove to be both unrealistic and unreliable, because the individual's emotional energy will soon be depleted, and he will not have effective ways to restore it.

When hiring specifically for oncology units, assessment of an applicant's personal experience with cancer is important. The interviewer should be aware that personal experience with a cancer patient, e.g., a relative or close friend, can have both positive aspects (e.g., increased empathy and understanding) and negative aspects (e.g., an increased potential for overinvolvement due perhaps to identification of care given a patient with care given the friend or relative) (Vachon, 1978).

## Staff Training and Orientation

New staff members should be given thorough and extensive orientation to provide them with a solid background in the physical and psychosocial care of the terminally ill. During the orientation period, the presence of positive staff role models (i.e., individuals who function effectively and provide good patient care) who can teach and provide support for new staff members is crucial. The use of a "buddy system," whereby an experienced staff member provides support and help to the new staff member on a one-to-one basis, or the use of a well-organized team approach can be very valuable in introducing new staff members to the most effective ways of dealing with the practical problems and stresses inherent in caring for the terminally ill.

The needs of more experienced staff for continued educational programs must also be acknowledged. Discussions focused on recent advances in the field and opportunities to attend and participate in workshops are effective methods for providing senior staff members with the intellectual input necessary for maintaining a high level of patient care; such programs also can help alleviate stress by providing a break in routine.

*Social Supports*

Staff members must have well-integrated social support systems both within and without the patient care setting. The stress of work with the dying can place severe pressures on personal relationships and on marriages and may even cause marital breakups. For example, one oncologist said, "I have no patience listening to my wife's complaints about the kids when I've been busy dealing with the threat of death all day." And a nurse remarked, "My husband doesn't want me to talk about my work because he finds it too depressing. Yet, at the end of the day, I have to unwind with someone."

The sense that only other people in the same field can really understand the pressures that work with the dying entails has led many units to develop staff support groups. There are, however, advantages in encouraging staff members to develop staff support groups with people outside their own unit or hospice setting, because contact with people in other disciplines can help the staff member maintain a perspective that extends beyond his job. Groups for oncology nurses or thanatologists, women's groups, prayer groups, and support groups composed of people from a variety of disciplines or hospital units can provide effective support systems for some people in the field. For staff members who work in relative isolation, such as psychotherapists or counselors working primarily with the terminally ill, continuing individual peer support and supervision or regular meetings with an outside therapist can help staff members maintain objectivity. Educational groups for the spouses of staff may also be worthwhile.

*Working Conditions*

One of the most effective ways to decrease staff stress is through the use of a well-organized multidisciplinary team approach to the care of patients. Communication between staff members is enhanced, responsibility is more effectively shared, and no one feels totally alone in caring for the patient; as a result, staff cooperation and effectiveness are usually increased.

Many hospice units also have psychiatrists or other mental health professionals available to the staff for weekly team support meetings, case consultations, assistance with program development, educational back-up, and staff support in general. This system works particularly well if the consultant is physically present often enough to acquire a real sense of the problems that staff members experience. The consultant must be readily available to the staff, both individually and collectively.

Some hospice units have begun to experiment with a variety of work patterns aimed at decreasing staff stress. One hospice has found that a four-day work week with an occasional night or weekend on duty improves staff attitude and level of efficiency (Lamers, 1978). Another hospice uses an occasional "day away," a corps of volunteers, and a carefully monitored workload to prevent staff exhaustion. Part-time staff also provide important relief (Lack, 1978). Other units strongly suggest that their staff members involve themselves in outside "life-oriented" activities and ensure that staff members have enough time off to take courses and pursue outside interests.

Staff in the general hospital setting may benefit from occasional rotation through hospital clinics for set periods so they can see patients who are responding well to treatment. It may also be helpful to assign staff members to units outside the hospice unit for a few weeks. This should decrease the feeling of isolation staff members may experience if they are involved only with those in the hospice.

## Conclusion

Good care for the terminally ill presents health care professionals with many challenges. To ensure the best possible care for dying patients, adequate attention must be paid to providing support for the caregivers—the hospice staff.

## References

Artiss, K. L., & Levine, A. S., "Doctor-Patient Relationship in Severe Illness," *New England Journal of Medicine*, 1973, *288*, 1210–1214.

Beszterczey, A., "Staff Stress on a Newly Developed Palliative Care Service: The Psychiatrist's Role," *Canadian Psychiatric Association Journal*, 1977, *22*, 347–353.

The International Work Group in Death, Dying, and Bereavement, "Assumptions and Principles Underlying Standards for Terminal Care," *American Journal of Nursing*, 1979, *79*, 296–297.

Lack, S. A., "New Haven (1974)—Characteristics of a Hospice Program of Care," *Death Education*, 1978, *2*, 41–52.

Lamers, W. M., Jr., "Marin County (1976)—Development of Hospice of Marin," *Death Education*, 1978, *2*, 53–62.

Rabkin, J. G., & Struening, E. L., "Life Events, Stress, and Illness," *Science*, 1976, *194*, 1013–1020.

Selye, H., *The Stress of Life*. New York: McGraw-Hill, 1956.

Shubin, S., "Burnout: The Professional Hazard You Face in Nursing," *Nursing '78*, 1978, *8*, 22–27.

Vachon, M. L. S., "Motivation and Stress Experienced by Staff Working with the Terminally Ill," *Death Education*, 1978, *2*, 113–122.

Vachon, M. L. S., Lyall, W. A. L., & Freeman, S. J. J., "Measurement and Management of Stress in Health Professionals Working with Advanced Cancer Patients," *Death Education*, 1978, *1*, 365–375.

Vachon, M. L. S., Lyall, W. A. L., & Rogers, J., "The Nurse in Thanatology: What She Can Learn From the Women's Liberation Movement," in A. M. Earle, N. T. Argondizzo, & A. H. Kutscher (Eds.), *The Nurse as Caregiver for the Terminal Patient and His Family*. New York: Columbia University Press, 1976, 175–194.

# IV

# Bereavement

*Just as dying is a natural part of life, so too are bereavement, loss, and grief. Both situations involve stress and coping; neither is in itself a mental aberration or a psychiatric illness. Obviously, there can be abnormal, dysfunctional, or even pathological modes of coping. We must be alert to these possibilities and ready to respond to them appropriately (often by referral to skilled professional resources). But by their very nature, they do not fit the norm. What are required for successful coping in the vast majority of cases are sound inner resources, plus the friendship and support of a concerned community.*

*Pity is not appropriate, for that suggests superiority and disequity. Instead, most people need a willingness to listen (both to the overt expression and to the underlying feelings) and empathy or compassion—the sincere attempt to enter into the feelings of others and to share with them. It is presumptuous to say: "I know how you feel." As has been pointed out above by Patricia Downie in Chapter 12, we never really do know precisely how another person feels, for we are not them. If we have endured similar experiences in life, we may sense what their experience might be like. And we can acknowledge that they must be coping with strong feelings. "This must be a difficult time for you, isn't it?" Or we can ask how they are feeling—and really mean it, so that we are willing to stay and hear the answer. Or we can express our own honest doubts and hesitations, and ask for guidance: "I don't know what to say or do. How can I help you?" Bereavement care within the hospice approach is not a treatment program in the sense of an intensive, long-term, and often hierarchical relationship addressed to pathology. Rather, it is an offering of support and concern in simple yet effective ways to those who need them in our inexperienced and in many ways alienated societies.*

*In the first of the following selections, Mwalimu Imara reminds us that grief is based in interdependence and loving relationships. It is hard to lose those whom we love and to be deprived of their company through death. Mourning or grief work is our way of "realizing" what has happened—making it real in our inner world, coming to terms with the external facts, so that we can achieve a way of living with the new present and future. In so doing, we also retain from the past the good memories that can never be taken away. The grief process—like life itself—is one of adaptation and growth. Both Imara and Bonnie Lindstrom, in a more programmatic way, show how friends and helpers can facilitate such growth. Simple confirmation that many others have faced similar trials and come through them successfully can be very reassuring. When it seems as though "I am losing my mind," it is important to know that this is a familiar experience in what for many these days is an unfamiliar situation.*

# 19

# Growing through Grief

*Mwalimu Imara*

Blessed are those who mourn, for they shall be comforted.

—*Matthew 5:4*

Talk to me about the truth of religion and I'll listen gladly. Talk to me about the duty of religion and I'll listen submissively. But don't come talking to me about the consolations of religion or I shall suspect that you don't understand.

—*C. S. Lewis,* A Grief Observed, *p. 28*

The human spirit seems inherently allergic to isolation. It cannot abide a sense of being permanently alone or stranded in all the vastness of the universe or lost in the midst of the complexities of personal experience.

—*Howard Thurman,* The Creative Encounter, *p. 31*

## Human Biology and Communion

You and I are bound together as fellow persons. We are connected through our genes, through our history, and by being born and nurtured in a human family. Human life is in its very essence interdependent, for "mutual interdependence is characteristic of all of life" (Thurman, 1971, p. 3). If this were not so, you and I would not know grief, and there would be no dramas and rites of mourning.

The need to care for and the need to be cared for is another expression of the same idea. It is unnecessary to resort to moral or religious authority for a mandate or for injunction. Such needs are organic, whatever may be their psychological or spiritual derivatives. Therefore, whenever the individual is cut off from the private and personal nourishment of other individuals or

249

from particular individuals, the result is a wasting away, a starvation, a failure of his life to be sustained and nourished. (Thurman, 1971, p. 3)

The grieving process that follows our separation from important others is a normal, human response. It is neither neurotic nor pathological. The fear and trembling following a separation from a significant person is appropriate because the separation does constitute a primary threat to our lives. Much of our psychology has been tightly focused on a person's mind, with far less emphasis on the influence on behavior of the transactions *between* people.

The ethos or dominant urge of Western culture is toward self-sufficiency or autarchy—while denying or suppressing the fact of personal, familial, communal, and even national dependence and interdependence. The very word *dependence* has come to imply pathological behavior. We are carefully tutored in this myth of the self-sustaining system where nothing need come in or go out. Judgments about what is the appropriate expression of grief come out of that unchallenged cultural norm: "She's taking it well, isn't she," means that she is showing no expression of pain or anguish following the death of someone she loves. This cultural denial of our essential relatedness to our human (and natural) environment has now to give way to the facts of our biology.

Our actual survival as human beings is directly dependent upon our being "attached" or "bonded" to other human beings. Among adult populations, this fact can now be demonstrated through epidemiological studies such as Berkman and Syme's examination (1979) of Alameda County, California, in 1966–1967. But the most potent support for this assertion is evident in the care of young children who do not have a close relationship with a mother figure who cares for and nurtures them. Such children will waste away and die in a very short order for no "apparent" reason (Spitz, 1945). This strongly suggests to me that there is an *"x* factor" called *caring, relatedness,* or *love,* without which isolated human adults or children will languish and be more likely to die than their bonded fellows. John Bowlby, in his pioneering three-volume work, *Attachment and Loss* (1969–1980), has shown that separation, especially between children and their parents "is dangerous and whenever possible should be avoided" (Vol. 2, p. 22).

The grief process on the biological level is an adaptive reaction genetically imposed on us individually to insure the survival needs of the species. As we isolate ourselves, we pine and pain; when we come together, we feel secure and confident. If this were not so, we would not have survived as a species, since the human "cub" is the most defenseless of young animals. Human beings are made to be in relation, to be bonded with each other. When these bonds are severed or strained, we become distressed and we grieve. We experience ourselves as being whole when we feel that we belong to someone in particular.

The human spirit cannot abide isolation, the sense of being permanently alone or stranded. Social bonding is so essential that without it, our life expectancy diminishes and our potential increases for the harmful health consequences associated with stressful living. As noted earlier, Berkman and Syme (1979) studied the relationship between mortality and social and community ties in a large population for 9 years and found that

> people who lacked social and community ties were more likely to die in the follow up period than those with more extensive contacts. The association between social ties and mortality was found to be independent of self-reported physical health status at the time of the . . . survey, year of death, social-economic status, and health practices such as smoking, alcoholic beverage consumption, obesity, physical activity, and utilization of preventive health services, as well as a cumulative index of health practices. (p. 186)

It appears that we were created to be in relation to each other. Relatedness, communion, or fellow personhood is nature's norm. If that is so, then a process of grief that follows the ending of the relation is a natural response. Let us now look more closely at the grief process itself.

## Grief's Journey

Jesus, in his Sermon on the Mount, taught "Blessed are they that mourn, for they shall be comforted." The meaning of that statement can easily escape us. In my own bereavement for people who have died and for others whom I have left behind as I moved on to other cities, I have not experienced a "blessedness." My experience, like that of my friends and family around me, was more one of "cursed" suffering. Let us look more deeply into the meaning of that statement. *Blessed* in modern currency has come to mean "happy." As a matter of fact, one modern translation of the New Testament renders *blessed* in just that way. But if we take *blessed* in its traditional sense to mean "highly favored of God," and the word *comforted* to mean "recover," the Biblical statement then speaks to bereavement behavior as we know it. "Blessed are they that mourn, for they shall be comforted," can be restated, "Highly favored are they that mourn, for they shall recover."

There is a typical set of psychological and physiological reactions to a traumatic loss that most people experience and display. The loss may be real or fantasized, but as long as it is sufficient to create a persistent inter-ference with our basic daily patterns of life, and is disruptive to the extent that it cannot be managed in our usual way of going about business, this typical grief pattern or syndrome follows. We can allow the process to travel its course, or we can try to suppress it. Engaging the mourning pro-cess promises recovery. Trying to resist this process can create physical and psychological illness. I have more to say about what helps the process a little later on. In the meantime, it is important to begin with the realiza-tion that the grief process is a gift from God, a given of our natural endow-ment, which promises us that no matter how painful our loss and deep our suffering, we can recover.

I see the bereavement process as a journey, a passage, a rite encoded into our biological and psychological makeup that moves us from the traumatic ending of one life stage into another. Geoffrey Gorer, an English anthropologist, writes: "Typically, a mourner goes through . . . a *rite de passage*—a formal withdrawal from society, a period of seclusion, and a formal reentry into society" (Gorer, 1967, p. xxxiii). The rite of passage as seen by the anthropologist begins with the person's being disengaged from the social order and experiencing a symbolic death. In the second phase, "the person must wait for a time in the nowhere between what was and what will be, in the gap, in emptiness; third, the person is born anew, as-sumes new roles and relations, and returns to the social order as a funda-mentally different person" (Bridges, 1977, p. 32). We do not just break a significant relationship and move on to "business as usual"—which is the popular expectation about grief. When someone important to us dies, something in us that was part of the other person dies too. We then go through a series of ordeals, trials, and sufferings, and a bone-crushing loneliness until the body and mind, it seems, can hold on no longer and we let go. Frightened to emptiness by our ordeals, refined by our anger's emo-tional fire, we feel the tentative stirrings of new birth. And we make new relationships and a new life. This is an ageless passage as old as the human race, as old as death, suffering, birth, and rebirth. It is in living this drama of passage that we grow in spiritual stature and become more human. Grief is a passage, a growth process.

Bereavement behavior—grief and mourning—is frequently ap-proached by outsiders from the perspective of mental illness. Even though lip service is often given to bereavement being a "normal" process, writings on grief tend to emphasize the aspects of grieving that *look like* pathological behavior. But expressions of anguish, depression, hostility, excitement, and guilt, as well as immobilizations and lethargy, following a major loss are *not* psychopathology. If these expressions were part of an ongoing pattern of living, that is, if they were enduring characteristics of one's life style, that would be another matter. There is a vast difference between depressive behavior that maintains an ongoing need to avoid social interaction, and the depressive response to a death that allows the bereaved person time to reintegrate and to achieve the wholeness that became broken by death.

Most people, about 80% to 90%, move through grief to recovery in a satisfactory manner within 2 to 4 years following the death. I believe that each of us could move through our grief, doing our grief work far more effectively, if we had an understanding of the process and of what facilitates it. Fewer people would then develop chronic psychological and physiological health problems. On the individual level, the natural and automatic grief response keeps us from pining away and dying when a loved person separates from us or dies. It moves us forward in our grief work to (1) complete the process of separation from the dead person; (2) readjust our living space and activities to the absence of the person; and (3) move toward reviving existing relationships and making new investments in other people.

Before I go on to discuss a model of bereavement as a growth process, I would like to clarify what I mean when I use the words *grief, mourning,* and *bereavement. Grief* refers to the characteristic pattern of psychological and physiological responses a person makes following the death of a significant person. *Mourning* is the behavior that is socially prescribed following the death of someone close. Patterns of mourning behavior vary from culture to culture, but the grief process is part of our human biology and is, therefore, a fairly consistent pattern among peoples. Mourning is conventional bereavement behavior. *Bereavement behavior* refers to a person's total response pattern, involving mental responses, somatic responses, and social interactions.

The grief passage normally involves a number of transitions. I have divided them into five phases. They are shock, work, emptiness, commitment, and recovery. As Figure 19.1 indicates, these five phases in some ways parallel the five stages set down by Elisabeth Kübler-Ross (1969) for coping with dying, but not exactly. In Figure 19.1, there are several parallel metaphors for the grief process and a line (C) indicating a time span of 2 years, the average minimum length of time for a grief resolution. Remember that this presentation is a typical or generalized picture of the grief process. No one grieves in quite the same identical way or for the same length of time, but there are common tendencies—and these are what is represented here. Line A is a span indicating the anthropologist's rite of passage, going from death through suffering to rebirth. Line B is an adaptation of

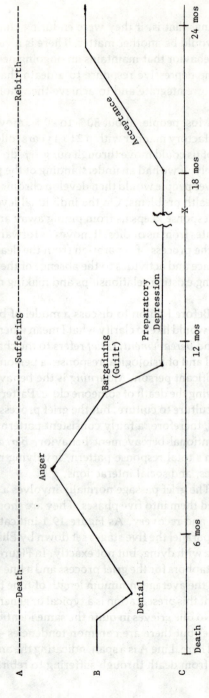

Figure 19.1.   Elmu's Journey: The Ross-Imara Bereavement Growth Curve

| | I. SHOCK | II. WORK | III. EMPTINESS | IV. COMMITMENT | V. RECOVERY |
|---|---|---|---|---|---|
| D | Disbelief<br>Cold feeling<br>Numb<br>Dazed<br>Empty<br>Confused | Anger<br>Guilt<br>Obsessional review<br>Search for meaning of death<br>Search for deceased | End of mental and physical struggle<br>Feeling spent, disorganized<br>Selective attention, disinterested<br>Life seems flat | Active will<br>Making an effort to be involved<br>Tired of feeling out of it<br>Struggling against feelings of disinterest to become involved<br>Moments of joy and happiness<br>Occasional moments of sadness. | Feeling--<br>*More aggressive<br>*Stronger<br>*More capable<br>*Amazed at own recovery<br>*Acquiring new skills<br>*Sense of competency<br>*Self confidence |
| E | EMOTIONAL & PHYSICAL REACTIONS<br><br>Crying<br>Conflicted feelings<br>Fear of emotional breakdown<br>Sighing<br>Empty feelings in abdomen<br>Sleeplessness<br>Irritability<br>Aches and pains<br>Lethargy<br>Headaches<br>Decreased symptoms<br>Tightness in throat<br>Visitations<br>Menstrual Irregularity<br>Shortness of breath | | | | |

my earlier plotting of Elisabeth Kübler-Ross's five stages as a growth curve (Imara, 1975, p. 161). Line D represents the usual sequence within the grief process and some common experiences in each phase.

What I am trying to do is to present a picture of what frequently happens to someone following the death of an important person in his or her life, such as a husband, wife, or close relative. This picture is meant to be descriptive and explanatory, to give insight into our own human grieving process. It is not prescriptive in the sense of being a criterion for "good" grief. Carl Jung has some wise words of caution about theories: "Learn your theories as well as you can, but put them aside when you touch the miracle of the living soul" (Jung, 1954, p. 7). A theory can apply to many people in all of its aspects, but it may touch on individual experiences only in a few places. This is but a very rough map for the challenging journey that will be thrust upon most of us somewhere on our path between birth and death.

## Phases of the Grief Process

### Shock

We cannot prepare ourselves for it. We may have been waiting for weeks or months, but when labored breathing stops and that leaden stillness comes to the person who is no more, we shriek aloud or silently, "No, it can't be!" The anticipation may have been long, but the finality of the actual death commonly deals us a crushing blow.

For the first several days or sometimes a week or two, we do not feel the blow. We feel numb, dazed, empty, confused, or have no sense of any feelings at all.

> It feels like being mildly drunk, or concussed. There is a sort of invisible blanket between the world and me. I find it hard to take in what anyone says. (Lewis, 1976, p. 1)

> Related to these circumstances, immediately following my husband's death I just stopped. Stunned beyond emotion, and unwilling to take any medication because of my pregnancy, I sat in bed or on a living room chair for hours on end—doing nothing. (Moro, 1979, p. 15)

This numbing is a natural shock absorber putting an insulation between the full force of our feelings and the conflicting ideas racing through our minds. We know the person we love is gone, and yet we don't believe it. We frantically want to do something, but we feel paralyzed, frozen. This initial period of natural avoidance is necessary and inevitable. It should be lived through without well-meaning attempts to "break through" to face reality. If immediately following the death the reality of the magnitude of our loss were to become strongly figural, it might be more than our systems could stand, and it could result in lasting damage. For example, a young woman felt concerned about not being able to cry for several days following her husband's death. She went to an introductory encounter group program and was there confronted until her protective veil cracked. The intense guilt and remorse following the session was so great that she had to be hospitalized for fear that she would take her life.

The shock and denial will open in its own time and should not be forced. It needs to be experienced fully. If we are numb, we should feel numb; if we feel like being quiet and sitting, we should do so. Sometimes we try to fight our shock with excessive activities; we keep going at full tilt, trying to avoid the unpleasant feelings of numbness or confusion. This "evasive preoccupation" can be very costly. We only have a finite amount of energy, and the grief process itself is draining. Impose on that a frantic schedule and something is likely to break down—our bodies, our minds, or both.

Occasionally, the raw panic of grief comes through following death before the curtain of shock can be raised. Then our initial response to the death may be to explode into a panic or rage. These episodes usually subside in a matter of minutes, and grief's natural anesthesia takes over. At moments like that, friends are likely to become upset and want to *do* something. That something often involves giving the bereaved person a sedative. However, the best sedative at those moments is someone who can be with us while remaining calm themselves.

The body has a wisdom of its own. In its own time, the veil of numbness lifts gradually and we move to the next phase of our grief "passage," the working phase. The phases of the grief process are not discrete. They tend to flow into each other with considerable overlap.

## Work

The work of grief begins when we begin to feel the fear, anger, and frustration of the assault on our minds and bodies by the death. Usually, by the end of the first month, a sense of sorrow pervades every corner of our being. We try to fend it off, but without success. The feelings come. We cry; we weep; we feel uncertain about whether to let others see our pain. We don't know whether we should be controlled around others as they tell us "how well you're handling it," or whether we should let down. We need them, we don't want to lose them, we want them around, and at the same moment we wish they would go. We begin to wonder if we are going crazy. We are so frightened of the feelings threatening to overwhelm us; the dam breaks and the anger, the fear, the body aches begin. The protective veil has lifted.

Grief work is the recognition and acceptance of the pain as part of the natural process of adjustment to a life without the deceased. The transformations are taking place in our bodies, in our minds, and in our social space. On the physical level, we frequently experience "sensations of somatic distress occurring in waves lasting from 20 minutes to an hour at a time, a feeling of tightness in the throat, choking with shortness of breath, need for sighing, an empty feeling in the abdomen, lack of muscular power . . . " (Lindemann, 1944, p. 141). These physical symptoms with accompanying mental distress can be brought on by the mere mention of the person, and quite naturally, we try to avoid such thoughts, hoping that we will not experience the distress. But the painful process is helpful to us. The death of a spouse is one of the most stressful events in our life. These episodes of distress are the means whereby we are able to release the pent-up pressures, thereby reducing our inner tensions. Drugs should not be used routinely just to relieve the distressing symptoms. Grief work needs to be done for healthy recovery.

Sleeplessness, which next to weight loss is the most disturbing symptom, is seldom severe enough to warrant the use of sleep-inducing drugs. Usually when people say that they are not sleeping, what they mean is that they are sleeping irregularly, but they are getting enough sleep to maintain themselves. There are occasions when we are close to exhaustion and need a night or two of drug-assisted sleep to restore ourselves. But pills should not become a habit for regular sleeping.

Much of our problem in coping with the mental anguish of grief comes from our lack of understanding about it and our consequent unpreparedness for the experience. The greatest stresses are those that we do not anticipate.

Grief is fundamentally a biological adaptive reaction to loss that is imposed on us by our very genes. The consequent anguish does not depend on our "ideas" about the loss. "Grief may occur in relative independence of higher mental processes. That is, the bereaved may not always expect or understand the potency of his reactions" (Averill, 1968, p. 738). We seldom expect our reactions to the loss to be as strong as they usually are, and we are often surprised by strong feelings of anger and guilt. The strong, unpleasant feelings are there, often much stronger than our feelings of connection before death to the deceased. They include blaming God, the doctors, a work environment, and even ourselves for what we could have or should have done or not done. This is our attempt to make sense of powerful feelings. Feelings come before meaning; we first feel our situations and then attempt to comprehend them by labeling. If adrenalin is high in my bloodstream and someone nearby is acting in an angry, aggressive manner, I will feel anger. If, on the other hand, I am at a party with music and happy voices, I will experience my adrenalin rush as a high or euphoria. Much of the guilt of grief is a product of using an interpretation of self-blame to make sense out of the impersonal, biologically triggered suffering.

This irrational blaming, a normal part of grief, can become a serious problem when two people in the house are grieving at the same time. We see this most often after the death of a child. Two grieving people are seldom able to be supportive of each other in their pain without assistance from a third party not in grief. Couples will find reasons why the other is to blame for the death of the child. When added to the already existing guilt and anguish, this is usually too much to bear, and they end up separating within 2 years of the child's death. Couples who lose a child should try to get professional help if their relationship is not weathering the strain of family grief. Men are usually the parties most resistant to outside help, and yet they often are the first to move toward separation.

During the working phase of grief, we are mentally trying to hold on to the dead person. We review in our minds, sometimes continuously, our experiences with the deceased. We may talk to the person, forgetting that he or she is not there.

> I knew Martin was dead, but somehow it took a long time for the reality to seep in, become part of me. I would go to the supermarket and think, "Oh, they have endive today. I'd better get some. Martin likes it so much." I would pick out an avocado for him, a fruit I've never really liked. Then I would realize, "My God! He is dead!" and put the avocado back as if it were burning me. (Caine, 1974, p. 101)

On occasion we may even "see" the person in a favorite chair or doing a familiar task. I have never known one of these "seeing" experiences to be upsetting to the bereaved. They usually produce feelings of reassurance. The deceased during the first year is seldom ever out of mind very long.

This work phase is a time of disorganization where the bereaved is required to go through the daily routine without the deceased. Many of the friends who were available to us as a couple are no longer there. They are frequently as unavailable to us as we are to them. New presenting demands, new economic conditions all contribute to the general confusion. There is no cure except to manage as best we can while keeping other major changes to a minimum. During this first period of grief we tend to make poor judgments, so decisions such as selling major investments, moving, or changing jobs should be done only with considerable caution and competent consultation. Children desperately need as stable a situation as possible following the death of a parent.

As we suffer the loss of a spouse or a child we ask the question, "Why did he die?"/"Why did she die?" again and again. It is helpful to know the actual circumstances and causes of the death, but even if we know, the question "Why?" is always there. I saw a woman holding the head of her dead husband as she softly intoned "Why?" like a ritual prayer. I had the urge to try to give her an answer, but I knew that was not what was needed. Months later at home she was still weaving that "why" into her conversation with me. We search for the meaning of the death—but there is no answer, except the living through the process itself to recovery. The death of a child or an adult has a natural explanation, but we experience it as a cosmic slap and we want to know why we were so badly treated.

*Emptiness*

The struggle to remain who we were when the deceased was with us comes to an end. We still think about the person often, and there are periods of intense painful recall, but they come and go. At this point, life may be going along rather well. The children are adjusting to school, and we may have taken steps toward a new career. But that is all on the surface. Deep down there is a feeling of being nowhere and going nowhere. Life seems flat and tasteless, but tolerable. We may attend a meeting only to find that we can't remember what someone has just said to us, and what's more, we don't particularly care. At times we will forget why life is so tasteless and depressing—and then remember, "Oh yes, he died."

> I see the rowan berries reddening and don't know for a moment why they, of all things, should be depressing. I hear a clock strike and some quality it always had before has gone out of the sound. What's wrong with the world to make it so flat, shabby, worn-out-looking? Then I remember. (Lewis, 1976, pp. 40–41)

*Commitment*

This sense of being no one, nowhere, and generally out of tune remains for several months or many years. But there comes a point, often in the middle of the second year following the death, when we realize and say to our friends that we are tired of feeling out of it, the way we have been feeling, and we begin to make an effort to be involved. We struggle against our lack of interest. While we may feel like calling up to cancel that dinner engagement, we bite the bullet and go. At first, we feel as though we are just going through the motions in our new involvements. But now and then we catch ourselves laughing a real laugh, having a good time. We are on the way.

There will be moments when our eyes will fill with tears. "My God, won't it ever end?" we say. But the grief is enduring. We are walking the final stretch of our passage. Although we may feel moments of sadness with tears, the physical and mental anguish of the early days are gone.

When the pain subsides and we are no longer so totally involved in our own pity, we are ready to reinvest in new relationships. We have something to give again. The work is finished and we are ready to cross the threshold from suffering to rebirth. We will always feel connected to our dead loved one. The bereavement process only detaches those bonds from the dead that keep us from making new attachments. Much of the treasures, the remembered joys and painful learnings that were shared, remain.

*Recovery*

We made it, but we never thought we would. We feel as though we have been saved for something special, that life has a special purpose for us. We are saying "yes" to life. We stand confidently with a sense of quiet amazement at our own recovery. We are energized, but unlike the energy of our long passage, it is free to flow in directions we choose instead of being squeezed painfully through a narrow channel in our soul. We are new people. We feel new. There will be occasional brief periods of flashback when the old feelings are played over again like old tapes. (Remember, they are *old* tapes.)

# Factors Influencing the Duration and Intensity of Grief

On the bereavement growth curve chart (Figure 19.1), I have given a 2-year span to the average bereavement. While a great many people do resolve their grief along the lines of that chart, many others take much longer, and an occasional few resolve their grief earlier. The period of intense mourning is frequently a year or a little less, but there are people in normal grief who have spent 3 or 4 years passing through these phases. The model is a general statement of what often happens, a statistical depiction that *cannot* apply without variation to each individual. Still, it does have value as a broad guideline to the key elements of the process.

The intensity and duration of the grief passage is determined by a host of factors, including our relation to the deceased (whether the deceased is a member of our immediate family or a distant relative or friend); our adult and childhood experiences with loss; the degree of material and emotional dependence on the person; our ages; the nature of the dying process (whether it was sudden or prolonged); the condition of the body (whether it was disfigured); the whereabouts of the body (whether it was reclaimed, as from an accident or war zone, or is still missing); suicide as a factor; the quality of our relationship just prior to death; the circumstances of the death (whether it was a result of carelessness or was inevitable); our need to hide our feelings; social support; opportunities opened or closed by the death; religious beliefs; and other life crises prior to death. All these factors and more determine the duration and intensity of grief that a particular individual experiences (Bowlby, 1969–1980, Vol. 3, pp. 174–196; Parkes, 1972, p. 121).

The grief process is normal. Most of us manage to traverse it without becoming stuck along the way. However, should we find that the intensity of our experience keeps us from functioning for extended periods of time or causes us to feel more than we can bear, professional consultation is indicated. How long grief lasts depends also on how well the grief work is done—that is, on how well we have been able to live with and adjust to the new realities that death has brought while allowing the pain to be pain. This is hard, almost impossible to do alone. We need the support of a *caring friend* who is not dealing with his or her own grief at the moment.

## Kara: I Will Sorrow with You—I Care

Because most people are not accustomed to having others express their grief in their presence, they often respond with alarm to their first encounter with the power of those emotions. The first impulse is to send the grieving person to the nearest professional therapist. However, most of us can and do move through our grief on our own, without professional intervention. The road is easier if there is someone who will care for us by (1) helping us keep a check on our reality frames—for example, asking us the right questions when we plan to sell the house, put the kids in boarding school, and take a trip around the world; (2) supporting our need to express our pain— to cry if we wish, talk about the deceased, go over the story of the death again and again, call on the telephone at night in panic or wretched loneliness, or disclose those crazy-sounding fantasies; and (3) standing by while we attempt to make meaning out of our madness—for example, assuring us that because we go out with someone, we are not unfaithful, or that we are really not a jinx even though we feel like one after having two husbands die on us.

A caring friend can be of inestimable value in helping us get through the first major holiday without the loved one. It is hard to understand if a person has never experienced it. As a hospice family member once said to me,

> Everything was OK until the kids went to bed leaving me alone with my memories of the little rituals we celebrated together past Christmas Eves; wrapping gifts, having a drink together . . . it was so painful . . . I thought I couldn't bear it and the telephone rang and D_____ was on the phone. I was able to go to bed after we talked. I cried and I felt much better.

Care allows grief to move through the rough spots without getting bogged down. We really need support after the first month when the practical matters of funeral and burial are over. As Lawrence Lanzissero, a bereaved parent, remarks in the movie *When a Child Dies*, "it's the aftershock . . . when you get back home and everything is over . . . then you need someone. And everybody just seems to disappear and go back to living their own normal lives." We cannot and will not ask others to call, but are happy to get the call, although we may not realize it or be able to tell them so at the time. Grief work keeps us busy; we don't even think of a "thank you." Friends go to listen to us in their grief because they care. Their reward comes many months later when they witness the radiant transformation of the journey completed. "The word 'care' finds its roots in the Gothic 'Kara' which means lament. The basic meaning of care is to grieve, to experience sorrow, to cry out with" (Nouwen, 1974, pp. 33–34).

I have found that the nonprofessional makes a better support person for the bereaved than the professional in normal grief situations. It is easy for the trained eye to find pathology in every word and deed of the bereaved. Normal grief can look very biazarre. We often look and sound morbidly depressed, but the last thing we need is an antidepressant or an intervention calculated to "mobilize" our frozen energy. Our sensations are often so distorted during grief that our report of our experience can sound like that of a borderline psychotic person in the process of decompensating into psychosis. Most of us experience these distortions with intense grief, yet few of us have any undesirable aftereffects unless we are inappropriately supported. Clearly there are instances where the duration and intensity of the bereaved's experience suggests intervention, but the existence of morbid grief cannot *always* be assumed. Very few people find their grief to be so abnormal as to be incapacitating or to require institutional treatment. Yet many cases of normal grief are inappropriately overtreated by drug therapy or hospitalization.

The lay person does not see many of the "symptoms" and puts most of his or her efforts into relating to the grieving person as a friend and peer, giving the bereaved a sense of being heard, of companionship—just what grief needs. Besides, these "friends" are usually more available at odd hours than the professional therapist is.

Many professionals have psychologized the normal and made natural human behavior sound sick. Within very broad limits, to be dependent on someone is a normal healthy state. Yet the mere mention of dependency, to many of us, suggests mental illness. Feelings of religious surrender are given such pathological interpretations that we would rather say that we "meditated" than "prayed" for fear of being labeled as religious freaks. People have been dying, survivors have been acting out the drama of grief's readiness, and friends have been giving support to their bereaved neighbors since the dawn of the species. But this century has forgotten how to care, so it calls the normal "sick." At our hospice, we visit the bereaved as friends, informed about grief of course, but more concerned with meeting and getting to know the person and not the symptoms.

> I share with you the agony of your grief, the anguish of your heart finds echo in my own. I know I cannot enter all you feel nor bear with you the burden of your pain;
>
> I can but offer what my love does give: the strength of caring, the warmth of one who seeks to understand the silent storm-swept barrenness of so great a loss.
>
> This I do in quiet ways, that on your lonely path you may not walk alone. (Thurman, 1953, pp. 211–212)

# References

Averill, J. R., "Grief: Its Nature and Significance," *Psychological Bulletin*, 1968, 70, 721–748.

Berkman, L. F., & Syme, S. L., "Social Networks, Host Resistance, and Mortality: A Nine-Year Follow-up Study of Alameda County Residents," *American Journal of Epidemiology*, 1979, 109, 186–204.

Bowlby, J., *Attachment and Loss* (3 vols.). New York: Basic Books, 1969–1980.

Bridges, W., *The Seasons of Our Lives*. Rolling Hills Estates, CA: Wayfarer Press, 1977.

Caine, L. *Widow*. New York: William Morrow, 1974.

Gorer, G., *Death, Grief, and Mourning: A Study of Contemporary Society*. New York: Anchor, 1967.

Imara, M., "Dying as the Last Stage of Growth," in E. Kübler-Ross (Ed.), *Death: The Final Stage of Growth*. Englewood Cliffs, NJ: Prentice-Hall, 1975, 147–163.

Jung, C. G., *The Collected Works of C. G. Jung* (H. Read et al., Eds.) (Vol. 17, *The Development of Personality*). Princeton, NJ: Princeton University Press, 1954.

Kübler-Ross, E., *On Death and Dying*. New York: Macmillan, 1969.

Lewis, C. S., *A Grief Observed*. New York: Bantam, 1976.

Lindemann, E., "Symptomatology and Management of Acute Grief," *American Journal of Psychiatry*, 1944, 101, 141–148.

Moro, R., *Death, Grief, and Widowhood*. Berkeley, CA: Parallax Press, 1979.

Nouwen, H. J. M., *Out of Solitude*. Notre Dame, IN: Ave Maria Press, 1974.

Parkes, C. M., *Bereavement: Studies of Grief in Adult Life*. New York: International Universities Press, 1972.

Spitz, R. A., "Hospitalism: An Inquiry Into the Genesis of Psychiatric Conditions in Early Childhood," in *Psychoanalytic Study of the Child* (Vol. 1). New York: International Universities Press, 1945, 53–74.

Thurman, H. *Meditations of the Heart*. New York: Harper & Row, 1953.

Thurman, H., *The Search for Common Ground*. New York: Harper & Row, 1971.

Thurman, H., *The Creative Encounter*. Richmond, IN: Friends United Press, 1972.

# 20

# Operating a Hospice Bereavement Program

*Bonnie Lindstrom*

## Philosophy and Goals

The ultimate goal of any hospice bereavement program is to assist families in their acceptance of and coping with the loss or death of a loved one. Why do this at all? In setting up bereavement programs, some assumptions are made from the relatively little data that is available. One fundamental principle that seems to underlie hospice work in general is that improving care for dying persons and their families before the death occurs is likely to have a positive influence upon its aftermath. Even though we do not know a great deal about the phenomenon of anticipatory grief itself or about its relationship to postdeath grieving, some careful analyses are beginning to appear (e.g., Fulton & Gottesman, 1980), and we believe that the former facilitates the latter.

Specifically, the phrase *preventive mental health* would seem to be applicable to hospice bereavement programs. Certainly, those who have worked in psychiatry can testify that many of their clients are dealing with the emotionally painful scars of past losses. A bereavement program, while not attempting to remove the pain of loss, can ameliorate the profound guilt, anger, and stress that individuals face while coping with the loss of a significant person in their lives. It may be hoped that this will improve quality of life in the present and prevent some long-term deleterious effects on mental and physical health in the future. It must be said, however, that hospice bereavement support is not a treatment program. Short-term individual counseling is available from the professionally trained

266

members of the bereavement team, but when intensive psychotherapy is appropriate, either for preexisting problems or for pathological grief reactions, a referral must be made to private psychiatry or mental health services.

One of the principles inherent in hospice care is that the whole family is to be cared for, not only the patient. Over and over again, I have seen how helping families and patients talk openly together prior to death can promote peace, dignity, and comfort for the whole family. It naturally follows, then, that a relationship with the family must look toward and continue into the bereavement period.

What are we actually doing when we offer support to a bereaved person or family? I believe there are four major goals that any bereavement program should address:

1. *Feeling the hurt.* Encouraging the individual to "feel" the pain or grief, working with it and not against it. When the pain is faced it becomes less fearful. The hurt is necessary to the recovery.

2. *Facing reality.* Assisting the bereaved person to engage in the process that Colin Murray Parkes (1970) has called "realization." This entails making real in one's inner life what has already come about in the external world. It also means that the bereavement counselor must act as a reality base, assisting with some of the day-to-day problems a bereaved person faces (e.g., problems involving finances, social relationships, possible relocation). Most often, this depends upon having appropriate resources and referral sources at hand.

3. *Achieving a positive memory.* Helping in the creation of a positive memory of the lost person. This most often occurs through talking about "the good times and the bad times," looking at old picture albums, "remembering" with other family members, and so forth. It is important to allow bereaved persons to talk and remember, even if they become repetitive. This is necessary to the process of resolution.

4. *Gaining a sense of meaning.* Aiding a bereaved family member spiritually so that he or she may gain a sense of purpose and meaning in life itself. We want to acknowledge that the relationship was important and that what was can never truly be lost. The aim is to help the bereaved person reach an understanding of the meaningfulness of the dead person's life and of how that life may have touched others in positive ways.

## Program Development

When should a hospice bereavement program intervene? Bereavement programs in hospices should intervene at the time of the initial referral interview. Because of the nature of hospice work, time is of the essence in assessing and meeting patients' and families' emotional and spiritual needs. "Now" is the time for "efficient" counseling, because by "tomorrow" the patient may have died. Intervention in the anticipatory phase of bereavement, as stated previously, can have a profound effect on an individual's coping after the death.

The following paragraphs outline elements of a bereavement program in the anticipatory and postdeath phases.

### Anticipatory Phase

Funeral and estate planning should be dealt with as soon as possible, usually in the referral interview with the family. This frequently means encouraging families to talk openly about something they have all thought about already. If appropriate, the patient may even be brought into these discussions. To deal with this subject early is frequently difficult, even for professionals, but if it is opened up tactfully, families are almost always grateful and relieved. For example, we might say, "I know this is a painful subject, but one I am sure you've thought about." Of course, we must be sensitive to those families who have difficulty even coming to a hospice, much less talking about funeral planning.

Taking care of "unfinished business" simply means resolving those issues that have caused anxiety and conflict in the family unit. It can mean facilitating the return home of a close relative for one last visit, or perhaps a mutual forgiveness for things that happened in the past. For some, it means reaching a spiritual sense of peace. Often it just involves saying "good-bye" and "I love you" to one another.

To accomplish the above in the anticipatory phase, individual sessions, as well as family and group sessions, are helpful. The frequency of these depends upon individual needs, but each family should have at least one contact per week. In our program in Tucson, family group sessions with an emphasis on helping families to support one another are held once per week. Attendance varies considerably, depending on the current needs of families in the program. Spiritually, an afternoon prayer group led by the chaplain is supportive and meaningful to many families.

At all times, it is important to assess high-risk factors in families.

This will assist in planning family intervention in the postdeath phase of bereavement. I will discuss these high-risk factors later on in the chapter.

## Postdeath Phase

In our bereavement program, we have decided that a minimum of five contacts will be made with families within the course of the first 13 months after the death of the patient. These include the following:

1. *Funeral.*   Attendance at the funeral always makes a firm statement of continuity to the family: The hospice still cares. It sets the tone for further follow-up. The person attending the funeral might be a nurse who had cared for the deceased individual or a member of the bereavement team who is supporting the family.
2. *First month.*   A personal home visit during the first month, usually after other family members and friends have withdrawn, is helpful in assessing the style of the griever. It allows the bereaved person needed time to ventilate, discussing and perhaps sharing again the events leading up to the death and through the funeral. This is also a time for education and guidance about what might be expected in the next few months. Referrals to other appropriate community resources may be helpful (e.g., legal aid or widow-to-widow groups).
3. *Third month and sixth month.*   At the third month and the sixth month, phone contacts are made, primarily for a friendly hello and assessment. If there is any question as to how a family member is coping, a home visit is made. We have noted clinically that during this period many people experience a "letdown" or depression, which we feel is related to an affective confronting of the loss and pain at that time.
4. *Thirteenth month.*   At 13 months, a final home visit is made to assist the family in gaining a sense of perspective and insight into what they have experienced during that initial year of bereavement. If there are unresolved or long-term issues requiring further counseling, appropriate referrals are made.

A survivors' group is an additional source of strength and support. Typically, this sort of group meets on a weekly, biweekly, or monthly basis. It is usually facilitated by members of the bereavement team, but in reality is run by the survivors themselves, who will have set up a telephone network and will plan dinners and other social events on their own.

A continuation of the spiritual dimension of hospice care can add to the bereavement program. For example, a monthly memorial service might be held by the hospice to honor those who have died during the previous month. Friends and families can be invited back for this service. Followed by a social gathering, this brings families and staff together again for further sharing and support.

At any time, should additional contacts or sessions be indicated or requested by a family, these are provided. If the problem is rooted in more serious psychological difficulties, a referral is made to skilled professionals within the hospice team or to private and community mental health agencies.

## High-Risk Assessment

Families can be assessed for their probability in having a greater psychological and physical morbidity during the bereavement period through both objective and clinical means. In our program, we have not used objective data in determining families at high risk. Other hospices do employ objective tests such as the Holmes-Rahe stress scale to assist in identifying high risk.

To determine high-risk families clinically, we look at the following variables:

1. *Reactions and coping styles to previous losses.* This would include numbers of losses and timing of their occurrence. A wife whose husband died in the hospice program had lost her son 2 years previously. This had a profound impact on her coping with her husband's death. She had never accepted the loss of her son, and was only beginning to do so now through the loss of her husband.
2. *Dysfunctional family relationships.* These are families in which either one spouse is completely passive and dependent on the other, or one exerts an angry controlling influence on the family. We are all familiar with these kinds of relationships. Serious adjustment problems can also occur when spouses are so mutually dependent on each other that other supportive outside relationships are excluded. Additionally, experience has taught us that in

marriages that have endured over 50 years, the surviving spouse is at high risk. Truly, in these instances, it is more than difficult for the one remaining to survive such a loss.

3. *Support that the bereaved person receives from family and community.* The amount and quality of this support is quite important in determining high risk. In the anticipatory phase, it is crucial to assess where the family gets its support and what supports can be mobilized. This includes learning where children live and how to reach them. It means learning who the friendly neighbors are. Church and organizational affiliations can also be extremely helpful in times of need.

4. *The personal style of the survivor.* This will also often determine how many supports are available. Did the family members tend to isolate themselves, or did they reach out to others in the community? In our clinical experience, those with greatest outside supports have tended to reintegrate themselves into a meaningful life with fewest problems. Those families with extreme anger and hostility in the anticipatory phase have rarely done well in the postdeath stage of bereavement. Indeed, one of the most angry and hostile spouses I have worked with died 3 months after his wife's death.

5. *Denial.* Another keynote to a high-risk bereavement period is extreme denial. This kind of denial is so strong that the spouse or other family member has difficulty visiting the hospice and refuses to discuss the possibility of death with the hospice staff. Of three examples that come to mind, one husband refused to tell his friends for several weeks that his wife had died, and secluded himself from everyone but his daughter. Another wife has joined an extreme religious sect and withdrawn from family and friends. And in one final instance, a husband became an alcoholic and eventually died.

## Who Should Receive Bereavement Follow-Up in Hospice?

Several hospices have opted to provide bereavement support only to those families identified as at high risk. This does make sense in light of the large number of families that might be included in any hospice bereavement program that has been in operation over a year. Nevertheless, we in Tucson have attempted to follow all families. This, as I discuss later, poses many problems. However, we have found that brief interventions can have a profound effect in lessening anxiety and stress in those not identified as high-risk survivors.

Interestingly, a study conducted by Colin Murray Parkes (1975, 1977, 1979) at St. Christopher's Hospice in London suggests that intervention of the hospice bereavement team does not significantly lower the incidence of morbidity and mortality of those survivors identified as at high risk. The discussion above of our experience in Tucson would seem to support that conclusion. However, clinical evidence and subjective statements by survivors demonstrate that intervention and support during bereavement can have a profound effect on the quality of grief and, indirectly, on the morbidity and mortality of survivors not at high risk. Further research in this area is needed.

## Staffing a Hospice Bereavement Program

Ideally, direction of the bereavement team should be the responsibility of one key family-service-oriented staff member in the hospice program. This person could be a social worker, a counselor, a psychiatrist, a chaplain, or even a professional volunteer. I feel that this should be minimally designated as a half-time position. Other members of the team might include nurses (particularly home care nurses who may wish to follow their own families in bereavement), social workers, chaplains, volunteers, students, and a consulting psychiatrist.

Volunteers are essential to the follow-up of families in bereavement. They maintain contact with the majority of families. We have found it helpful to team a volunteer with each staff member. After the first month, the volunteer makes the family contact under the supervision of the staff member. Graduate students in counseling, social work, or related areas also make excellent bereavement team members. However, I would not suggest accepting undergraduate students, as the training and supervision they require are greater than what they can offer the program.

A consulting psychiatrist or psychologist is a must. It is not unusual for a family member to become suicidal or severely depressed, and having psychiatric consultation available within the hospice program is extremely helpful. The psychiatrist can also be useful in evaluating the need for additional referrals in unclear situations, as well as in educating the staff in appropriate techniques for intervention with specific families.

Recruitment of volunteers and students is an ongoing process. Most newspapers have sections in which volunteer advertisements can be placed. Speaking to church groups and other volunteer organizations offers an excellent source of volunteer personnel. In recruiting students, I have found it helpful to elicit the support of department heads of various counseling and psychology programs. Subsequently, I visit classes to discuss the bereavement program in our hospice. This frequently results in many students' requesting practicums and internships with the hospice program.

Selection from those volunteers and students who are interested requires an in-depth personal interview, addressing such issues as motivation, loss experiences, communication skills, and commitment. Less than a full semester's commitment from a student is not acceptable when the training and supervision required are considered, as well as continuity in the follow-up of families. For the same reasons, a minimal commitment of 6 months from volunteers is requested. Those volunteers and students being selected must be made aware that confronting the losses of others frequently will force them to review their own, perhaps unresolved, losses. These issues are explored during training sessions.

The training of staff and volunteers in bereavement should include an initial in-depth introduction to the field, as well as ongoing education in special seminars and as part of the bereavement team meetings. Specialized training in bereavement should follow an extensive orientation to hospice philosophy and practice. In our hospice, staff and volunteers receive 20 hours of orientation to the general program.

The initial bereavement course should include a balance of theory, discussion, and group exercises. A brief outline of the 14-hour program that we offer is as follows. Each session is two hours in length. Approximately half of each session includes discussion and a group exercise.

I. Introduction and Overview of the Field
II. Basic Theories of Grief and Bereavement
    A. Erich Lindemann—Symptomatology of Acute Grief (1944)
    B. Colin Murray Parkes—Defined Stages of Grief (Bowlby & Parkes, 1970; Davidson, 1979; Parkes, 1972)
III. Types of Grief
IV. Approaches to Helping the Bereaved
V. Discussion of Children and Bereavement
VI. Visit to a Mortuary
VII. General Review and Discussion/Role Playing

It must be mentioned that each time I teach the course it never seems to cover as much material or include as many opportunities for discussion or role playing as it should. It is very basic, and I view it as providing a stepping stone to further experience and education in bereavement. It is offered every 3 months, as there is a continual need for training new staff and volunteers.

## Record Keeping

Probably the most frustrating task of the bereavement team coordinator is to develop and maintain an efficient, workable record-keeping system. Accurate documentation is essential for accountability, continuity, supplying statistical data when making grant applications, and myriad other reasons.

From our experience, the following system seems to work best. On admission to the program, a 5″ × 8″ card is typed for each patient, including the following:

1. Name of patient and significant other or key person.
2. Address and telephone number.
3. Date of admission and (inserted later) date of death.
4. Family service staff member who processed the referral (facilitator).
5. Bereavement counselor.
6. Required contacts and dates when they were made.
7. Comments.

This card is placed in a loose-leaf notebook. It is kept in the front of the notebook until the patient dies. At that time, it is placed in the body of the notebook in alphabetical order. Each month, all cards are reviewed and assignments made of those requiring follow-up during that month. Following the 13th-month visit, the card becomes a part of the permanent bereavement file.

Prior to the death of the patient, documentation of each contact is recorded in the family service portion of the patient's record. Following the patient's death, the family service portion of the medical record becomes a part of the permanent bereavement file. Contacts during the period of bereavement are recorded on a simple bereavement form especially designed for this purpose. As these forms are completed, they are charted on the bereavement card and placed in the permanent file. At the 13th-month visit, we do a more extensive assessment of the family for research purposes.

A weekly bereavement team meeting is necessary for adequate coordination. At this meeting, new families are assigned to individual members of the bereavement team, and problem cases are reviewed. Families are assigned to a bereavement team member on admission in order to provide continuity through both the anticipatory and postdeath phases of the bereavement program. A part of the meeting is also set aside for educational purposes. This is helpful in improving the skills of individual team members, as well as in promoting and monitoring the interest and motivation of team members.

## Discussion of Other Program Models

As I have previously stated, each hospice must develop a program that will meet its needs and be possible within the limits of its resources. Hospice of Marin, in California, holds monthly meetings for families. Each month, 30 to 40 families attend to share and support one another. Individual counseling is offered by a marriage and family counselor, and by their medical director, who is a psychiatrist. This is on an as-needed basis. Every 6 months, Hospice of Marin holds educational seminars for families, offering material on such things as money management and theories of grief. Nurses follow up families they have cared for on an informal basis.

Boulder County Hospice, in Colorado, has a unique approach (Lattanzi & Coffelt, 1979). Following the patient's death, the hospice staff present the family history to the interdisciplinary bereavement team, who then assume the responsibility for follow-up. Members of this hospice program have found that this new relationship with the family reinforces the importance of assisting the family through grief. It also offers them the opportunity to begin a relationship that is unencumbered with any problems from a past relationship with the patient and family. The Boulder County Hospice bereavement team also offers a Bereaved Persons Group, as well as a Bereaved Parents Group.

Both of these programs are extremely effective in their communities, and they demonstrate that there are several approaches to consider when developing a hospice bereavement program.

## Problems Common to Bereavement Programs

One of the greatest problems that any hospice bereavement program will face is a rapidly increasing caseload, which can become overwhelming for members of the bereavement team if not dealt with efficiently. Generally, each staff member on the bereavement team has another role within the program, and, as responsibilities increase in their primary roles, it becomes more and more difficult to follow through on bereavement families.

It is for this reason that I recommend funding for at least a half-time to full-time position of bereavement director.

Another problem undermining the cause of bereavement programs is that funding sources often do not reimburse hospices for bereavement support. Consequently, in times of organizational crisis or monetary insufficiency, bereavement can become a low-priority program. Therefore, energy must be spent in applying for funding through grants and other resources. For this reason, as well as for those indicated above, the use of volunteers as members of the bereavement team is invaluable.

On a more concrete level, a problem facing many bereavement coordinators is deciding within what limits to provide service to families. Nurses particularly can feel totally responsible for the bereaved person. It is essential to assist staff in understanding and accepting the limits of their responsibility and in knowing when referrals to other agencies are necessary and appropriate to the family's needs.

## Experiences in a Bereavement Program

Through all the problems of developing and implementing an effective bereavement program, I feel we have learned a great deal. It is difficult to describe the feeling of closeness that grows when you are sharing one of the most intensely personal times that families experience. If we have learned anything at all, it is because our hospice families have taught us. One of the insights we have gained through our clinical experience is that somewhere between 3 and 6 months after the patient's death, there seems to come an emotional confrontation of the loss. It is a time when families usually feel they should be "getting on with things," even though they may in reality be experiencing more tears and depression—which can be frightening and immobilizing. This is usually short-lived, and, with one or two counseling sessions, their feelings improve markedly. We feel it is a necessary emotional facing of the loss.

An example of this is the experience of Ann. Ann's husband, a respected physician, died of cancer. He had been on our hospice home care program. At the time of her husband's death, Ann was her usual vivacious self, grieving but managing to keep everyone else's spirits up as well. She refused any visits from the bereavement team and busied herself with volunteer work. However, 4 months after her husband's death she called me, saying, "I think I am losing my mind." Every afternoon on her return home from volunteer work, she would spend most of the afternoon crying. I made two home visits during which Ann grieved openly, expressing much of her sadness and loneliness at losing her husband. Following this brief intervention, she began to feel better, crying less but allowing herself to cry when she needed to. She made the decision to get a job and now—months later—is really doing quite well.

## Conclusion

A bereavement program is an essential component of hospice care. What I have attempted to do here is to demonstrate one approach that can offer some alternatives in the development of bereavement programs. Hospice literature frequently attends to the problem of "burnout" and "stress" in staff who continually work with patients who are dying. Personally, I have found great hope and satisfaction in being a part of the growth that can occur when families face and cope with a profound loss.

## References

Bowlby, J., & Parkes, C. M., "Separation and Loss Within the Family," in E. J. Anthony & C. Koupernik (Eds.), *The Child in His Family*. New York: Wiley, 1970.

Davidson, G., "Hospice Care for the Dying," in H. Wass (Ed.), *Dying: Facing the Facts*. New York: McGraw-Hill/Hemisphere, 1979, 173–179.

Fulton, R., & Gottesman, D. J., "Anticipatory Grief: A Psychosocial Concept Reconsidered," *British Journal of Psychiatry*, 1980, *137*, 45–54.

Lattanzi, M., & Coffelt, D., *Bereavement Care Manual*. Boulder, CO: Boulder County Hospice, 1979.

Lindemann, E., "Symptomatology and Management of Acute Grief," *American Journal of Psychiatry*, 1944, *101*, 141–148.

Parkes, C. M., "The First Year of Bereavement: A Longitudinal Study of the Reaction of London Widows to the Death of Their Husbands," *Psychiatry*, 1970, *33*, 444–467.

Parkes, C. M., *Bereavement: Studies of Grief in Adult Life*. New York: International Universities Press, 1972.

Parkes, C. M., "Determinants of Outcome Following Bereavement," *Omega*, 1975, *6*, 303–323.

Parkes, C. M., "Evaluation of Family Care in Terminal Illness," in E. R. Prichard, J. Collard, B. A. Orcutt, A. H. Kutscher, I. Seeland, & N. Lefkowitz (Eds.), *Social Work with the Dying Patient and the Family*. New York: Columbia University Press, 1977, 49–79.

Parkes, C. M., "Evaluation of a Bereavement Service," in A. De Vries & A. Carmi (Eds.), *The Dying Human*. Ramat Gan, Israel: Turtledove, 1979, 389–402.

# V

# Implementing Hospice Principles in Various Settings

*Throughout this book, we have attempted to make clear that if hospice is a broad approach or outlook regarding care for dying persons and their families, its principles can be applied by many people in many settings. Implementation of hospice principles is not limited to units bearing that title, much less to medical institutions or professional caregivers. Hospice offers a program for helping ourselves and others as we struggle with basic experiences of life and death. Efforts to enhance quality of life should not be confined to particular circumstances or individuals. They are a responsibility and an opportunity for us all.*

*Even among health care contexts or hospice programs themselves, the diversity of possibilities for implementation is staggering. We cannot address every possibility here, nor would we be able to anticipate all of them. In the final analysis, particular individuals or groups must adapt the basic approach and principles to what is possible, needed, and appropriate in their own specific situations. Our goal in Part V is not to be comprehensive, but to illustrate three basic possibilities as a springboard for further thinking.*

*Because the hospice approach stresses an effort to permit those who can and who wish to do so to remain at home for as long as possible—even through death itself—we begin with home care programs. Claire B. Tehan offers a balanced assessment of both advantages and limitations to such programs, and of central elements in planning for and operating a hospice home care service. As Tehan recognizes, however, some dying persons or their families need the services of an inpatient facility, and the mere presence of backup beds may provide the security for many that enables them to remain longer at home. Free-standing inpatient hospice facilities have led the way in this regard, and are often the basic model that comes to mind when many think of the hospice-as-institution equivalence. But such institutions are more and more difficult to establish and to operate, and less and less likely to be the model of the future. Instead, hospice leaders are moving to rein-tegrate with the mainstream of their health care systems. In terms of in-patient facilities, this most often means a program based in some sort of hospital or medical center. Again, there are advantages and disadvan-tages—or, more precisely, important considerations to bear in mind when setting up and running such programs. These are reviewed here by Susan Grinslade and Ruth Reko.*

*Finally, a comprehensive implementation of the hospice approach should consider possibilities inherent in a day care program. In many ways, such programs are a bridge between home care and inpatient operations. More importantly, they enable many people to remain in the community who could otherwise not do so. And they combine all of the best elements of physical, psychological, social, and spiritual care that hospice represents. At this stage, few have given much attention to day care hospice programs—a fact that is a bit surprising in view of rather broad interest in geriatric day care in general. Our chapter by Eric Wilkes, Anthony G. O. Crowther, and Cyril W. K. H. Greaves de-scribes the pace-setting day unit at St. Luke's, Sheffield, England; they demonstrate both that such a program is feasible and that it can be a relatively inexpensive addition to existing hospice or other sorts of ser-vices.*

# 21

# Hospice Home Care Programs

*Claire B. Tehan*

## Introduction

The purpose of this chapter is to explore those significant aspects involved in providing hospice services to terminally ill patients and their families in their own homes. Home as a "setting" for dying is discussed in its broadest sense. Basic considerations for developing hospice home care programs are briefly presented, followed by a review of the major hospice home care models and specific operational details.

## Home as a Setting for Dying

It often comes as a surprise not only to patients and their families, but to health care professionals as well, that it is possible for patients to remain comfortably at home even while they are suffering from a terminal disease; it is even possible to die at home. Whether or not the health services are provided by a hospice team or a public health nurse, the advantages of being at home remain the same.

### Advantages

The control of pain and other symptoms (such as nausea, vomiting, constipation, diarrhea, and decubiti) that accompany a terminal disease can be managed well in the home. Hospice teams have demonstrated that through regular visits and communication, institution of pain control and bowel regimes, and instruction of patient and family, many symptoms can be prevented and/or minimized. Comfort care does not require high technology; most symptoms respond to persistent follow-through and scrupulous attention to details.

Even as death becomes imminent, a dying patient can be kept quite comfortable with simple measures: glycerine swabs and crushed ice for dry mouth, suppositories or injections for pain control, careful positioning or turning, and addressing the patient in a reassuring voice.

✳ The major advantage of the home as a place for dying is that most people prefer to remain in their own homes, amid familiar surroundings with friends or relatives. There, the patient can determine his or her own routine of when to arise, bathe, and eat, or whether or not to get dressed. Most institutions cannot tolerate the luxury of such self-determination, and the patient must conform to hospital routines and regimens. Also in the home, it is much easier to remain a participant in family life; often the patient is situated in a family room, which may be the center of activity. This helps to lessen two common fears of dying patients: the fear of being abandoned and a feeling of isolation. In addition, when the patient is at home, the family is able to participate actively in the giving of care. Many families talk of the therapeutic effect of physically tending to the needs of the dying patient. Although most families are not experienced in caring for a seriously ill person, they are eager and able to learn. The love and concern with which the family attends to the patient are of inestimable value both to the patient and the caregivers.

Another advantage of home care is the potential for economic savings to the family as well as to insurance companies. Daily hospital costs are escalating rapidly, and the average daily rate in a metropolitan area is now $400.00. In addition to the basic charge, hospitalized patients are "subjected" to myriad tests and procedures, which further escalate the costs. By contrast, visits by health care professionals, such as nurses, social workers, physical therapists, and home health aides, rarely cost more than $50.00 a visit.

*Limitations*

Obviously, there are limitations in regard to home care for the terminally ill patient. "Not everyone has a family, not all families can support this sort of care and, even among the most willing and cooperative families, physical problems demanding admission may outweigh all other considerations" (Saunders, 1978).

Caring for a dying person is not an easy job, for even through a hospice team provides 24-hour/7-day-a-week on-call coverage, the main burden falls on the family. It is a 24-hour job, with little respite. The hospice team can offer relief by providing (1) home health aides who can relieve the primary caregiver of the details of personal care (bathing, shampooing, and skin care); (2) a homemaker for light housework; and (3) volunteers to run errands or provide respite care for several hours.

Many families do not want the death to occur at home and may be frightened even to bring the patient home from the hospital. In such situations, the hospice nurse works with the members of the family, instructing them as to the signs of impending death and thereby enabling the patient to be transferred back to the hospital just before death. Although a home care program is designed to maintain a patient in the home, we must recognize the fact that death at home is not the sole measure of success. Death should occur wherever the patient and family wish. This attitude removes the family's sense of failure when a patient enters the hospital or another institution.

In reviewing the limitations of hospice care, it is safe to say that home care for terminally ill patients is not for everyone. Some families are unable to manage, while others prefer the security of the hospital. Still others need to pursue the aggressive cure-oriented treatment available only in a hospital setting. A key to the success of home care is the appropriateness of the setting for a particular patient and family.

Another point to consider is that home care may only work well on a short-term basis. Many patients welcome the opportunity to return home for a short period of time in order to enjoy their own environment one last time or to finish business that they must personally complete.

## Considerations in Developing a Hospice Home Care Program

Initiating the development of a hospice home care program requires the assessment of several basic factors. Planning for a hospice program is a complex process and could easily be the subject of a full-length book. The purpose of this section is to highlight some of the more obvious points. To facilitate this review, this section is divided into a discussion of *external factors* (those considerations in the environment external to the organization) and *internal factors* (those considerations that reflect the internal environment of the organization).

### External Factors

An obvious first step in planning a hospice home care program is to determine the number of deaths due to cancer in your area within the past year. Experience has shown that, given no restrictions of disease, the vast majority of all hospice patients are cancer patients.

It is essential to assess the existing community resources that are available to terminally ill patients and to determine the rate of their utilization and effectiveness. Exactly what services are available for terminally ill patients and their families? Where are the gaps? Should a new organization be formed to provide these services, or is it more appropriate for an existing organization to develop a hospice program?

Community support is crucial if hospice is to succeed. It should be ascertained whether or not hospice is a recognized or accepted concept in the community. If the concept is not well known, then an intensive educational program should be developed. The professional and lay communities should be targeted, and the hospice coordinator should be prepared to spend significant amounts of time developing community support. This is an ongoing task, but particularly crucial in the initial stages of development.

*Communication to community for support*

### Internal Factors

Anyone who accepts the responsibility of developing a hospice program (particularly in an existing agency) should recognize and be able to distinguish between hospice care and more traditional modes of terminal care. A common objection raised to hospice care is that there is no clear-cut difference between it and terminal care. Some of the unique features of hospice care include the following:

1. The patient and the family unit as the focus of hospice care.
2. Bereavement follow-up with the family.
3. Provision of volunteer services.
4. 24-hour on-call coverage.

Other differences are more subtle: (1) development of an interdisciplinary team to provide this care; (2) the emphasis on process; (3) inclusion of the patient as a member of the team; and (4) individualized care that reflects the patient's and family's own wishes.

The National Hospice Organization has developed a booklet titled *Standards of a Hospice Program of Care* (1979), which delineates very clearly the essential elements of a hospice program. The standards also allow room for individual community needs and preferences. Eventually, in order to be considered a "bona fide" hospice program, there must be an attempt to meet these standards. Developing a hospice program is an evolutionary process, and certain basic components must be "in place" in order to deliver hospice care. As the program grows, other dimensions and "extras," such as consultants (pharmacists, psychiatrists), may be added.

Before a hospice program is started in an existing home care agency, it is essential to determine the willingness of the staff to participate. Not everyone is prepared, able, or willing to work with dying patients. The commitment, temperament, and abilities of individual staff members must be addressed; careful screening is mandatory.

The final basic consideration for the development of a hospice program is administrative support and financial commitment for a minimum of 1 year. Experience has shown that at least 1 year is needed before a hospice program can begin to meet its expenses.

## Models of Hospice Home Care

There are three basic organizational models whereby home care is provided: the certified licensed home health agency; the hospital-based home care program; and the community-based hospice program. A brief description of each model follows.

### Certified Licensed Home Health Agency

Home health agencies have been offering services to patients in their own homes since the late 1800s. In order to be reimbursed by third-party payers for their services, a home care agency must be licensed by the state and certified (for payment) by Medicare. Within this framework, there are two variations: a home health agency caring exclusively for terminally ill patients (e.g., Hospice of Marin) or a home health agency caring for medical-surgical patients with a separate or integrated hospice program as one of its services (e.g., Hospital Home Health Care Agency). A home health agency that accepts only terminally ill patients tends to have a higher operating cost than that of an agency with a mixed caseload, because it costs more to deliver care to hospice patients than to medical-surgical patients.

A major advantage to this particular model is the stability and security that reimbursement affords. Experience indicates that a significant number of hospice programs begin as a community-based effort, offering "free" service. Within a period of roughly 2 years, many such hospice organizations have found it increasingly difficult to survive, let alone to expand, on grants and donations alone. A concomitant responsibility of being licensed and certified is the necessity to adhere to defined standards and regulations. Many hospice programs have viewed these regulations as restrictive and narrow, and thus have not sought to obtain a home health agency license.

### Hospital-Based Hospice Home Care Program

The hospital-based model is not significantly different from the model of the licensed certified home health agency, described above. However, there is an important economic factor: Providing service out of a hospital-based home care program is usually more expensive than providing service out of a private home health agency. This is due in large part to the fact that the home health agency is considered a cost center of the hospital and absorbs many indirect costs attributed to all cost centers.

### Community-Based Hospice Program

The third model is that of a community-based hospice program. Often, this sort of program evolves out of several individuals' concern and interest in the care of terminally ill patients. There are two main variations within this model:

1. A largely volunteer staff provides medical, nursing, psychosocial, and spiritual aspects of care. This is done either "free" of charge or on a sliding-scale basis.
2. The hospice contracts with the Visiting Nurse Association or other home health agencies for nursing services, and the hospice staff provides/coordinates support services of volunteers, clergy, psychologists, and bereavement follow-up care (e.g., Hospice of Santa Barbara).

A community-based program that extensively recruits professional and lay community support and involvement ensures its survival, because the needs of the particular community will have been taken into account.

## Operational Details

As with any program, there are a multitude of operational details to consider when developing a hospice home care program. I have selected eight significant areas for special consideration.

### Who's In Charge?

The interdisciplinary team is the foundation of hospice care. It is essential, therefore, that one person should coordinate the efforts of individual team members in the delivery of care. A hospice coordinator definitely facilitates communication between staff, patients, families, and the attending physician. In addition, my experience demonstrates that it is necessary to have one person responsible for responding to the needs of clients, staff, and the community. Another factor to consider is the percentage of time that the coordinator can allot to that particular job. Initially, a hospice coordinator may function on a part-time basis; however, within a relatively short period of time (6 months), it usually becomes apparent that a full-time commitment is essential if the program is to expand and attain long-term financial and program stability.

Individuals from a variety of disciplines can certainly serve as hospice coordinators; the choice depends upon the primary function outlined. The hospice coordinator does not have to be a nurse. This is obviously a controversial issue, yet one worth considering. Coordination of an interdisciplinary team of nurses, physicians, social workers, physical therapists, volunteers, home health aides, and clergy does not necessarily require the skills of a nurse. An individual with a generalist perspective (public health, management) often is better equipped to manage the efforts of this diverse group. A coordinator from one of the disciplines represented on the core team *may* not be able to be objective in his or her dealings with other disciplines. There is a natural tendency to be influenced by the perspective of one's own discipline, which can make teamwork more difficult.

If the coordinator is also solely responsible for the quality of nursing care, then, obviously, it would be wise to select a nurse for this position. Consider, however, the option of utilizing a nursing supervisor (from within the agency) to insure a high level of nursing care. If the hospice program subcontracts with a home health agency for nursing services, it may be advantageous to select a social worker as coordinator, since he or she would be able to perform psychosocial evaluations to supplement the home health agency appraisals. Regardless of discipline, the coordinator must be able to manage a diverse group of staff members, to support the staff members from all disciplines, and to relate effectively to the professional and lay community.

## Admission Criteria

A basic operational detail for all hospice programs is that of the admission criteria. Although there are very few universal criteria, a number of standard criteria must be considered. A medical prognosis of 6 months or less to live is usually a minimum requirement for a patient's admission to a hospice program. In addition, the geographic area to be served must be defined. Other criteria include the following:

1. *Restriction by disease.* Many hospice programs restrict admission to patients suffering from cancer alone. Often this is a direct result of the requirements of a particular funding source; at other

times it reflects the nature of cancer as a progressive disease with a relatively clear and identifiable terminal phase. Even with the absence of disease restrictions, approximately 98% of hospice referrals are cancer patients.

2. *Restriction by age.*   A hospice program may decide that it can care only for adult patients, and therefore may set a minimum age of 18 years. In making this determination, it is important to consider the skills of the hospice team in caring for pediatric patients. Most important is the attitude of the staff toward caring for young children; often staff members may express doubts about their emotional ability to care for children. If this is to be an option, a hospice will find it necessary to hire individuals who are willing to care for patients in this particular age group.

3. *Requirement of a primary caregiver.*   One of the most difficult tasks for hospice is that of caring for a patient who has no primary caregiver available. Often, the availability of a primary caregiver is a basic requirement for admission to a hospice program. If a primary caregiver is not required, the hospice team must be prepared to play a much more active role by arranging and coordinating friends and volunteers for assistance. Usually the person who is alone can benefit tremendously from the full range of hospice services; in fact, he or she may be unable to remain at home without the team's assistance. If there is no single caregiver available, the safety of the patient must be carefully evaluated at all times; often, the patient is transferred to the hospital prior to death.

4. *Priority to patients in need of pain/symptom control.*   Not all terminally ill patients need hospice care; therefore, it is helpful to identify those factors that will establish priorities in admission. The particular skill of the hospice nurse is the control of pain and symptoms associated with a terminal disease. For this reason, patients with problems in either of these two areas are most appropriate for immediate admission. In addition, patients and families experiencing severe psychosocial problems related to the disease process can benefit significantly from the support of the hospice team.

5. *Aggressive therapy.*   Hospice care is designed to be palliative and supportive; consequently, most programs have developed a policy stating that aggressive, curative treatment is not appropriate. We must clarify the distinction between chemotherapy and radiation for palliative treatment as distinct from curative treatment. Increasingly, patients who are being maintained on hyperalimen-

tation are referred to hospice programs. This is one of those "gray areas" that must be interpreted in the light of existing medical/nursing policies.

### Exclusive Caseload versus Mixed Caseload

When an agency offers both medical-surgical nursing and hospice care, there are two major ways of delivering hospice care. One may be through a separate hospice staff with a caseload comprised exclusively of terminally ill patients. The other may be through a staff that has a mixed caseload comprised of medical-surgical and terminally ill patients.

A staff working exclusively with terminally ill patients is apt to be smaller, which may be more conducive to the building of a team. A strong, supportive team is one of the single most important factors in delivering quality care. With an exclusive caseload, the development of appropriate skills occurs rapidly, as the staff person is totally focused on the needs of a select population.

Concern has been voiced that this approach leads to a high turnover or "burnout" rate, because the hospice staff person is working only with patients on one end of the health-illness continuum. This has not been my experience. Nevertheless, a staff that is responsible for both medical-surgical patients and hospice patients has more of a balance and may be able to "last longer." If there is a very small staff, a mixed caseload might be just as advantageous because a sense of "team" already exists.

An important consideration is that not everyone wants to, or should, care for dying patients. If all staff members are expected to see hospice patients, their appropriateness and ability to care for dying patients should be carefully evaluated. However, the home care nurse who cares for a mixed caseload has the opportunity to utilize his or her "hospice" knowledge in the care of medical-surgical patients as well, thereby integrating the hospice concept into the larger health care system.

### On-Call Coverage

On-call coverage is probably one of the most important services offered to patients and families. It also strains the staff, because it is a tremendous burden for the hospice nurse to work a full day and then be "on call" for the evening. There are ways to minimize the burden.

1. Rotate the on-call duty among several staff members. It is far too much for one nurse to be responsible for 24-hour on-call coverage, day in and day out. If at all possible, a nurse should not be

on call more than one night per week. If the staff is small, consider augmenting the staff, with additional nurses trained only to take call. This may be an effective measure, but it necessitates close communication, coordination, and backup.

2. Weekend call should be scheduled as a block of time, (e.g., Friday night to Monday morning). Extra staff members for this purpose are particularly helpful.

3. Determine who actively participates in the on-call rotation. Some hospice programs include social workers or clergy as primary (first-call) or secondary on-call staff. Experience has shown that most calls are related to physical nursing needs, and it is most appropriate for nurses to rotate this responsibility. Backup coverage by physicians, social workers, and clergy is extremely helpful to staff.

4. If at all possible, staff should be paid for this responsibility. At the very least, monetary compensation is recognition of the importance of the service.

5. Build in provision for time off for nurses who have been up all night. To expect them to work the next day is often unrealistic.

## Burnout Prevention

Regardless of the manner in which it is provided, hospice care entails considerable stresses that increase the probability of burnout. Burnout occurs when the staff person is not able to cope successfully with feelings of stress. There are interventions that can be implemented in an attempt to prevent or alleviate burnout in a hospice home care setting (Friel & Tehan, 1980). One should not assume, therefore, that burnout is inevitable.

In order to be effective in this area, the individual organization of each hospice and the personal needs of the hospice team necessitate very specific and tailored approaches. There are several ways to approach burnout prevention: through administration, through education and training, and through development of professional and social support systems. Top administration sets the tone and creates the staff work environment. Administration must be supportive of the hospice concept and willing to build mechanisms to control burnout into the system. These policies may entail a great amount of flexibility, as well as extra cost to the hospice, but they are essential to a program's success. An example of this flexibility includes the supervisor's authority to grant time off or personal leave when it is obvious that the staff member needs a break.

Evaluation and training in interpersonal skills constitute another key aspect of burnout reduction. This will (1) increase the nurse's realistic perception of stressor(s), and (2) strengthen the communication and counseling skills that are required in hospice care. This approach is based on the assumption that the interpersonal skills required for effective intervention in hospice care are difficult to achieve without intrapersonal strength and insight.

Professional and social support systems influence the staff member's perception of stress and ultimately its occurrence. Clinical experience indicates that energy and strength are generated when team members are able to depend upon and support one another. A regularly scheduled support group, led by a facilitator, is one approach that may be successful. Professional support encompasses both administration and the entire health team; social support includes one's family, friends, or both.

## Development of Internal Standards

It is the experience at the Hospital Home Health Care Agency that hospice nurses see half as many patients in a given day as their medical-surgical counterparts do. It is obvious that attending to the multiple needs (physical, emotional, spiritual, and social) of not only the patient, but the family as well, takes considerable time.

A significant amount of time each day is spent updating team members on changes in condition of various patients. This is essential if continuity of care is to be provided; it is particularly crucial for the nurse who is on call in the evening to be updated on all patients. In addition, a weekly conference attended by all team members is an integral part of the delivery of hospice care.

Given the demands on the staff person's time, it is important to establish some guidelines concerning expectations about numbers of patients to be seen per day. In addition, the roles and skills of individual team members should be clarified. Without some guidance, a particular staff person may try to solve all the problems with which he or she is confronted —an unrealistic goal. Instead, staff members should understand that they are not solely responsible for this patient and family; all appropriate team members must be involved in resolving difficulties as they arise. The social worker, psychologist, pharmacist, and volunteer all may be able to contribute significantly to an understanding and/or resolution of family difficulties.

## Bereavement Services

Bereavement services constitute a unique component of hospice care, and they may be instituted in a number of ways. Most often, the staff member closest to the family makes a bereavement visit shortly after the death has occurred. This offers the family and the staff member the experience of closure or completion; it is important for both of them to review the last few months, weeks, days, or hours of the deceased's life. Often, this is a very emotional visit with the expression of much grief and sorrow; however, it is an important phase of the family's bereavement process, for it aids in establishing the reality of the loss.

If a volunteer has been assigned to the family, it may be appropriate for that person to maintain contact. Often a support group for the bereaved is valuable. In addition, a bereavement team, composed of volunteers who are experienced in bereavement follow-up, can make regular phone or personal contact with individuals who wish this continued support. It is helpful if a mental health specialist (psychologist, psychiatrist, clinical social worker) is also available for counseling those who are experiencing a particularly difficult bereavement.

Another aspect of bereavement follow-up that does not require skilled personnel is the sending of a card on the anniversary date of the death. This reminds the family that the hospice is still thinking of them and, likewise, is still available for support. In recent years, we at the Hospital Home Health Care Agency have hosted a Holiday Open House at Christmas, which offers the family an opportunity to be with the hospice staff for an evening. All of these practices can be a hospice's way of "reaching out" to the bereaved, making it easier for the individual to seek or receive support.

## Community Outreach

One of the basic tenets of hospice care is that it reflects the needs of the community it serves. Therefore, there should be continuing dialogue between a hospice program and the community. Initially, the hospice concept may encounter resistance from the professional community; in this case, repeated educational programs and individual contact with health care professionals will be necessary. Without the support of these professionals, the hospice program will flounder.

Often it is helpful to concentrate initially on developing a core group of professionals who are respected by their peers. This group then participates with the hospice team in presentations to professional groups and organizations. Because of the high number of referrals, oncologists are a natural group to cultivate. In addition, discharge planners in general hospitals play a critical role in determining the appropriateness of home care in general. If they understand the services offered by a hospice program, they can be a major source of referral.

Development of strong relationships with professionals is particularly important, because a home care hospice program must provide for continuity of care. Many patients require intermittent hospitalization, and it is extremely important that the hospice team develop a close working relationship with the hospital(s) to which patients will be admitted.

The hospital staff should understand the approach employed by the hospice and be willing to continue those pain regimes or interventions that have proven effective at home. Likewise, it is helpful when the hospital staff shares their observations and knowledge with the hospice team prior to a patient's discharge to home.

There must be mutual recognition that both the hospital and the hospice home care program play an important role in providing high-quality, comprehensive care to the patient and family. This is only possible when all health care professionals involved understand and recognize the value of one another's work.

The lay community also requires significant attention. Education is an important function of all hospice programs; it should be consistent and continuous in the community. Support from community organizations, church groups, and individuals is invaluable. In addition, because volunteers are an integral part of all hospice programs, it is important for the program to maintain high visibility so that it will attract interested individuals.

## Summary

The primary focus of hospice care has been, and will continue to be, in the patient's own home. Pain and symptoms of terminal disease can be readily controlled in the home; the patient and family often prefer the familiarity and comfort of their own environment. In addition, the economic savings of, and third-party reimbursement for, home care make it advantageous to continue to support the development of hospice home care programs.

## References

Friel, M., & Tehan, C. B., "Counteracting Burn-Out for the Hospice Care-Giver," *Cancer Nursing*, 1980, *3*, 285–293.

Saunders, C. M., "Hospice Care," *American Journal of Medicine*, 1978, *65*, 726–728.

National Hospice Organization, *Standards of a Hospice Program of Care* (6th revision). Unpublished booklet, 1979.

# 22

# Hospital-Based Inpatient Hospice Units: Planning Considerations

*Susan Grinslade and Ruth Reko*

Dying in a hospital has been characterized as a desolate experience, undignified at best and demoralizing, degrading, or detached from human contact at worst. Yet dying people are brought to hospitals for care each day, in large measure because of the types of caregivers and services that are concentrated in such settings. Clearly, there is a need to establish new standards of appropriate care for these dying people and for their families within the context of the institution to which they look for aid. Here, we address this subject by examining the place of inpatient hospice units within the general hospital and by exploring some of the advantages and disadvantages of the hospital as a setting for hospice. Our discussion is based on several years' experience with the development of a hospice program as a separate unit offering inpatient and home care services within an existing urban medical center, along with observations of other programs, conversations with many hospice planners, and the few relevant items in the literature (e.g., Ajemian & Mount, 1980; Mount, 1976; Walter, 1979). We recognize that this is not the only context for hospice inpatient care, but we judge that it is one of the most likely settings for the future development of hospice work; we hope that our analysis will have application to free-standing inpatient units, as well as to those hospice programs that operate in affiliation with or within a larger inpatient setting (e.g., systems involving "scattered beds" or consultation teams).

## Predetermining Factors

Certain predetermining factors in the decision to develop a hospice program within a medical center constitute a background for our discussion. Unless there is a demonstrable need for a hospice program in the community served by the hospital, hospice proponents may face significant obstacles. One of the difficulties in surveying such needs lies in developing an adequate research methodology to undertake the task and prove the thesis. If a given population of bereaved families is asked whether they would have preferred to have their relative die in a hospice, and the hospice is described as an ideal, the majority would most likely respond positively. But of what value are such results? Looking at cancer death rates in the hospital or in the surrounding community as a means of assessing need may not necessarily yield any more definitive proof.

However, some combination of factors may lead a given hospital to the conclusion that a hospice program could be incorporated into its institutional structure even before all the results of possible research could point to the hospice's becoming an unqualified success. A survey of the demographic features of the broad community served by the hospital may yield evidence, for example, of a high incidence of cancer, a significant percentage of the population over age 55, and a large proportion of people who participate in or have available to them a well-developed, extended family system. Statistics regarding the percentage of deaths in a given time period from cancer and the place where most deaths occur are easily obtainable and might be compared with specific data from the hospital considering the question.

Another method of demonstrating need has been to conduct an in-house study of the types of care given by hospital personnel to dying patients within the current structure. This sort of study was undertaken at the Royal Victoria Hospital in Montreal in 1973 (Mount et al., 1974). The results may establish evidence of gaps in services that could be filled by a hospice program. One potential difficulty with this approach is that hospital staff might become defensive, viewing the study as intrusive and as an indictment of existing services. If so, there might be poor acceptance of any new hospice program that is later proposed. This difficulty can only be avoided or minimized by emphasizing the shared goal of achieving optimal care for patients and their families.

In a community where some hospice services may already be available, the hospital contemplating the development of a hospice program must assess the unique contribution that it can make on the basis of a thorough study of the program(s) already under way. It certainly behooves all hospice providers to develop patterns of cooperation, even in an area where competition among health care providers is the accepted norm. Provider rivalries can weaken the impact of hospice, thereby undercutting individual efforts and leading to negative effects on patients and families.

For the administration of a hospital to initiate a study process of any type with the intention of developing a hospice program, there must be at least a modicum of knowledge, interest, and even willingness to give support to the effort. This intention may be motivated by a key individual's highly personal experience, a general desire to be the first with the new or the newly popular in the area, a response to a request from a community interest group, a perception of the hospital's philosophy as being consistent with the hospice philosophy, or any of a number of other factors. Whatever the initial stimulus has been, the study group or the developers will bring the process to full flower only if there continues to be strong administrative support and a substantial willingness to venture into the unknown.

A major influence on entering into plans for an inpatient hospice program will be the response of the medical staff. Obviously, hospice care has many implications for physicians and for their patients. Some planning groups have spent valuable time devising questionnaires, tallying or publishing results, or personally surveying physicians, only to find that their ultimate decision to proceed must depend on lukewarm comments by physicians who indicate only vaguely that they might admit patients to a hospice.

Support from physicians representative of the broad spectrum of the medical staff is a crucial factor in hospice development, whatever the setting, even though it may not always be possible to achieve full acceptance by the medical staff before implementation. On the other hand, a strongly vocal resistance movement may be a deciding factor in delaying plans for the hospital-based hospice program. Such resistance indicates the need for an educational campaign and for visible leadership from carefully selected physician advocates of hospice. Even then, physician understanding and acceptance may come only after a patient urgently petitions his or her physician to make hospice services available.

Should the medical center decide to offer hospice care to the community it serves, it begins a journey into a new and at this point largely uncharted area of health care delivery for the acute care setting. This endeavor will encounter both advantages and disadvantages, but it will be sustained by the deep, caring commitment for quality of life that hospice represents. In the following discussion, we explore many of the elements essential to the development of an inpatient hospice program.

## Physical Setting

The hospital as a physical setting has several inherent advantages for the establishment of a hospice. The patient care areas within the facility may be considered by some to be ready-made for housing hospice patients. Various models provide data on the advisability and patient acceptance of the effects of room configurations, and the debate is still going on among hospice team members as to private versus semiprivate versus ward-type rooms. Economics may be the final determinant in this matter, balancing adaptability of existing rooms against costs to be borne in altering major structural features, loss of bed capacity, and projected future uses of the designated area.

Utilization and availability of space for a variety of family needs may be a positive or negative factor with regard to decision making. The areas needed to allow privacy for family groups of varying numbers may make use of converted patient rooms, storage areas, or other spaces. Proximity to patient care areas must be achieved for these families. However, the conversion of floor space to footage not producing revenue may be a severe drawback from the standpoint of hospital administrators who are asked to establish a segregated hospice setting. Nevertheless, patterns of usage by families and enthusiastic response in consumer surveys are documentable and tangible factors to consider when confirmation is needed of a decision to continue allocation of living, eating, and sleeping spaces for families.

Designing a modern health care facility implies attention to a myriad of details to make the setting comply with building codes, governmental regulations, and accreditation standards. By appropriating an area of an existing hospital, the hospice team has achieved this compliance with minimal exertion. On the other hand, there may be certain built-in features or sophisticated technological equipment that are of little value in the care of hospice patients and that may be difficult to remove.

Standardized decorating regulations may be seen as an obstacle in remodeling an area to create a more homelike atmosphere for the hospice area. Large institutions tend to prefer standardized paint colors for simplicity of maintenance. Drapes or bedspreads may have been purchased in such bulk lots that no pattern variations can be considered. However, ways can be found to introduce a more intimate touch even in such circumstances by attention to details—tropical plants in abundant variety, pictures, wall hangings, afghans, seasonal decorations, fish aquariums, and the like. Many of these can be maintained through assistance from caring volunteers. Patients can also be permitted to bring their own possessions from home to personalize the areas around their beds. The trade-off for remaining within house regulations is the availability of a large maintenance and housekeeping staff, whose members can be called upon to use their skills and tools to keep the hospice functioning.

The availability of equipment choices within a large medical center may contribute to the hospice team's ability to meet specific needs of individual patients with rapidity and ease. By no means will all of the patients in the hospice need an overbed trapeze, for instance. However, the ability to get such equipment quickly by making just one in-house telephone call can satisfy a specific felt need on the part of a patient and contribute to the establishment of a positive, caring relationship early in his or her hospice stay.

In the same vein, the availability of a linen service and a dietary department can be an advantage. Frequent linen changes are the rule rather than the exception with hospice patients—a fact of life that might prove taxing in a small, independent facility. Likewise, the range of diet selections may be a boon in the care of many patients. Special diets for those with secondary diseases such as diabetes, and a variety of ways to prepare food, can enhance mealtimes in the hospice. Here a responsive dietician can be invaluable in interpreting to the kitchen staff the frequency of diet changes and the reasons for many special requests. A vivid example of the benefits of this special understanding is the dietician who, upon hearing that a patient had announced a taste for rabbit, organized a shopping expedition to procure this for the next meal—to the absolute delight of the gentleman.

## Financial Responsibilities

An important area of protection and recognition for the hospice is the established agreements with third-party payers negotiated by the hospital and most likely of long and solid standing. These can afford the hospice program a distinct advantage if managed properly, with all parties fully informed of possibilities and limits. A fair portion of the care provided in the hospital-based hospice may well be covered by existing hospitalization insurance policies. New benefits are also being added for licensed home health care.

However, some aspects of hospice care are not recognized in current standard reimbursement packages. Examples include family support and education, or bereavement follow-up services. As a consequence, these services must be offered in one of three ways: solely by unpaid staff and volunteers; by paid staff members who perform these functions on their own time; or by staff and volunteers whose salaries and training respectively are paid for by the hospital. Furthermore, hospice precepts consistently favor making care available without regard for ability to pay. Hospice patients are often those who have expended sizeable sums in lengthy courses of treatment, inpatient stays, and consultants' fees before coming to the hospice. For such people, medical benefits may be severely depleted. Difficulty in predicting the length of inpatient hospice stays needed for symptom control and pain management may mean that the hospital could experience a financial loss in such care.

Even in small inpatient hospice facilities, the average daily census of patients may fluctuate dramatically. Extended periods of low census can present major problems in maintaining full staff to provide full service. Since productivity is a real concern in this decade, there may be pressure to utilize hospice beds for other types of patients in order to minimize loss. For example, when hospice beds are empty, the admitting office may arbitrarily notify the hospice staff members that they will receive several new patients who are accident victims receiving aggressive treatment. This can constitute a challenge to the integrity of the hospice. Staffing patterns and morale could be affected, and volunteers may be lost as well. Challenges such as these may embody the most potentially destructive issues for hospital-based hospices.

Adherence to utilization review practices within the hospital can create a major problem in the care plans for many hospice patients. For instance, sometimes acute care criteria are employed, using severity of illness and intensity of service as the sole standards for inpatient admission and continuation of stay. In these circumstances, the hospice program will be severely limited, and hospice patients will suffer from having inappropriate criteria dictating terms and conditions of service. To deny care or benefits can have significant implications for a patient's emotional well-being and for his or her family as they face a need to go elsewhere or to assume large out-of-pocket expenses. Furthermore, from the hospital's standpoint, the fiscal responsibility for continually aiding patients whose benefits have been denied can reach the proportions of a major problem.

Sound planning for a workable inpatient hospice program in the hospital setting will dictate intense negotiations with the relevant review and funding agencies to establish realistic criteria for parameters of care unique to the palliative treatment of terminally ill patients. The hospital's past and current history of lengths of stay can have a significant bearing on any willingness to negotiate new criteria for the hospice unit.

## Standards and Licensure

Establishing a recognized basis for operating the hospice program may be made more problem-free in the hospital setting. Functioning within a licensed and accredited institution may provide freedom and protection to the hospice. If the hospital-based hospice offers home care through the hospital-based home health agency, this license is also of great significance. The bearing of licensure upon hospice reimbursement is a definite advantage. Similarly, the relationship of the hospital with the local health systems agency may be an important factor if a certificate of need for the hospice is required.

The medical center is already familiar with standards established for acute care. Consequently, it may be difficult also to adhere to a new and different set of standards when providing hospice care. Presently there are no binding standards of care imposed on institutions providing hospice services. In North America, the National Hospice Organization has adopted a document outlining standards of care to which participating members adhere, and various other criteria have been proposed. However, the present uncertainty can be threatening in that current programs may need in the future to adapt or significantly alter their services when a universal standards document is enforced.

## Presence of Multiple Disciplines

An important advantage to the establishment of an interdisciplinary hospice team within a hospital is the diversity of professions already represented in the staff. Since a new hospice program is often unable to predict with total accuracy the needs of each of the families it will serve, it is beneficial to be able to call upon the expertise of many individuals to attend to rare but vital concerns. From an administrative standpoint, it is helpful to be able to offer a broad range of services from the opening day when initial census will be low, realizing that the burden of salarying the whole team does not depend solely on the success of the hospice program. If the hospice is to be regarded as a hospital department, a referral process for bringing in needed expertise is available with the ancillary services. Computation of staff budgets may include consideration of a given department's employee working on a shared-time basis with the hospice.

Orientation to hospice principles of care can be accomplished for the entire hospital staff, department by department, in anticipation of certain individuals' participating in the hospice team. Mechanisms are already in place for this, such as a training and development department or in-service schedules in various departments; these can be considered as part of an overall staff development program. Because these programs are offered on site, expenses are not great. Established working relationships between departments and within departments can be assessed by the hospice team leaders so that existing strengths can be maximized for the benefit of the hospice program.

Should a hospice need be identified for a particular discipline not represented within the hospital's current staffing, it may be an involved process before a new team member can be brought on. Development of a part-time or consultative position may or may not conform to standardized procedures, but that can offer one possible way to expand the team. Another related issue could involve a needed discipline that constitutes such a small department within the hospital that time for hospice team participation is precluded. Furthermore, within a small department there may not be a predisposition on the part of any of the employees to participate in hospice care. Recruitment of specialized volunteers may offer a solution to these problems.

For some large medical institutions, the concept of an interdisciplinary team may be widely touted, but time and effort may not be devoted to implementing the concrete aspects of helping the team to function. For the hospice program faced with the need to develop a smoothly working team, justifying the actual time needed for formal and informal team meetings may be a challenge. When the team members function in a number of areas of the institution, finding a mutually agreeable conference hour can also constitute a hurdle. On the other hand, once a schedule is established, the accessibility of the common meeting place to all of the team members is an asset.

## Primary Caregivers

Another significant issue is the need for providing sufficient numbers of personnel to achieve high-quality, humanistic care for patients and families. Because dying persons and their families have needs that go beyond basic physical care, additional staff members are required above what may be standard in a general acute care service area. This need for additional staffing is particularly evident among primary caregivers, such as professional nurses. The desired ratio of patients to staff in hospice work is generally cited as one nurse per shift for every three patients in the inpatient setting (or one to one over the 24-hour day). This staffing ratio is equivalent or similar to staffing ratios for intensive care settings and is a significant factor in budgetary concerns. The medical center is thus faced with valuing the services it wishes to provide for dying patients and their families.

The need for comprehensive nursing care for the hospice patient places a heavy burden on the hospice provider, but this is a burden that may be shared when the hospice is within the medical center. The presence of an established department of nursing facilitates selection of available staff members, a factor not to be taken lightly. Ultimately, the effectiveness of the hospice program is determined largely by the competency and sensitivity with which care is delivered. The department of nursing can suggest to persons already employed that they might have the qualifications for hospice work and encourage them to interview for available hospice positions. This provides an opportunity for caregivers who are frustrated by the limits on their practice imposed within the acute care areas—where time and staffing ratios may fragment their care—to explore a service area where personalized care is the rule and not the exception. Should the medical center convert an existing service area to a hospice unit, staff previously assigned to this area can be given the opportunity to work in the hospice setting or to transfer to another area. This mutual retaining and/or transfer of staff will protect the individual's employment and at the same time benefit the medical center.

During periods of time when occupancy within the hospice is high, the medical center offers the advantage of providing additional staff, just as the reverse can be true with low hospice occupancy when staff are needed in other service areas. Although there are problems when staff members are working in an area that is unfamiliar to them, there are also distinct advantages to this type of arrangement. For the hospice staff member who is working in another unit, the opportunity is provided to develop and/or maintain technical skills that are not utilized when providing care to hospice patients. In addition, the hospice staff member is presented with the opportunity to share the hospice philosophy with other employees who remain skeptical or unclear about the program's purpose or goals. In this way, hospice-type care is modeled for others to see. Another advantage to this arrangement is the opportunity for potential patients and families to be identified and evaluated as possible recipients of hospice care.

Similar benefits are available to the staff member coming from another unit to work in the hospice. This person is able to experience and participate in the delivery of hospice care. The experience may enable the person to renew or further develop psychosocial skills that may not be fully utilized in the acute care unit. Also, such staff members become more knowledgeable about the needs of patients with a terminal illness, as well as those of their families, and can incorporate this knowledge into work elsewhere. The hospice team working with these staff members can help diminish or alleviate any misunderstanding that the hospice is a "death ward." Generally this mutual sharing of experiences enhances the interaction among units and minimizes any feelings of isolation felt by persons working within the hospice.

Typically, the community medical center has an existing corps of volunteers who provide many valuable services within the institution. Once again, the hospice unit may draw on this existing resource to aid in the delivery of its care. Selection of volunteers is a process that needs careful attention so as to obtain volunteers with a wide variety of suitable skills. Especially within the inpatient hospice, the volunteer brings an additional touch of "normality," which may otherwise be inhibited by institutional routines and trappings. Training mechanisms and aids exist within the institution to introduce volunteers to hospice and to facilitate volunteer education.

Established hospice units are increasingly aware of the stresses experienced by caregivers working within their programs. These stresses are directly related to the intense relationships developed between patient/family units and caregivers, and to subsequent loss. Caregivers, whether salaried or volunteer, are subject to experiencing a wide range of intense emotional responses. These feelings have the potential of becoming so overwhelming that caregivers may develop defensive mechanisms to enable them to cope. Not all of these mechanisms are desirable; some may directly affect relationships between caregivers and patients or families. In an effort to prevent this from happening, many hospices have developed formalized team support systems to facilitate caregivers' awareness and understanding of their emotional responses. Such systems may require an uninterrupted period of time when members of the interdisciplinary team can meet together. This time may be viewed as nonproductive if there is no administrative sensitivity to the potential for staff burnout. Moreover, it is sometimes beneficial to recruit a person whose sole responsibility is to facilitate staff support meetings. This may generate an additional operating expense that is nonreimbursable and that may appear unjustified to the medical center. However, it cannot be overemphasized that staff support is an integral need for the hospice unit that wishes to retain and develop its personnel.

## Home Care

Despite the thrust of much hospice literature toward the preferability of home care and the fact that the inpatient service may be linked with the hospital's own home health department or through a contract with a home health agency, in many instances inpatient care seems to receive more attention and emphasis. This may be due to the convenience of a centralized location and the higher revenue associated with inpatient care. Even with the best of intentions, the inpatient staff has a great investment in keeping patients and often creates such a remarkably protected environment that motivation on the part of the family for the patient to return home can diminish. The hospital-based home health department may also have an institutional bias, which can set the stage for the patient to return to the shelter when the illness seems to be reaching a difficult stage. Lack of awareness of other community resources to call upon in addressing the multitude of needs families encounter when caring for a terminally ill person at home plagues the hospital-based hospice. The impetus to develop methods for assuring continuity of care for discharged patients is not particularly strong in the medical center as a whole, and it is only natural that this situation can become a disadvantage to the full-service hospice.

The success of the inpatient hospice with or without a home care program is dependent upon adherence to the hospice concept that the patient and family together are the unit of care. The perception and willingness to embrace a philosophy of care that includes both patients and families may be difficult for the acute care medical center. Delivery of services within the institution has principally been directed toward the patient, and services for the family or significant others have not been major priorities. Utilization of staff and time specifically to address the needs of families, especially to permit them to assist in the giving of care or to teach them methods to be used at home, may not be seen as the best allocation of resources. This may stem from an unfamiliarity with the precepts of humanistic health care. Once again, lack of knowledge or misunderstanding of goals can directly affect the acceptance and effectiveness of the hospice unit.

## Nontraditional Role

The medical center that has provided a consistent and expected presence within a community needs to be aware that it may encounter a negative response when it proposes to alter its existing realm of services. Involved in the medical center's decision to provide hospice services is an understanding of the level and kind of commitment being made in undertaking this work. Presently, the medical center's role is traditional in the types and levels of services it provides. Given the general taboos and fears surrounding the care of dying patients, the provision of hospice services may be viewed by many as very nontraditional. The hospice itself may come to be viewed as the hospital's "death ward." By venturing into this unknown area, the medical center may run the risk of being misunderstood by its local community and by its own employees. This potential for misunderstanding should serve as a caution to the medical center to fully explore and develop an understanding of the hospice philosophy, and to examine its own relationship to that philosophy so that the full implication is comprehended by planners and executors of plans.

The primary emphasis of acute medical care in recent years has been on "all-out effort" to sustain life. This has been encouraged by technological advances and increased specialization of medical services. Resulting fragmentation of care delivery has led to the perception of the patient as composed of many separate parts that each need specialized attention, rather than as an integrated whole with physical *and* psychosocial needs. Further, litigation against physicians has understandably made them wary of choosing to withhold any aspect of care that is technologically available. This whole issue is further complicated by disagreements about what constitutes "viable life" and a medically acceptable definition of death. Fortunately, consumers of health care services are becoming more aware of their own rights, and this is requiring a higher degree of accountability by health care providers. By bringing into focus the issues of death and dying, Elisabeth Kübler-Ross has identified a distressing lack of caring and concern by providers of medical services for individuals for whom cure is not a reasonable goal. It is difficult to look at one's own weaknesses, and this is compounded when the weaknesses are shared by many disciplines professing to attend to health care. Because these providers invariably have differing perspectives as to what health care should be, their understanding and acceptance of the hospice philosophy may also be expected to vary significantly.

Major opposition to the hospice unit by a particular discipline within the parent organization can alter the hospice's initial or continuing success. In particular, lack of peer group support and understanding from physicians will undermine the ultimate effectiveness of the hospice. For example, a medical center with a hospice medical director who is not receiving support from his or her peers in the center and the community may find itself operating a unit without patients. While lack of support in other disciplines is also felt, it is felt less acutely because of the key role of physicians in the medical hierarchy.

The resistance to change that accompanies any new human endeavor is yet another factor to consider in departing from the traditional hospital role. Human beings are creatures of habit, and changes in life styles involve feelings of uncertainty and insecurity. These feelings can interfere with educational efforts to develop understanding of the hospice philosophy and its benefits to the members of the community. These feelings may also be complicated by a "show me" kind of attitude. Concern about the unknown is a universal aspect of human behavior; it should not be ignored when proposing the delivery of any new service, especially one touching on such a sensitive issue as care of the dying.

## Community Outreach

The well-established medical center has a position in the community by virtue of its governing board, its auxiliaries, a reputation of long-standing service, and in some cases the delegate body or religious affiliates. These are all beneficial to the hospice program in its infancy, lending credibility to the effort. The availability of concrete support and advice from individuals who have a strong understanding of the community's needs and response to new health care programs can be invaluable to the hospice team when planning strategies to present their services to the public. Also, the hospital's public relations department should have well-established contacts and effective channels for developing media campaigns to keep the community abreast of hospice developments. Natural opportunities exist for publicizing the hospice program by means of the hospital's customary marketing strategies (e.g., health fairs, annual reports, newsletters, fund-raising appeals, and special anniversary celebrations). All of these provide significant advantages in terms of savings for the hospice budget and its human resources.

The consumers of a hospital's services typically have been a fairly consistent population during the history of most such institutions. Geographical proximity, need for specialties offered, or ideological similarities with the hospital's founding group may lead people to identify themselves as patrons. Of course, a strong reason for use of a given medical center is the personal physician's position on the medical staff. This often results in a broader service area than might at first seem logical. All of these factors may influence many consumers to make use of the hospice services at the hospital with which they feel a certain identification. Geographical distance or a religious bias may, on the other hand, be barriers with which hospice team members need to deal as they attempt realistically to address the broader needs of the entire community.

## Conclusion

The reader may have a sense of unease at this point, because the variables present in each individual hospital considering the development of a hospice program cannot be simply totaled on a ledger, and an easy guarantee of success for a particular program probably cannot be drawn. As we have attempted to demonstrate in the discussion, the ledger page shows an unbalanced list of assets in some areas and debits in other aspects of any given setting, taking into view the various items covered.

There are undeniably wide variations in hospitals—in styles of management, in general philosophy, and in recognition by the community—and these have great bearing on whether or not hospice can become a part of the service offerings of a particular institution. Hospitals can be nurturing and sustaining environments for hospice care, for the caregivers, and for patients and families if the hospital can be found to be a compatible host in a given setting. In this era, when we realize that human and financial resources are not limitless, it seems most appropriate to develop cooperative efforts to make the wisest use of the resources that we do have in our health care system to serve the widest range of needs, including those of all confronted with the crisis of dying.

# References

Ajemian, I., & B. Mount (Eds.), *The R. V. H. Manual on Palliative/Hospice Care.* New York: Arno Press, 1980.

Mount, B. M., "The Problem of Caring for the Dying in a General Hospital: The Palliative Care Unit as a Possible Solution," *Canadian Medical Association Journal,* 1976, *115,* 119–121.

Mount, B. M., Jones, A., & Patterson, A., "Death and Dying: Attitudes in a Teaching Hospital," *Urology,* 1974, *4,* 741–747.

Walter, N. T., *Hospice Pilot Project Report.* Hayward, CA: Kaiser-Permanente Medical Center, 1979.

# 23

# A Different Kind of Day Hospital—For Patients with Preterminal Cancer and Chronic Disease

*Eric Wilkes, Anthony G. O. Crowther, and Cyril W. K. H. Greaves*

## Introduction

Most day hospitals are for geriatric or psychiatric patients. We run a day hospital catering for patients with preterminal cancer and chronic disease, which has been developed (mainly through the generosity of the Nuffield Foundation) as an integral part of a terminal care unit; and we discuss here its first 26 months.

## The Background

The 25-bed unit for patients with terminal cancer and the chronic sick is supported by an independent charity, but most of the beds are financed by a contract with the area health authority. It takes 350–450 patients a year,

*From:* Eric Wilkes, Anthony G. O. Crowther, and Cyril W. K. H. Greaves, "A Different Kind of Day Hospital—For Patients with Preterminal Cancer and Chronic Disease," *British Medical Journal*, 1978, 2, 1053–1056. Reprinted by permission from the publisher and Eric Wilkes.

mostly suffering from disseminated cancer; some 12% of the local cancer deaths occur in the unit, the average stay being about two weeks for men and three for women (Wilkes, 1974). In a series of 500 patients the nurses judged the quality of life to have been excellent in 29%, satisfactory in 70%, and poor in only 1–2% (Wilkes, 1977).

Nevertheless, we had five grounds for concern: (1) Each year over 100 patients with terminal illness on our waiting list died before we could find them a bed, some of them in most unsatisfactory conditions. (2) We were discharging some 15% of our patients (who were most commonly admitted to give respite to their families or for the control of symptoms), but they and their families were still under stress and we wanted to keep in touch with them. (3) We were increasingly taking in spouses to share in routine care, but there were many who wished to carry on at home and yet to have help. (4) Most patients die in acute hospitals among strangers, having been at home until near the end (Ward, 1974); but we hoped that a day unit with a rota of nurses common to the terminal care unit would mean that patients could be later admitted—if admission were needed—to the care of familiar and trusted staff. (5) Many of the chronic sick, while not bad enough for admission, needed far more than consultations in an outpatient department or with the general practitioner.

We therefore started a day hospital for patients with advanced but not yet terminal cancer and the chronically sick, to enable both patients and their families to live less restricted and unsupported lives.

## The Unit

The day unit is purpose-built and contains baths, showers, and toilet facilities suited to the disabled. It also has a physiotherapy department, an occupational and recreational therapy room, an area for lunch, and a hairdressing and beauty salon that is very popular.

The unit has a social worker and trained volunteers working under qualified physiotherapists and occupational therapists. But basic nursing also looms large, and there is a sister-in-charge assisted by three other nurses.

Patients attend from 10 A.M. until 3 P.M., and volunteer drivers (some of whom work in the unit) are invaluable in saving frail patients from delays or circuitous routes. The unit is open five days a week for about 42 weeks a year. When volunteers are short and we close the unit at holiday times, we keep contact with those most in need by home visits. In this the community nurse seconded as a liaison nurse is of great value.

## The Patients

In the first 26 months, 197 patients with preterminal illness and 66 with chronic illness attended the day unit (Table 23.1). As with the inpatients, more were in their sixties than any other decade. Attendances totaled 3,528, 32% of them being by men and 68% by women—there are more women patients, and the long attenders (Table 23.2) are mostly women. Whereas nearly 60% of the women are widowed or single, only 22% of the men are, and their families are therefore more likely to need support. In 1976 an average of seven patients a day attended and in 1977 10; recently we have had as many as 17 on some days. The increase is due entirely to patients with preterminal cancer.

Patients with preterminal illness are accepted by the day hospital with little delay and attend for as long as they need. Eighty-five per cent come once a week, but some with special problems two or three times a week. The relationships that develop are often kept up after patients are admitted to the terminal care unit, with inpatients visiting their friends in the day unit and joining in activities even from their beds.

We try to limit the chronic sick to about 20% of the total. They attend once a week for eight weeks but they are accepted for another eight weeks, when space permits, nine to 12 months later.

## Diagnosis and Duration of Attendance

Breast cancer is common and is also a lengthy illness (Table 23.2); such patients account for 38% of attendances. Patients with lung cancer account for 17%. Prostatic and brain tumours often have a prolonged course and patients may attend for many months, whereas those with other common tumours of the genital and gastrointestinal tracts attend for about two months. Patients with cancers in the 12 most common primary sites attend on average 13 times (Table 23.3).

Despite the support of the day hospital, 14 patients (three men and 11 women) had to be admitted as inpatients—in all, 43 times, 21 of the admissions being for breast cancer. Thirty-seven patients attended the unit only once (Figure 23.1), most being then speedily admitted as inpatients. The main difficulties were pain control (17 cases) and family problems (13).

Half of the chronically ill patients had had strokes (20) or suffered from multiple sclerosis (14), and there were seven cases each of Parkinsonism and rheumatoid disease. Among the less common diseases were motor neurone disease, severe chronic respiratory disease, presenile dementia, and cervical arachnoiditis.

Table 23.1

Patients with Preterminal Cancer and Chronic Disease by Age and Sex during the First 26 Months of the Day Unit

| Age (y) | No. with cancer | | | No. with chronic disease | | | % of total patients | % of total attendences |
|---|---|---|---|---|---|---|---|---|
| | M | F | Total | M | F | Total | | |
| ≤50 | 3 | 15 | 18 | 2 | 6 | 8 | 10 | 12 |
| 51–60 | 16 | 22 | 38 | 6 | 5 | 11 | 19 | 17 |
| 61–70 | 30 | 39 | 69 | 10 | 16 | 26 | 36 | 33 |
| 71–80 | 22 | 30 | 52 | 9 | 9 | 18 | 27 | 26 |
| >80 | 5 | 13 | 18 | 1 | 0 | 1 | 7 | 11 |
| Not known | 1 | 1 | 2 | 0 | 2 | 2 | 1 | 1 |
| Total | 77 | 120 | 197 | 28 | 38 | 66 | 100 | 100 |

## Table 23.2
### Details of Patients with Cancer (3 Men and 14 Women)
### Attending for 50 or More Weeks

| Primary site or type of tumour | No. of patients | Duration or mean total duration of attendance (weeks) | Main problems |
|---|---|---|---|
| Breast | 7 | 74 | Social support (4), pain control (5), dressings (2), nausea (2), depression (2) |
| Bronchus | 3 | 65 | Social support (3), depression (2), dyspnoea (1), pain (1) |
| Prostate | 1 | 68 | Social support, depression |
| Astrocytoma | 1 | 97 | Mobilisation |
| Non-Hodgkin's lymphoma | 1 | 50 | Social support |
| Stomach | 1 | 68 | Pain, anxiety, cachexia |
| Bladder | 1 | 56 | Nausea, cachexia |
| Unknown | 2 | 67 | Social support, incontinence |

## Table 23.3
### Attendances by Patients with 12 Most Common Cancers

| Primary site or type of tumour | No. of patients | No. of attendances | | | |
|---|---|---|---|---|---|
| | | M | F | Total (with % of all attendances) | Mean |
| Breast | 52 | 1 | 1015 | 1016 (38) | 20 |
| Bronchus | 38 | 354 | 93 | 447 (17) | 12 |
| Prostate | 6 | 146 | 0 | 146 (5) | 24 |
| Bladder | 10 | 23 | 97 | 120 (4) | 12 |
| Stomach | 10 | 31 | 61 | 92 (3) | 9 |
| Rectum | 10 | 34 | 47 | 81 (3) | 8 |
| Colon | 12 | 23 | 55 | 78 (2) | 7 |
| Cervix | 9 | | 63 | 63 (2) | 7 |
| Ovary | 6 | | 51 | 51 (2) | 8 |
| Uterine body | 5 | | 43 | 43 (2) | 9 |
| Brain (cerebral primary) | 3 | 47 | 0 | 47 (2) | 16 |
| Others | 29 | 86 | 227 | 313 (12) | 11 |
| Unknown | 7 | 28 | 176 | 204 (8) | 29 |
| Total | 197 | 773 | 1928 | 2701 | |
| % | | 29 | 71 | 100 | |

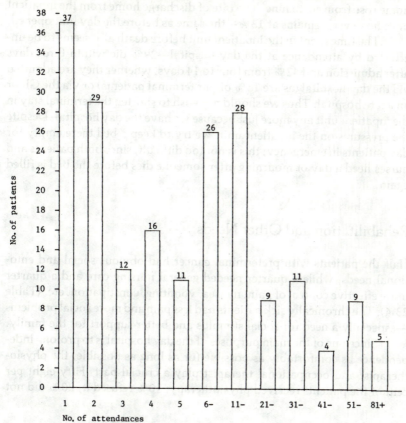

Figure 23.1. Attendances at the Day Unit over 26 Months

## Absences, Deaths, and Patient Flow

There were 442 absences, a rate of 12.5%. Only 2% were due to defaulters who did not like the unit. Nearly half of the absences were because patients were too ill to attend, and a quarter because they had been admitted to our hospital or elsewhere.

Four of the 66 chronically sick patients and 140 of the 197 cancer patients died; of the latter, 116 died in our inpatient unit, 17 at home, and 7 in other hospitals. Thus there were about six deaths a month among the day unit patients, with new patients making up from a quarter to a third of those attending.

In the first year we discharged from the inpatient unit 32 patients who had attended the day hospital and in the second year 45, and deaths at home rose from six to nine. The rate of discharge home from the inpatient unit, however, remains at 13% —the same as before the day unit opened.

The time spent in the inpatient unit before death also seems to be unaffected by attendance at the day hospital—29% die within three days after admission and 42% from four to 14 days, whether they are admitted via the day hospital (as are 16% of our terminal patients) or via the GP or an acute hospital. Thus we should not wish to shorten the terminal stay in the inpatient unit any more just because we have the day hospital. Despite the pressures on the inpatient unit, we try to keep a bed there empty for day patients in emergency; this is not too difficult, since both patients and nurses need a day of mourning after someone dies before the bed is filled again.

## Rehabilitation and Other Needs

Half the patients with preterminal cancer had obvious social and emotional needs, while a quarter needed general nursing care and a quarter more effective control of pain, nausea, vomiting, constipation, etc. (Table 23.4). The chronically sick patients had less pain and more social problems —especially a need for social stimulus and better support for the family.

Since one of the main purposes of the day hospital is to prolong independence as comfortably as possible for as long as possible, the physiotherapist and occupational therapist play a crucial part. Fifty-eight per cent of the patients received physiotherapy, 10% refused it, 20% did not

Table 23.4
The Patients' Main Problems

| Problems* | No. (%) of patients | |
|---|---|---|
| | Cancer | Chronic Disease |
| Social problems (isolation, poor housing) | 59 (14) | 20 (16) |
| Emotional needs (depression, anxiety, poor emotional support) | 65 (16) | 20 (16) |
| Lack of social stimulus (bored, frustrated, given up trying) | 42 (10) | 27 (21) |
| Inadequate family support (relatives tired, not coping well) | 40 (9) | 26 (20) |
| General nursing needs (baths, dressings, catheter or stoma care) | 107 (25) | 17 (13) |
| Specific symptoms (pain, nausea, vomiting, constipation, etc.) | 110 (26) | 18 (14) |

*Many patients had several major problems.

need it, and 12% were too ill for anything more than undemanding group exercises that could be performed if necessary in a wheelchair. The most common need, in 28% of patients, was help in mobilisation.

The occupational therapy transformed the atmosphere of the day unit. Sixty-two per cent of patients were very keen on it, 19% were not so keen, 6% refused it, and 4% were too ill. By selling the products at a small charge, the cost of materials can be largely recouped.

The most unlikely people enjoyed simple, repetitive tasks such as making plant-pot holders and sticking shells on wine bottles for table lamps, or showed enthusiastic talent for painting, pottery, or making mosaic trays. Items made by dying patients must be treated with respect. However humble and badly made (some need tactful revision by staff), they are very important to relatives. The men especially enjoyed growing sweet peas and tomatoes on the verandah. Those who took less part in occupational therapy often enjoyed music or bingo (which should be organised to provide a lot of cheap prizes). The needs of more intellectual patients must not be neglected, and some of them particularly appreciated the chapel services.

## Survey of Patients and Relatives

Since our day unit was costing over £20,000 [ca. $36,000] a year, we attempted to assess its usefulness further by sending a questionnaire to the bereaved relatives of the patients with cancer and to the chronically ill patients who had attended. Not surprisingly, only half completed the forms and the results cannot be statistically valid, but some interesting facts emerged.

We received replies from 65 relatives of patients who had died. Of these, 51 graded the unit as excellent, seven as good, and one as satisfactory. Fifty-eight families had been greatly helped by having a day off. One relative wrote, "I felt supported at last," and many made similar remarks. Forty-four of the patients were said to have greatly enjoyed their visits, and 16 to have enjoyed them a little; seven had attended as a duty. Patients had apparently liked the company, the change of scene, and the occupational therapy; the visits had given them something to look forward to. One relative said that they had been "always pleased to see how much more cheerful she was after a day unit visit." At least 45 had found relief from physical problems; some of these could have been more easily helped by admission but had preferred to battle on at home. Most had enjoyed the journey to the day hospital, but some found the work and the pain of getting ready a burden.

Of the 23 chronically sick patients who replied to the questionnaire, all but one had much enjoyed their visits and found they helped their own and their families' morale and also their physical problems. Most of all they enjoyed meeting people, but feeling useful and having something to look forward to were also important. Twenty graded the unit as excellent and two as good.

## Discussion

A day unit for those with terminal cancer, though it does not necessarily postpone the final admission to hospital, does provide a rallying point for the patient and family that is beyond the scope of routine hospital and general practitioner services. Clinical and social needs cannot be disentangled, and the administrative separation of the resources of social services, hospital, and primary care is unhelpful to our patients.

Despite the difficulties of transporting sick people across a city, the value of such a unit, in circumstances such as ours, seems clear. Even chronically ill patients with their symptoms mostly under control benefited, and we were surprised how much we could help their long-standing disabilities.

In those urban areas where supportive medical care seems most difficult to organise, such a unit could be grafted onto existing day hospitals to avoid capital expenditure and large running costs. Certainly a day unit or domiciliary service represents a relatively easy way to start to meet the needs of dying patients and their families; but a backup of beds and hospital facilities is also needed—83% of our patients died as inpatients. Moreover, patients seem to find it convenient and reassuring to have the day hospital integrated with the inpatient unit. We believe that this should be the arrangement of choice and the pattern of the future.

## References

Ward, A. M. W., "Terminal Care in Malignant Disease," *Social Science and Medicine*, 1974, *8*, 413–420.

Wilkes, E., "Some Problems in Cancer Management," *Proceedings of the Royal Society of Medicine*, 1974, *67*, 1001–1005.

Wilkes, E., "Effects of the Knowledge of Diagnosis in Terminal Illness," *Nursing Times*, 1977, *73*, 1506–1507.

# VI

# The Hospice Movement

*Hospice is more than an abstract philosophy or point of view. It is also a widespread, grassroots movement with a history and present status around the world. As a modern movement, its history is short, though it has antecedents in a long tradition of humane care for sick, dying, and grieving persons. As a relatively new phenomenon, the specific contexts from which hospice arose—especially in Great Britain and North America—are not well appreciated by many people. Yet the nature of those contexts and their differences help to define what hospice is today in its concrete manifestations. And they are the background for what it may become in the immediate future.*

*The two chapters in Part VI trace the history of the hospice movement in the United Kingdom and North America. E. Richard Hillier and Inge B. Corless are well acquainted with the strengths and limitations of hospice on their respective sides of the Atlantic Ocean. They define the character of the hospice movement and the issues that it faces in Britain, Canada, and the United States. Explicitly and implicitly, they point out directions in which hospice might go forward in its next years of development.*

# 24

# Terminal Care in the United Kingdom

*E. Richard Hillier*

> There is a tide in the affairs of men,
> Which, taken at the flood, leads on to fortune;
> Omitted, all the voyage of their life
> Is bound in shallows and in miseries.
> On such a full sea are we now afloat,
> And we must take the current when it serves,
>     or lose our ventures.
>
> —*William Shakespeare*, Julius Caesar, *Act IV, Scene iii, ll. 218–224.*

## Introduction

The quotation above was never more true than in the care of the dying, for although through the centuries individuals have emerged to do this kind of work, there has been more help for the terminally ill in the past 10 years than ever before. In 1967 Cicely Saunders opened St. Christopher's Hospice in London, and the dramatic changes that have occurred since then are impressive by any standards.

Why was she successful? What was so special about 1967 that made the mustard seed grow to the tree we see today—the development of a handful of hospices into the hundreds that exist all over the world and hundreds more in the planning stage? I propose to look at the historical background of these hospices and to describe how the movement has grown. I wish to examine their strengths and weaknesses, and finally to take a glimpse at the future of the hospice movement in Great Britain.

But before examining the present-day hospice's link with the past, we need to know the political and social environment that provide the fertile ground on which St. Christopher's could grow. A hundred years ago, doctors cured only a few patients because they lacked the powerful medical tools that exist today. With the advent of safer surgery and the enormous advances in therapeutics, doctors have apparently developed the power to remove problems and effect cures. This seductive world has obvious dangers. The relentless pursuit of cures for more and more diseases can lead the blinkered into believing that care of those who are incurable is less important. After all, the child severely injured in a road traffic accident first requires competent surgeons; compassion comes later. The urge for cure, therefore, is reasonable and right, but as in all things a balance is required. Technological medicine can go too far, and when this happens the incurable can too easily be neglected. It is no coincidence that the promises of Prime Minister Harold Macmillan in the 1960s, summarised in the famous slogan "You've never had it so good," were beginning to turn sour. The growth of materialism was outstripping the more spiritual and caring aspects of society, which seemed to be declining. Thus, the message proclaimed from St. Christopher's in 1967 was what many people wished and needed to hear.

But there were other matters in Saunders' favour. For thousands of years doctors, philosophers, and others had been writing about death and dying, but more was published on the subject in the 1960s than ever before. Some of the earlier writing was outstanding, but much was ineffectual, unimpressive, and based on little practical experience. In the 1960s a rash of outstanding publications appeared (Feifel, 1959; Glaser & Strauss, 1965, 1968; Hinton, 1963; Saunders, 1959, 1967; Weisman & Hackett, 1961). At the end of this decade a building appeared that exemplified all that these writers spoke of. Above all, it demonstrated for everyone to see the ideas of these writers working effectively in a practical everyday approach to the pains and suffering of the dying and their families. Thus, St. Christopher's showed by example what had been learned, and the testimony of patients, relatives, and visitors confirmed that this was good. Moreover, doctors who found the dying and their problems difficult to manage were now able to obtain help and advice that worked.

Finally, any pioneer must be dedicated. Saunders and her staff gave everything they had to make St. Christopher's and what it stands for successful. This requires knowledge, strength, tactful persuasion, and action. Although these pioneers are the first to admit that others have done or said precisely what they have done, it is undoubted that the great catalyst in the growth of the hospice movement was born.

From this beginning the movement has spread. Symptom control has become increasingly professional, and its minutiae have been analysed and researched with care. The first hospices were established in the private sector, but similar care is now being given under the British National Health

Service in the continuing care units and by support teams working in the community and in district general hospitals. Just as in medicine itself, professionalism has now been born and points the way to a future where care is as professionally respectable as cure and is the hallmark of the balanced doctor.

## History

The hospice movement is a microcosm of human physical and spiritual development throughout the centuries. To provide sojourn and a rest for earthly travelers as well as for those on life's pilgrimage—these aims attractively represent humans as physical and spiritual beings in the way they are seen by today's hospices. But what of the past? From where did this revolution come? To find out, we must go back centuries to Roman times when civilisation in Britain began.

Fabiola, a Roman matron and disciple of St. Jerome, opened a place of refuge in the time of the Emperor Julian the Apostate. She and those with her gave food and rest to the healthy traveler, tended the sick, and also cared for the dying pilgrim. She thus recognised active, resting, and dying man—and cared for all three together, in contrast to today when each apparently needs a host of specialists in health and disease. Fabiola's approach has characterised hospices throughout the ages, and at different times and in different places some hospices have provided more physical comfort while others have thought more of spiritual needs. The movement can be traced throughout Europe from the Knights Hospitallers of the 11th century to the numerous monastery-based hospices of the Middle Ages. They increasingly acted more as stopping places for travelers and less as refuges for the sick. With the dissolution of the monasteries in Britain, even this ceased. The idea of the hospice died, and in its death gave birth to the humanitarian and scientific approach to illness as developed by the professional doctor (and, much later, the professional nurse).

Following the upheaval of these chaotic times, the seeds of the present hospice movement were planted. In the 17th century a young French priest, St. Vincent de Paul, founded the Sisters of Charity in Paris and opened a number of houses to care for orphans, the poor, the sick, and the dying. A century later, Baron Von Stein of Prussia visited these Roman Catholic nuns and was so impressed by their work that he encouraged a young Protestant pastor named Fliedner to found Kaiserswerth, the first Protestant hospice also staffed by nuns. An interesting historical coincidence is that nuns from both these groups accompanied Florence Nightingale to the Crimea, where the competence and compassion of professional nurses was born. From this unbelievable training ground, the Irish Sisters of Charity founded Our Lady's Hospice for the care of the dying at Harold Cross in Dublin. The need for such a place had become particularly acute because of the horrors of the potato famine in Ireland and the Poor Law establishments in England, where the needy and the sick suffered appalling privations and indignities. At a time when many of the English believed that pain and sickness were punishment for sin, the hospitals in England were also selecting outpatients for teaching and research, and encouraging the disposal of the incurable to other institutions even less sympathetic than themselves. *Caritas* had become charity, and a charity meant cash — or lack of it.

In 1900 five of the Irish Sisters of Charity founded St. Joseph's Convent in the East End of London and started visiting the sick in their homes. In 1902 they opened St. Joseph's Hospice with 30 beds for the dying poor. The only other establishments caring for the dying in London at that time were the Hostel of God, run by Anglican sisters, and St. Luke's in Bayswater, managed by a Methodist committee.

Fifty years later, Cicely Saunders arrived at St. Joseph's to work there for 7 years, developing the technique of pain control and total care for dying patients that, as everyone knows, has become the cornerstone of hospices all over the world. Yet in the religious houses a person's developing relationship with God is as important as his or her physical treatment, and the daily routine of the nuns and their patients includes spiritual care. But the world's priorities are different. So Saunders, who was a qualified nurse and social worker as well as a doctor and a Christian, envisaged a centre that would be an oecumenical religious and medical foundation combining the best care for dying patients with opportunities for teaching and research in the fields of medicine, nursing, and allied professions. She opened a building fund in 1964, and in 1967 St. Christopher's Hospice opened in London. As time has gone on, her original aims have been abundantly fulfilled and new ones achieved. Many of the results are reflected in her recent book (1978), and their worldwide impact was demonstrated at an International Hospice Conference in London in 1980 when 16 countries were represented.

## Development of the Hospice Movement in Britain

St. Christopher's Hospice was the culmination of many years of evolution and planning. Its impact on the care of the dying has been dramatic both in terms of the number of patients helped and of doctors and nurses inspired. In the past 13 years, this has led to an expansion of services for the dying in four main areas: (1) more facilities for the dying in private foundations, nursing homes, and non-National Health Service hospices; (2) the development of continuing care units by the National Society for Cancer Relief, which are subsequently maintained by the National Health Service; (3) the development of home care teams designed to support patients at home by cooperating with family doctors and district nurses; and (4) the emergence of hospital support teams involving a part-time doctor, nurse, social worker, and chaplain, who advise on the care of patients dying in acute hospital wards. The essence of all these groups is to work with others caring for these patients rather than to take over from them—an essential ingredient in any effective education. In addition, and of equal importance, the influence of all these groups has raised the standard of terminal care for patients who never come into contact with them.

Table 24.1 shows the development of hospice services in Great Britain over the past 20 years. Each hospice is listed under the group that provides the majority of its funds. The first of the modern hospices was St. Christopher's. But before this, private foundations were caring for the dy-

Table 24.1
Development of Hospice Services in Great Britain

|  |  | 1960 | 1965 | 1970 | 1975 | 1980 (Jan) |
|---|---|---|---|---|---|---|
| PRIVATE FOUNDATIONS AND NURSING HOMES | Inpatient | 5 | 7 | 9 | 11 | 16 |
|  | Community + Home Care | - | - | - | - | - |
|  | Hospital Support Team | - | - | - | - | - |
| NON–NHS HOSPICES | Inpatient | 3 | 3 | 5 | 10 | 17 |
|  | Community + Home Care | - | - | 1 | 2 | 10 |
|  | Hospital Support Team | - | - | - | - | - |
| NATIONAL HEALTH SERVICE | Inpatient | 3 | 3 | 3 | 3 | 22 |
|  | Community + Home Care | - | - | - | - | 13 |
|  | Hospital Support Team | - | - | - | - | 5 |

*Adapted from:* B. Lunt and R. Hillier, "Terminal Care: Present Services and Future Priorities," *British Medical Journal,* 1981, 283, 595–598.

ing, including the Marie Curie Foundation, with homes for cancer patients of all types, and the Sue Ryder Foundation, most of whose beds were used for the chronic sick. The increase in the number of all services during the 5 years from 1975 to 1980 is dramatic, especially those financed by the National Health Service (Ford, 1979).

The surge of interest in terminal care posed considerable problems for the government. Not only was the public attracted by the idea of hospices, but as different parts of the country developed their services in different ways, increasing pressures developed upon those areas that were poorly served. Britain is divided into 14 Regional Health Authorities, with Scotland and Wales considered separately. Table 24.2 shows the population of a selection of these regions and the number of beds available in each region for terminal care. The beds per 100,000 population are shown in both the National Health Service and the non-National Health Service units, as are the number of home care services in each region. This table, showing the situation in January 1980, indicates the wide discrepancy of available services in the different regions of a relatively small country. It is not surprising that the North of England, with its dense industrial population, fares far worse than London (the Thames regions) or the South and that the public pressure on the regions in the North to provide a service equivalent to their better-off counterparts in the South is considerable. What, therefore, can the government do but review the services available and comment upon them? The *Report of the Working Group on Terminal Care of the Standing Sub-Committee on Cancer*, chaired by Eric Wilkes (1980), concludes:

> We do not consider therefore that there would be any advantage in promoting a large increase in the number of hospices at present, and we recommend that the way forward is to encourage the dissemination of the principles of terminal care throughout the health service and to develop an integrated system of care with emphasis on co-ordination between the primary care sector [the general practitioner, district nurse, and associated team], the hospital sector and the hospice movement. (p. 11)

The report goes on to warn against overenthusiastic planning of hospices and continuing care units which cannot be financed satisfactorily. It encourages existing units to undertake day care, teaching, and high-quality research, and to look toward voluntary funding as a source of finance. The recommendation that major cities "should have a service for terminal care which fully involves the primary care sector, and the hospital service and includes a special unit" (p. 13) points to the advantage of linking such units to nursing and medical schools, and clearly indicates a policy.

Table 24.2

Regional Differences in the Number of Hospice Beds and Home Care Services in England, Wales, and Scotland: January 1980

| Health Region | Population (1,000,000s) | Inpatient Hospice Beds | | Hospice Beds/100,000 population | | | Home Care Services |
|---|---|---|---|---|---|---|---|
| | | NHS | non NHS | NHS | non NHS | Total | |
| S.W.Thames | 2.97 | 6 | 138 | 0.20 | 4.65 | 4.85 | 2 |
| Scotland | 5.19 | 40 | 147 | 0.77 | 2.83 | 3.60 | 1 |
| S.E.Thames | 3.54 | – | 99 | – | 2.80 | 2.80 | 3 |
| Oxford | 2.28 | 45 | 14 | 1.97 | 0.61 | 2.59 | 2 |
| N.W.Thames | 3.46 | 86 | – | 2.49 | – | 2.49 | 3 |
| Wessex | 2.72 | 50 | 13 | 1.84 | 0.48 | 2.32 | 3 |
| North West | 4.05 | – | 72 | – | 1.78 | 1.78 | – |
| Wales | 2.77 | 16 | 29 | 0.58 | 1.05 | 1.62 | – |
| Northern | 3.09 | – | 45 | – | 1.46 | 1.46 | – |
| South West | 3.03 | – | 24 | – | 0.79 | 0.79 | 2 |

*Adapted from:* B. Lunt and R. Hillier, "Terminal Care: Present Services and Future Priorities," *British Medical Journal*, 1981, 283, 595–598.

This policy was independently pursued by the National Society for Cancer Relief before the 1980 report was published. The Society accepted that the capital and running costs of specialised units would be heavy and appreciated that a large number of new hospices would be difficult to staff. Furthermore, the National Health Service had reduced its spending for the first time since its inception in 1947, and the Society had to find methods of raising the quality of terminal care as inexpensively as possible. Hence the Society encouraged the development of home care teams working from the continuing care units it had already provided. A typical team works under the directorship of a doctor and includes nurses, social workers, physiotherapists, occupational therapists, and sometimes a chaplain. They visit patients' homes individually to support them and their family, and they work in close cooperation with the primary care team. Most patients prefer to die at home if adequate resources and support are available. This multidisciplinary and interdisciplinary approach gives the patient and family what they need where they want it, and thus relieves the pressure on hospital beds.

It is perhaps worth stating that though the National Health Service hospices do not admit patients on a religious basis, most of them would agree that they do not work well without such support. Indeed, many medical directors believe that it would be impossible to work exclusively with the dying for many years without a religious faith.

A more recent development is the hospital support team. These are similar to the home care teams, but the groups see patients in the wards of general hospitals at the request of other specialists. They often facilitate earlier discharge and then support the patients when they return home. Such teams are funded by the National Health Service exclusively.

At present the evaluation of these services depends on anecdotal material, apart from some comparative research concentrated on St. Christopher's. Hinton (1979) showed that this hospice provided better care than did radiotherapy wards of good reputation in a London teaching hospital, as measured by patients' level of satisfaction of care and degree of mental stress. Parkes (1977, 1979) has also shown that St. Christopher's patients received better pain control and that relatives suffered less strain during the patient's stay than was the case with patients admitted elsewhere.

Proper evaluation is needed urgently to establish whether special units provide the high quality of care claimed for them, and if so whether the same results can be achieved in other settings. A comparative study of this sort, which will include cost-effectiveness as well as quality of care, is in progress at Countess Mountbatten House in Southampton. Other studies are being planned in other areas, for factual evidence is vital if sensible planning is to be achieved.

## Hospice Strengths

Hospices and continuing care units have undoubted strengths. For the most part they provide good symptom control, a relaxed homelike environment, and a group of professionals whose sole aim is to care for those for whom curative therapy is no longer appropriate—a quite different approach from that of their general hospital colleagues, who quite rightly are committed to cure. No one forgives them for giving up. Most people do one job well, so that to carry out terminal care in an acute surgical ward with a quite different purpose is more difficult than it is in a specifically designed hospice. In addition, hospices adopt a goal-oriented approach. This means that the staff seek what patients want to do and then help them and their families achieve it. This may demand a variety of different interventions from all members of the interdisciplinary team; it recognises that humans are physical, psychosocial, and spiritual beings—the hallmark of hospice care. Not surprisingly, this approach produces practical results of great benefit to patients and families.

In hospices, families may be encouraged to help in the day-to-day care of their relatives—something not easily achieved on an acute medical ward, where they would undoubtedly interfere with its efficiency. Further, the terminally ill in general hospitals may languish in a corner bed or side room, or may even be inappropriately sent home to circumstances that are quite unacceptable. Here again, the hospice attempts to identify where the patient wants to be. If this is at home, then the house must be reorganised around the needs of the patient, and a member of the home care team will help the family make the necessary changes. While still in the hospice, the patient will learn how to overcome any difficulties that are envisaged; properly planned discharge is arranged so that methods of coping with problems are worked out in detail and the patient does not feel threatened in any way.

Hospices also have strengths from which the staff may draw. Many multidisciplinary teams are ineffective because each discipline has its own hierarchy and may be based some distance from the point of action. Staff, therefore, are likely to meet on formal occasions only, and relationships take longer to build. In the hospice, all staff are located under the same roof, have meals and coffee together, and frequently meet one another informally. Relationships form more quickly, informal consultations occur often, and a unity of purpose and even of community develops that is hard to replicate in less cohesive settings. All this naturally leads to better patient care and a broader, more mature approach to a wide range of patient and family problems. In addition, staff can draw support from one another and learn from colleagues in different disciplines so as to become a truly interdisciplinary team.

Nor should the attached home care team be forgotten. This team often works unsupported in the community. For example, one nurse may be helping an emotional young man whose problems are insoluble in the home setting, yet who refuses admission. To help him may need much time and not a little emotional involvement. This imposes considerable strain, and at such times a mutual trust among staff and the unspoken recognition of one another's difficulties may help them to cope successfully. Moreover, when patients are admitted, they are taken to a place they know, staffed by people who are their friends and who therefore provide vital continuity of care.

Staff support occurs at many levels. The nurse saddened by the death of some young man of her own age is sensitively helped by her colleagues. There is no simple answer; each situation is different. For some it might be to weep alone in the sluice (dirty linen room), while for others it might be right to confide in a friend. If the difficulty is more intense, the nurse may wish to consult more senior colleagues, the ward sister (charge nurse), social worker, chaplain, or visiting psychiatrist. Each will recognise the ward sister's problems and yet maintain the confidentiality she in turn knows that she can expect. Weekly support meetings or a discussion at coffee time may also indicate to the ward sister that others were similarly saddened by the same event, and she gradually learns to realise that sadness can be universal and is more often a sign of strength than of weakness.

Finally, the hospice provides a group of people with a rare wealth of experience. In one year, a hospice will see more patients with cancer than a family doctor sees in a whole lifetime. And because the staff on medical wards have a variety of patients to care for, the experienced hospice worker will be unrivaled. Experience is related to intensity, not duration. Such experience provides a unique setting for teaching. Only the bare bones of terminal care can be learned in a lecture theatre; to be effective, this form of caregiving must be experienced, and there is no better place to acquire such experience than in a hospice or with a home care team.

## Hospice Weaknesses

The weaknesses of hospice may arise through misunderstandings, too rapid growth of the movement, or the customary tendency in hospices to concentrate on those dying of cancer.

If hospices work well, there are bound to be misunderstandings of their role, which may lead to jealousy or hostility. Other professionals may view the hospice as a "holier-than-thou death house"—a place devoid of hope, from which their patients should be protected. They may concede that the doctors and nurses are "nice" to the patients, but may not regard them as otherwise competent. They may believe that they are already doing perfectly adequately the job that hospices claim to do.

Such views are understandable, for any small group is bound to be slightly defensive or even inward-looking. Moreover, the positive comments made by patients and relatives about hospices may imply criticism of previous medical care. New patients arriving at a hospice should not be told that "everything will be all right *now*," since this represents a subtle damning of previous management.

Dying patients frequently need more tolerance of the difficulties and anxieties of their relatives than relatives do for the patients. It is the same with hospices. The hospice staff cannot expect appreciation unless they have earned it. They have neither right nor justification to criticise other hospitals, but should gently and tactfully help them to improve their care of the dying where this is possible. If they respect what others do in far less favourable circumstances, that respect will be returned, and the criticisms to which hospices are subjected will gradually melt away.

The second weakness is the danger of overzealous growth. As has been seen in Table 24.1, the growth of hospices and other terminal care teams has been considerable. As of January 1981, there were already 50 more terminal care facilities being planned than have been shown in the table. But too rapid growth will lead to a lack of properly trained staff, so that there is a real danger of bad hospices. To hasten slowly is essential, and high standards of care must be rigorously applied. In the National Health Service, with its dwindling resources, the case for a new continuing care unit must be well thought out and the evidence clearly presented, showing what has happened in the past and what is planned for the future. Though frustrating for those trying to build in this environment, careful monitoring is essential—for if rigorous criteria are not satisfied, resources will not be made available.

In the private sector, those engaged in planning hospices will have to impose their own audits. The board of governors or the management committee must plan imaginatively and set crystal-clear objectives. Once established, these hospices must first prove their excellence and then offer contractual beds to their local Regional Health Authority. This will give them guaranteed funding and built-in safeguards to their quality of service, for if this declines, their funding will be revoked. However, they will retain one enormous advantage over the National Health Service continuing care units—namely, that of autonomy, in which staff can make their own plans, reach clear decisions, and initiate prompt action. Although continuing care units will never possess similar freedom, many seek some charitable finance in order to obtain some independence and develop particular interests.

The last great weakness of hospice is the tendency to specialise in those patients suffering from cancer. There are several reasons for this. In aiming to treat as many patients as possible with the resources available, cancer has the dubious advantage that life expectancy in the terminal phase is relatively short and relatively certain, and that pain and distress, though often acute, are amenable to treatment and can usually be relieved. In most other diseases, the uncertainty of survival would mean that hospice beds were rapidly filled by patients who might survive many years. Without denying the needs of the chronic sick, it is understandable and almost inevitable that cancer should have been singled out. In addition, cancer has a particularly formidable reputation. Patients regard cancer as more of a death sentence than they do any other chronic disabling disease, and this makes symptomatic treatment more difficult. Nevertheless, with cancer causing one-fifth of all deaths in the United Kingdom, hospices cannot possibly cope adequately even with cancer patients alone. In the area served by one continuing care unit in Southampton, there were 3,500 cancer deaths per year; yet this 25-bed unit and its home care service advise on less than 20% of these patients.

Despite such difficulties, the predilection for cancer must eventually change. Some hospices accept patients with long-term neurological disease—usually a maximum of two or three patients in a 25-bed unit. But it is arguable whether a cancer-oriented hospice is the correct place for them. The death of nearly every patient with whom they form a relationship becomes an unbearable pressure. Patients with other chronic diseases (e.g., renal failure, chronic lung or cardiac conditions) are often dealt with in their own specialist areas or by their general practitioners at home. The catalyst effect of the hospice movement must affect the care in those areas where the staff, perhaps more used to high-quality technological medicine, find themselves exposed to intolerable strains by the deaths of their younger patients. 1981 (the year of this writing) was the International Year of the Handicapped, and perhaps this is a good omen for the future as we urgently look at other ways of helping these patients and the staff who care for them.

## Future of the Hospice Movement

The future of the hospice movement must be based on a clear evaluation of what is happening in hospices, continuing care units, and the other teams engaged in caring for the dying. Only by such evaluation will it be possible to determine the resources required to produce an adequate national policy. Government policy is currently attempting to curb the overenthusiastic expansion of free-standing hospices. A few already regard such buildings as an anachronism, but this is a gross oversimplification of the problem.

A reasonable plan is for each region to have one or two hospices of 25 to 40 beds, staffed by full-time medical and nursing staff. Each unit must have its own ancillary services and have close links with a medical school and university. National Health Service continuing care units in Edinburgh, Oxford, and Sheffield are already linked with universities, and the Southampton unit is developing its own Department of Continuing Care as part of the medical school. Similar developments will undoubtedly occur elsewhere. From these units and other hospices, home care teams will work closely with general practitioners and family doctors. Wherever possible, units should provide some variant of a hospital support team.

Unsupported home care teams—that is, those who have no unit to back them, no beds of their own, and often no ancillary supporting services—must be critically examined. They exist primarily because of financial restrictions, and if they can provide a good service for the terminally ill, they will be a major advance. But there are considerable dangers here. Medical support is likely to be part-time only; ancillary support will probably be widely scattered; the nurses will have to face hostile colleagues without the help available to the home care team based on a hospice, and this will reduce their effectiveness. Undoubtedly some will founder, and this will put the clock back for a time. There is one other danger. It may be easy for them to become ineffectual; they may visit and listen to the dying and their families in a way more appropriately carried out by social workers and volunteer organisations. Should this happen, it will mitigate against the high medical standards such services can and should offer, and in the long run will reduce their credibility and their authority.

This leads to the growth in voluntary services both inside and outside hospices. Already in the United Kingdom, the National Organisation for Widows and Their Children (CRUSE), a society that supports bereaved adults, is a powerful source. The Compassionate Friends is an international organisation of parents who have had a child die and who offer friendship and support to other more recently bereaved parents. There is also a voluntarily run Children's Hospice about to open in Oxford. In addition to these formal groups, volunteers work in hospices, hospitals, and in the community. In the past, the unions have objected to volunteers' working in areas where people could be paid to do the same job. Now, with the shortage of resources and personnel, volunteer services are being actively encouraged within the National Health Service. Some churches form small groups of volunteers to help with the handicapped, the dying, and the bereaved, and although many fail through lack of support, this is a fascinating beginning that may have enormous implications for the future. The hospice movement can play an important role in advising these groups and providing them with practical professional help if necessary. The *Report of the Working Group on Terminal Care of the Standing Sub-Committee on Cancer* (1980, p. 12) states that the advantages of day care units should also be considered, particularly in relation to hospices and continuing care units. Some day care units have already opened, notably at St. Luke's Nursing Home, Sheffield, in the private sector, and the Macmillan Unit, Christchurch, in the National Health Service. These units provide an opportunity to give patients more concentrated attention than might be received at home and also give them a chance to meet others and join in group activities to alleviate isolation. Finally, this is an excellent way of establishing relationships with staff for a time when later admission is required. Relief of relatives in order to prevent breakdown in home care is also useful. It may be that all continuing care units and hospices should develop such a centre, but further examination of their role and effectiveness must first be made.

Although teaching is already occurring, education programmes need to be developed and systematised. Each hospice connected to a university must have a full and clear committment to the medical school. Unfortunately, with the gross overcrowding of existing medical curriculae, it is not easy to obtain teaching time. In Edinburgh, students are introduced to the hospice philosophy in their first year, when they meet patients and perhaps spend 2 or 3 days at the hospice. Throughout the course, they learn different aspects of terminal care, and in their last year they see and discuss an essay they wrote about terminal illness in their first year. Similar courses are being developed in Oxford and Southampton, and other centres will undoubtedly follow. In addition, the training of nurses, social workers, occupational therapists, and physiotherapists is occurring, and hospice doctors are also running courses for the clergy. The churches are organising seminars for lay people on death and dying, to remove the anxieties and taboos associated with death and to show the general public how to deal with friends and relatives who are seriously ill. Such courses tend to be popular and are an important part of health education. All this activity emphasizes that hospices themselves provide a wealth of practical experience from which teaching can develop.

Finally, it is vital that an educational programme is developed for the leaders of hospice teams. Doctors should undergo training programmes similarly to those available in other specialties, and a group in Britain is already examining the possible structure of such a programme (Lunt & Hillier, 1981). In the future, each district containing a thousand beds may well have its own specialist in continuing care to participate in pain clinics and to coordinate other terminal care services.

As already indicated, specialist units must engage in research. Research must evaluate what is happening at the moment, examine better ways of achieving pain and symptom control, and finally provide information for the planners of the future. Despite the increase in the medical literature on death, dying, and thanatology (the scientific study of death), there is still an enormous need for good-quality research. Work is currently proceeding in psychosocial research, the clinical pharmacology of analgesics, and alternative methods of pain control. A steady trickle of information about new drugs for the control of symptoms is appearing, and academic departments of medicine and pharmacology must be encouraged to work with hospices and to develop similar interests, since hospices alone cannot possibly study all that needs to be investigated.

There is little doubt that the hospice movement has more to offer than it is achieving now. By constant review and by developing new methods, progress is assured. Without it, the movement will stagnate and become unworthy of the great and gifted founders on whose shoulders we stand. Growth must be slow and steady—more rational and more a part of the main stream of medicine than it is at present. If the 1980s is a decade of cooperation among colleagues who are encouraged to become more involved in this work, the future is indeed exciting.

## References

Feifel, H. (Ed.), *The Meaning of Death*. New York: McGraw-Hill, 1959.

Ford, G., "Terminal Care from the Viewpoint of the National Health Service," in J. J. Bonica & V. Ventafridda (Eds.), *International Symposium on Pain of Advanced Cancer: Advances in Pain Research and Therapy* (Vol. 2). New York: Raven Press, 1979, 653–661.

Glaser, B. G., & Strauss, A. L., *Awareness of Dying*. Chicago: Aldine, 1965.

Glaser, B. G., & Strauss, A. L., *Time for Dying*. Chicago: Aldine, 1968.

Hinton, J., "The Physical and Mental Distress of the Dying," *Quarterly Journal of Medicine*, New Series, 1963, *32*, 1–21.

Hinton, J., "Comparison of Places and Policies for Terminal Care," *Lancet*, 1979, *1*, 29–32.

Lunt, B., & Hillier, R., "Terminal Care: Present Services and Future Priorities," *British Medical Journal*, 1981, *283*, 595–598.

Parkes, C. M., "Evaluation of Family Care in Terminal Illness," in E. R. Prichard, J. Collard, B. A. Orcutt, A. H. Kutscher, I. Seeland, & N. Lefkowitz (Eds.), *Social*

*Work with the Dying Patient and the Family.* New York: Columbia University Press, 1977, 49–79.

Parkes, C. M., "Terminal Care: Evaluation of In-Patient Service at St. Christopher's Hospice," *Postgraduate Medical Journal,* 1979, *55,* 517–527.

Saunders, C., *Care of the Dying.* London: Macmillan, 1959. (Reprinted from *Nursing Times,* 1959, *55;* 2nd ed., 1976.)

Saunders, C., *The Management of Terminal Illness.* London: Hospital Medicine Publications, 1967.

Saunders, C. (Ed.), *The Management of Terminal Disease.* London: Edward Arnold, 1978.

Weisman, A. D., & Hackett, T. P., "Predilection to Death: Death and Dying as a Psychiatric Problem," *Psychosomatic Medicine,* 1961, *23,* 232–256.

Wilkes, E. et al., *Report of the Working Group on Terminal Care of the Standing Sub-Committee on Cancer.* London: Her Majesty's Stationery Office, 1980.

# 25

# The Hospice Movement in North America

*Inge B. Corless*

In the latter part of the 20th century, we are reminded repeatedly of the finitude of both environmental and human resources. Exhaustion of fossil fuels and precious metals, as well as the limits of scientific knowledge in the curing of disease, are apparent. This is not to diminish the importance of the work of the biogeneticists; rather, it is to contrast the current Weltanschauung with the one that was present 20 to 40 years ago. That prior time was filled with hope and an unmitigated belief in the potential for scientific discovery and the resolution of the ills of the world. Chastened in the ensuing years, the public is beginning to engage in a variety of consumer movements to reclaim responsibilities so readily given over to experts. In situations where there are many questions and specialists limit their field of vision so as to increase their knowledge about a given phenomenon, generalists are also required. In recent years, generalists and those interested in holistic health have been involved in the demand for consumer control of two "once in a lifetime" events—birth and death.

The hospice movement was born out of a concern for "doing something" for dying patients. In a society typified by "mastery over the environment," the objective in standard medical therapeutics is mastery over disease and thereby death. When this is no longer feasible, it appears that there is "nothing more to be done." Those concerned with palliative care practice from this same Western philosophy of mastery, arguing that symptom control and a concern with the physical, psychological, social, and spiritual (née cultural) aspects of patient and kin *are* appropriate areas for action.

In this chapter, I briefly examine the historical context and development of the hospice movement in the United States and Canada, giving

particular attention to some of the key issues facing individual groups and
the movement as a whole.

## Historical Context and Development

Concern for those with progressive debilitating chronic diseases did not
begin with the advent of hospice. A long tradition of caring for the ill in
each community, as well as for travelers en route, exists from earliest recorded history. The cave dwellers, the Greeks, the Egyptians, women in
each community knowledgeable about herbs, the Knights Hospitallers in
Rhodes, the Sisters of Charity established by Vincent de Paul, Florence
Nightingale, the Protestant nursing sisters established by Pastor Fliedner
at Kaiserswerth in Germany—these are some of the individuals and
groups associated with caring for the ill and medically indigent. Around
the turn of the century in the United States, Rose Hawthorne Lathrop initiated a program of care for individuals with cancer. She started her work
by taking ill persons into her own home and caring for them there. Mrs.
Lathrop subsequently established a domiciliary facility for patients. Accepting no compensation from patients or their families, she relied on the
generosity of the community for support. This same tradition of caring is
embodied in the modern hospice movement, which began in the United
States and Canada with groups in Connecticut, New York City, and Montreal, and shortly thereafter in Boonton, New Jersey; Tucson, Arizona;
and Marin and Hayward in California. (Several of these programs are described in Plant, 1977, and Davidson, 1978.) In these and many other locations during the late 1960s and early 1970s, concerned professionals and
other citizens met to organize individual hospice programs (Foster et al.,
1978).*

These programs may be distinguished according to the base of their
activities. Community-based hospice groups have their primary locations
either in free-standing units or in offices that serve the members of the hospice care coordinating team. The "First American Hospice," Hospice, Inc.,
or as it is now named, The Connecticut Hospice, was founded as a coordinating committee to extend both the scope and quality of care rendered to
the dying and their families (Lack & Buckingham, 1978). With an emphasis on home care, nursing services were contracted from the Visiting Nurse

*Research by Florence Wald provided the basis for the development of Hospice, Inc. (i.e.,
The Connecticut Hospice); see "A Nurse's Study of Care for Dying Patients," USPHS Grant
NU 00352, Florence S. Wald, Principal Investigator, 10/1/69–9/30/71, and "An Interdisciplinary Study of Care for Dying Patients and Their Families," ANF Grant #2-70-023, 2/1/70–
1/31/71.

Association for care during the day. Volunteers extended these hours, making care available on a 24-hour-per-day basis. In June 1980, a 44-bed free-standing facility explicitly designed with the needs of dying persons and their families in mind (Chan, 1976; Kron, 1976) was dedicated and opened in Branford, Connecticut. Although this 44-bed unit is currently filled, there is some question as to the appropriate size of inpatient facilities, with some in the field recommending units of 4 to 6 beds. A perusal of the first directory of hospices by the National Hospice Organization (1978) suggests that most inpatient units fall within the range of 8 to 12 beds. To utilize their facility fully, The Connecticut Hospice has established satellite home care groups throughout Connecticut. The use of such community bases apart from the inpatient facility is supportive of a wider range of coverage by the home care teams, although it also necessitates longer travel by patients, relatives, and friends to the inpatient unit. The attendant costs and benefits of this satellite model will need to be evaluated.

Hospice of Marin in California is also a community-based hospice (Stoddard, 1978). The emphasis is on home care, and when this is no longer feasible, "backup beds" are available in the hospital with which the attending physician is associated. In effect, these beds are whichever ones are available at the time and thus are "scattered" throughout the institution. The Hospice of Marin team follows its patients into the various institutions and attempts to improve the quality of care received there.

Community-based hospice groups are also located in free-standing facilities—that is, facilities that are not physically proximate to an acute care institution. Two of the earliest free-standing units were the Riverside Hospice in Boonton, New Jersey, and the Hillhaven Hospice in Tucson, Arizona. The Riverside Hospice, the former home of the president of a major corporation, is beautifully situated in rural New Jersey. It is replete with a patio and pool; is adjacent to community playing fields and woods; and contains a wood-paneled library, a living room complete with fireplace, a dining area, and bedrooms (each of which has its own bathroom). Although the physical facility is one of the most esthetic in appearance, the narrow corridors and steps down to the living room are a physical barrier for individuals whose mobility is limited. Initially, Riverside Hospice was one of three units funded by the National Cancer Institute for a 3-year period of study. At the termination of the study, the administration of the Riverside Hospice has moved to space within a local hospital. Home care will continue, and the backup beds are now in an acute care institution rather than its former facility.

Hillhaven Hospice in Tucson, Arizona, was formerly housed in a wing of a nursing home (Hackley, 1977). It is distinctive in that it was one of the only hospices in North America offering day care to patients—although that service has not been much utilized. Hillhaven's program sought to bring the skills of various community members into the hospice to enhance the quality of life for all. Recently, however, the Hillhaven chain changed ownership, and the hospice program has now become a department of St. Mary's Hospital in Tucson.

Involvement of a large nursing home chain with hospice raises the specter of the "Kentucky Fried Hospice syndrome"—that is, will the field be beset by profiteers? This question is examined later in the chapter when the issue of regulations is addressed. It has been one of the persistent concerns of hospice leaders.

Institution-based hospice groups are typically located in acute care facilities. The consultation model, which is often found in hospitals, is the direct counterpart to the community-based coordinating group. The former has its base of operations in the hospital, the latter in the community. Both models utilize "scattered beds."

An example of the hospital-based consultation model is given by St. Luke's Hospital in New York City, which provides a multidisciplinary consultation team of professionals who visit patients throughout the hospital (Paige & Looney, 1977). Follow-up upon discharge from the hospital is available through the hospital's home care department. Consultation programs like St. Luke's have the potential for broadening the impact of the hospice concept of care among medical professionals. The question of continuity of care is more acute with this model in that after discharge home, readmission to some protected environment may be a necessity. Return to hospital is not always possible for patients whose presenting complaint is "dying." This necessitates admission to an extended care facility if one can be found, and in turn leads to one more change in caregivers and location at a time when the individual's resources are depleted.

Institution-based hospice groups may also be found in a discrete unit within an acute care facility. An illustration of this type is the Palliative Care Service in Montreal, Canada, which offers an integrated program of comfort care by providing consultation throughout the Royal Victoria Hospital; direct service within the inpatient Palliative Care Unit; a bereavement follow-up program; and home care rendered by nurses attached to the Service (Ajemian & Mount, 1980; Mount, 1976). Involvement of home care nurses as part of the hospice/palliative care service is a major difference from most programs in the United States, where home care is often contracted from existing agencies such as the Visiting Nurse Association. This is often done with the aim of utilizing existing agencies and avoiding duplication. At the Palliative Care Service, patients, wherever they are located, are cared for by members of one team with a central administration. The Palliative Care Service, which has been one of the premier programs in North America, is currently expanding its base of operations to two hospital-based units in Montreal. This is in keeping with the philosophy of providing care within the patient's community. The organizational and administrative questions inherent in this mitosis are a challenge to all involved in the endeavor.

The hospice program at the Kaiser-Permanente Medical Center in Hayward, California, was created to test the applicability of the hospice based in an acute care facility (Walter, 1979). Would a program like that of the Palliative Care Service of the Royal Victoria Hospital work in the United States, or was the community-based model the hospice of choice? In addition, the significance of this hospice was its inclusion as part of a health maintenance organization's program of care.

Other models of hospice/palliative care abound, ranging from hospice care organized by the Visiting Nurse Association, programs that are part of nursing homes, and community programs staffed by nurses "donated" from participant hospitals. Services range from education and family support, to coordination and consultation on a community basis, to inpatient care available in free-standing structures and in discrete units in hospital-based facilities.

Palliative care programs in Canada appear to show less variation than those in the United States. Most are hospital-based and are located in a discrete unit. This seems to be related in part to the organization and funding of health care in Canada via national health insurance. Nonetheless, there is the occasional program (e.g., Mount Sinai Hospital, Toronto) that establishes a consultation team or hires a nurse to coordinate care for patients.

Responses to a questionnaire on the development of the hospice movement in Canada indicate that there are many professionals who are interested in palliative care (Corless, forthcoming). The common concern seems to be funding.

The movement toward palliative/hospice care is clearly growing both in Canada and the United States. The development of the National Hospice Organization, state hospice groups, the biannual International Seminars on Terminal Care at Montreal, and the Forum for Death Education and Counseling are all manifestations of this maturing of the hospice movement. There has also been a growing recognition of the problems facing hospice and palliative care leaders.

## Issues

There is a wide range of issues facing the providers and consumers of hospice care. Among others, these issues include the desirability of the various models, questions of professional resistance, financial concerns, evaluation, and innovation and regulations (Osterweis & Champagne, 1979; Ryder & Ross, 1972).

## Which Hospice?

For groups examining the particular needs of their own communities, the question arises as to which hospice model to adopt. Proponents of free-standing units argue that they can provide a less institutional and more homelike atmosphere. Advocates of hospital-based units note the ready availability of medical technology and personnel, which eases problems of patient access to professionals with a variety of medical skills.

The crux of the argument, aside from the financial issues, which are considered shortly, is one of how best to influence medical care. Some suggest that change is most readily achieved outside the system—that careful attention to symptom management and the emphasis on the whole person and family are diluted by primary physicians who do not avail themselves of the expertise offered by hospice personnel. Involvement with a physician who requests hospice consultation but disdains the incorporation of hospice recommendations other than nurse and volunteer support at home vitiates the full potential of hospice care. Under these circumstances, the inclusion of the primary physician becomes a source of continuing irritation and frustration. Others state that change is more readily achieved within the system than it is from outside. Location of the hospice team within the hospital, particularly within a discrete unit, makes the hospice concept more difficult to banish from thought. Day-to-day achievements and problems are more visible than are those occurring in a facility further afield. The unit itself makes a statement as to alternative concepts of care.

## Resistance to Hospice

The questions of physician education and medical resistance emerged numerous times in a recent survey of the hospice movement (Corless, forthcoming). If these problems are not one and the same, there is indeed some overlap. The question of education is, on the one hand, as simple as apprising practicing physicians and medical students of the significant advances made in the knowledge about pain and symptom control in individuals with far-advanced diseases. On the other hand, it is as radical as treating the patient and family as a single unit rather than in a reductionistic mode, isolating and treating symptoms without an interpretation of their meaning (and that of the disease) to the person. It is also as innovative as suggesting that physicians are employed by patients to amass the facts and provide alternative solutions.

Physician resistance may result from a "wait and see" attitude about innovations. Some individuals don't get on the bandwagon until the parade is almost over. In other situations, there may be the feeling that holistic care is being given already, and therefore why all the fuss about hospice? Physicians desiring not to "abandon" their patients often use chemotherapeutic drugs and extensive laboratory services literally until the patient's last breath. The quality of life achieved under these circumstances is often miserable. The physician does this in the belief that it may help the patient and, if not that person, others in the future. These physicians are not "awful" men and women. They are faced with the dilemma of how to practice medicine with a credo that demands faithfulness to the preservation of human life. The question of when to recommend that treatment directed at cure be stopped is a very difficult one and demands the mind of the scientist and the heart of the artist.

Oncologists often find it difficult to comprehend the depth of appreciation by patients for palliative care. This appreciation is often manifested publicly as well as privately, financially as well as verbally. Often the time span of involvement in hospice care is relatively brief, as compared with the length of time the patient has been treated by an oncologist. Part of the explanation for the gratitude patients and families exhibit is related to the quality of the palliative care services. Another part is related to timing. Hospice care is rendered at a time when many people feel desperate. Anyone who shows concern is appreciated. Furthermore, hospice usually steps in at a time when physicians no longer can realistically hope for cure or even for significant prolongation of life. Doctors who no longer "hope" for cure are frequently concerned that the referral to hospice will take away the patient's "hope." Giving the verbal message that "We'll keep trying" and "We've got this new protocol," when the nonverbal cues indicate that cure is not likely, is a double message that connotes hopelessness and helplessness to the patient. Including the family in this conspiracy abets the patient's sense of loss of control and divides patient and family. Coming into situations like this, hospice groups assist patients and families with communication and connectedness with each other.

Resistance to the hospice movement in the United States is also evinced by public health nurses. In some situations, opposition occurs when the local Visiting Nurse Association is not the major provider of nursing services. In other instances, the necessity for extending the availability of nursing services to 24 hours per day is the problem. Taking call becomes another demand on the nurse. Many nurses elect to work in a visiting nurse service not only for the independent practice but also for the regularity of working hours. A requirement for weekend service transforms some of the working conditions to those more typically found in acute care facilities. Another reason for resistance is the difference in the approach to care. Although some visiting nurses are interested in caring for terminally ill persons, others prefer providing services of a restorative nature. Hospice nursing emphasizes communication, symptom management, care of and by family to the end of the patient's life, and bereavement care thereafter to the family. The concern with quality of life results in a focus on assisting the patient in making each day meaningful. Reviewing the past and completing any unfinished business is part of the process of bringing order to the patient's life. This, in turn, contributes to the individual's finding meaning in living and in dying. The varied work of the visiting nurse and the need to visit a larger number of clients each day often precludes the lengthier visits typical of the hospice nurse.

Resistance by some health professionals is a major problem for hospice groups. In the long term, the elimination of such opposition will be necessary to the survival of the hospice movement. The critical factor in the diminution of resistance may very well be consumer demand as much as professional education.

## Financial Considerations

Consumer demand may also influence the resolution of the major problem for hospice/palliative care in the United States and Canada—money. Although the problem has the same name in both places, its manifestations are distinctive to each country. In Canada, the problem seems to be one of raising initial funds and allocating resources. The Canadian National Health Service reimburses for services, once the decision to allocate funds for a certain program is made. In the United States, reimbursement is provided for designated services rendered in discrete locations—acute care facilities, skilled nursing facilities, private homes, and so on—by licensed providers of health care. Individuals requiring services available in those locales are eligible for reimbursement. Services not meeting these guidelines are not funded by third-party payers (Hollander & Ehrenfried, 1979). In Canada, programs not funded result in services not rendered. In the United States, services may be rendered, but when reimbursement is available only for specified services, facts may be manipulated to fit the case for traditional reimbursement. Thus, strict guidelines for reimbursement can serve both to control services offered and to inhibit innovation in health care delivery.

The lack of a specific reimbursement rate for hospice care has affected the development of palliative care in the United States. The paucity of reimbursement affects all components of hospice programs—consultation, home care, inpatient care, and bereavement care. The impact is not only on the type of service that is reimbursed, but also on the qualifications of the provider of care. There are strict limitations as to which professionals may be reimbursed for certain types of caregiving activities. Whereas physicians may charge a fee for consultation, nurses cannot do so unless they have established an independent practice. Thus, reimbursement for consultation is not available other than for that rendered by a physician.

Counseling and bereavement work may be reimbursed under traditional coverage by third-party payers under the provision for mental health. Here again only certain professionals are eligible for reimbursement—namely, physicians, social workers, clinical psychologists, and psychiatric nurses. Other nurses and members of the clergy are not eligible for direct reimbursement.

Home care is on a somewhat sounder financial footing, but here, too, there are difficulties. Reimbursement is available to nurses and in some cases to home health aides. Nurses must render "skilled nursing care," which typically is defined as a "hands-on" approach; counseling is not included as a service for which nurses may be reimbursed as purveyors of care.

As noted previously, hospice inpatient beds are either "scattered" (i.e., available throughout an institution) or are located as a discrete unit. Inpatient stays are not, for the most part, reimbursed on the basis of a discrete hospice rate. As a result, hospice groups in the United States are receiving higher rates for inpatient care than may be necessary. The question of inpatient costs for hospice as compared with patient charges requires further investigation. Preliminary inquiries suggest that costs for inpatient care may be less than or at least may not be more expensive than those for acute care (Walter, 1979, p. 150).

Depending on the patient population, labor costs may vary. If patients are referred to hospice in the last week of life, the need for all aspects of care is increased. This is above and beyond the increase in physical care that occurs with increasing dependence. The responsibility for meeting those needs is more likely to fall to a smaller cadre of paid staff members. Time constraints inhibit wider participation by members of the hospice team such as volunteers, perhaps due primarily to the numbers of strangers who can be incorporated by patient and family at this time of high stress. When patients and families have been involved in a hospice program, there may also be an increase in the care requirements during the last week of life, but family, friends, and volunteers, as well as staff, are all in place providing aid and comfort to patient and family. Aside from the fact of the longer involvement in the acute system in the first instance, the last week of life may also be more expensive because of requirements for paid staff.

To provide a graphic illustration of these points, consider the different situations of three patients, all of whom start in the acute care system. Patient A remains there and is referred to a hospice inpatient unit during the last week of his or her life. Not only does this patient have the cost of the long period of time in acute care; transfer to a hospice inpatient unit during the last week of life, while it may result in some cost savings, is still expensive because of greater staff and institutional involvement. Contrast this situation with that of Patient B, who starts in the acute care facility but is referred to hospice, is placed on home care, and continues at home until death occurs. Costs in this situation are noticeably reduced. Just as some patients in an acute care setting never are referred to hospice and thus continue to sustain higher costs, so, too, some hospice home care patients will be able to remain at home until they die. Other home care patients, like Patient C, may need to return to the inpatient unit, although to a hospice rather than to an acute care unit. Even if the worst economic case is assumed—that is, nearly identical inpatient costs for hospice and acute care inpatient services—there will still be a savings, due to the fact that the patient is in a continuous care system that attempts to maintain patients at home. The freedom that family members and friends have for visiting and for being with their loved ones in hospice care necessitates less intervention by staff. Hospice patients are not neglected by paid staff, but caregiving is not assumed to be the exclusive domain of professionals. Caring is a shared process in which all participate—patient, family, friends, volunteers, and paid staff.

It has been observed that longer involvement in the hospice care system enhances the probability of a more peaceful death by providing an opportunity for the resolution of the problems of living and dying (Corless, 1980–1981). Whether there is an optimal length of involvement is a matter requiring further inquiry. The relationship among length of hospice involvement, quality of living and dying, and costs of care needs to be investigated in a rigorous fashion so that facts replace assumptions and hypotheses.

It behooves us to examine the impact of a lack of hospice Medicare reimbursement on the development of the hospice movement. As it stands now, reimbursement is available through traditional channels by a third-party payer, such as Blue Cross/Blue Shield, Medicare, Medicaid, or other insurance programs. Unless a specific rate is set for hospice reimbursement, payments will be those available through rates currently set for other modalities. This is or becomes what has been referred to as "fitting the facts to the case." Very often, this means that professional notes are written in such a way that provision for reimbursement can be made. Often these "notes" are less than candid in portraying the reality of the patient and family's situation. Stringency of Medicare requirements in particular precipitates such action by hospice and other caregivers. Thus, the documentation available from a patient's charts may not reflect totally the situation of patient and family and the care received. How, then, may a true picture of the content of hospice care be obtained? This is a problem, given the current state of reimbursement.

## Evaluation

To answer this question and others, 26 hospice programs in the United States have been selected as pilot projects in an evaluation being conducted by the Health Care Financing Administration (HCFA). All other groups delivering hospice care will not be reimbursed by Medicare under a discrete hospice rate until such time as the evaluation has been completed. For most hospice groups in the United States, reimbursement is currently the major problem. Some groups have been able to obtain community and foundation support, but there is a concern about building programs on "soft" money. Others are faring less well. For the 26 hospice groups that have been selected as part of the demonstration program, immediate concerns about reimbursement have been alleviated.

The initial request for proposals by HCFA was so broad as to be an immense task for one research study. The request was the result of the collaboration of several agencies, including the John A. Hartford Foundation, the Robert Wood Johnson Foundation, and HCFA. Brown University was ultimately selected to carry out the evaluation and was awarded the contract on September 30, 1980.

Although the initial goal was to implement the evaluation 1 month thereafter, this goal was never realistic. The tasks involved in doing the evaluation are multiple and varied, and unless the research is carefully constructed, the results will be all but meaningless. The researchers will examine a number of interesting questions (Brown University Division of Biology and Medicine, Section of Community Health, 1980). These include the following:

1. What is the differential impact of hospice, waivered or nonwaivered, on the quality of life of terminal patients and their families as compared to "conventional" or "customary" care?
2. What are the differential costs of caring for comparable terminally ill patients in waivered hospices, nonwaivered hospices, and customary care settings?
3. What is the likely impact of Medicare reimbursement on the organizational structure, staffing pattern, and costs of hospices?
4. What is the likely national utilization and cost of Medicare-reimbursed hospice care?

Sensitivity of the researchers to issues touching on the quality of life is underscored by the placement of this item as the first of the four major questions. Concerns as to whether or not hospice is a better approach to caregiving may be overshadowed by questions regarding the cost of care and the impact of, or lack of, reimbursement. The cost analysis will be conducted by Abb Associates. The question of the comparative costs entailed in different types of care requires that an accurate measurement of the cost of care be obtained. There are, however, many barriers to such an accounting. Among hospice groups located in acute care facilities, there has been a real concern that they would have to bear the "step-down" costs of the availability of such services as laboratory, X-ray, operating room, and so on. While for the most part this has been avoided, the opposite problem may occur. That is, hospice groups located in an inpatient facility may receive "hidden benefits"—services for which they do not account. These may be as simple as some advice from a hospital accountant, suggestions from a pharmacist, or the assistance of a recreational therapist. These costs may not be charged to the hospice unit; nonetheless, the unit benefits from their availability. Under conditions of a free-standing unit, such services may need to be purchased if they are not donated. Perhaps an additional way to contrast hospice units in different locations is to tally the number, type, and frequency of donated services. While this is more readily apparent in groups located in the community, or in free-standing units, it may nonetheless also be accomplished in hospital-based hospice units. Information about volunteer services donated by professionals would give us a clearer idea of all the costs and assets of hospice care.

Another important question is whether volunteerism is reduced as hospice programs mature in their development. Many hospice groups owe their start to the voluntary contributions of professionals and other citizens in their community. Volunteers who initiated the needs assessments necessary to determining whether there was a role for hospice in a given area may or may not continue to be involved when the program is operational. It is conceivable that charismatic volunteers will be joined by those who are more comfortable with working in an organizational framework.

Volunteers make noticeable contributions to hospice programs. Volunteers who provide direct care to patients and families, as well as program volunteers, expand the potential of a given program and are of great benefit to all involved. Volunteers support those in key positions in hospice programs, as well as supporting patients and families through the last days of life. The question, however, as to whether the enthusiasm of volunteers can be maintained so that they continue to be a source of support is a crucial one and is the concern of both volunteer directors and hospice financial officers.

In preparing for the reimbursement for hospice services, HCFA officials have needed to make some determinations as to which services and which quantity thereof would be reimbursed. The constraints which HCFA has placed include limits, for example, on the number of Medicare-reimbursable bereavement visits. This restriction may change the nature of the programs being evaluated. By using control groups wherein bereavement care is not available, one can begin to obtain some measure of the impact of bereavement care. Ideally, there would be two types of control groups—those without a hospice program, and those with a hospice program but without bereavement aftercare.

Group A—No hospice program.

Group B—Hospice or hospice-like program, with no bereavement component.

Group C—Hospice program, with bereavement component (three visits).

Group D—Hospice program, with bereavement component (structured visits plus "as needed" visits).

Further study is required to determine how many visits are required on average in bereavement care; one study in California (*Report to the 1980 California Legislature on the Hospice Project,* 1980) has suggested that three visits are the norm. The work of Colin Murray Parkes (1975) and others in determining the population "at risk" will be useful in identifying those persons requiring additional professional intervention. In addition, Mary Vachon and her colleagues at the Clark Institute of Psychiatry and Community Contacts for the Widowed in Toronto, Canada, have examined the impact of a community bereavement service on the course of bereavement (Rogers et al., 1980; Vachon et al., 1980).

Another question that has been proposed for evaluation by HCFA and bandied about the hospice movement is one that has already been mentioned in somewhat different form. Essentially, it is the question of which is the "best" hospice model. The response has been that it depends on the community. Whether that is or is not so, the question needs to be addressed seriously. Given a set of specified objectives in a certain environment, is one model of hospice more efficient in meeting these goals?

## Innovation and Regulations

The sentiment in the hospice movement has been that freedom and flexibility are required, since we do not "know" which is the best approach to the organization of palliative care. This concern for the provision of an environment in the United States that encourages innovation in hospice models is markedly different both from England and Canada. In England and in Canada, palliative care programs of the past appear to be institution-based—either free-standing, such as St. Christopher's Hospice, or associated with an acute care facility, such as St. Joseph's Hospice or the Royal Victoria Hospital Palliative Care Service. Community-based groups are more likely to be found in the United States than in either England or Canada.

In the United States, the existence of community-based nurses who give "hands-on" care to bedridden individuals, as opposed to an emphasis on health teaching and clinic visits, may have provided the infrastructure and tradition of home care. Unfortunately, the reality of the current financing structure of most visiting nurse groups mitigates against these professionals' being able to devote the time to patients and families that they would wish. In addition, the society-wide emphasis on restoration and recuperation reduces the interest in giving care to those for whom cure is no longer a possibility. While there are "visiting nurses" in both England and Canada, they are attached to local governmental units rather than employed by private agencies.

In the United States, there has been a concern with making use of existing agencies to avoid duplication of services. As admirable an objective as this is, further inquiry is also pertinent—namely, is hospice merely the coordination of care obtained from existing health care providers? This is a very radical question. If hospice care is "coordination plus," what is the nature of the additive? Certainly it is important that the skills of an interdisciplinary team are utilized and that the patient/family is considered the unit of care. The availability of care 24 hours per day, 7 days a week, is also crucial. These characteristics of hospice care are also attributes of other health care programs. Even the addition of preservice training does not distinguish hospice care from other modalities.

Hospice care *is* more than coordination of care from a variety of caregivers. It is scrupulous attention to the physical, psychological, social, and spiritual aspects of the patient/family constellation. It is the involvement with clients from the last 6 months of illness through bereavement. It is the facilitation of resources to meet the concerns and needs of patient, family, and friends. And it is the catalyzing of communication and connectedness.

For caregivers, hospice care requires ongoing in-service training so as to increase the knowledge base. It also requires frequent formal and informal communication about client care and staff members' needs. When existing agencies provide these services, and they are of the quality of hospice care, then duplication of services will be a significant issue. In effect, the hospice movement will have achieved its stated aim—that is, to transform the care of individuals and families in current health care practice so that separate hospice programs will no longer be necessary. That goal is not yet at hand.

Currently, there is an interest in exploring a variety of hospice models with a view to enhancing innovation. The belief is that the hospice movement in the United States is too young to make determinations as to the definitive type of hospice. Such conclusions would result in premature closure on an issue that is far from resolved. The contravening pressure is the perceived need to prevent exploitation of hospice consumers. The thrust for legislation to license and accredit hospice providers arises from the concern that there must not be a repetition of the nursing home scandal.

Along with the tension between the desire to allow experimentation and the concern for the protection of consumers from hospice profiteers, there exists the question of how much regulation and by whom. Although unanimity prevails that regulation is necessary so that profiteering can be averted, the necessity of contending with current regulations is nonetheless a significant problem for developing hospice groups. It is feared that the promulgation of hospice legislation of a regulatory nature will inhibit the innovation necessary to the development of hospice. At the moment, hospice groups are attempting to meet regulations currently applicable to home health agencies, acute care facilities, and other related institutions, as well as to fulfill any requirements specified by special hospice legislation in particular locations. The need to satisfy numerous requirements impedes the development of young organizations. The regulatory phase by which society ensures the safety of its members against the unscrupulous also serves to inundate fledgling hospices with numerous bureaucratic obstacles. Many officials of regulatory agencies do use their offices to be of assistance to developing groups, while at the same time monitoring these groups to assure that the safety of the community is not compromised.

The regulations as delineated in legislation are often very specific. Those developed in Connecticut specify the dotting of each *i* and the crossing of each *t*. While such attention to detail can be meritorious, it also serves to safeguard groups from competition from parvenus.

There is greater clarity about the physical requirements for inpatient facilities than there is about the standards for hospice services and the credentialing of providers of care. Questions abound, including these: When does palliative care end and terminal care begin? Is chemotherapy an appropriate palliative therapy? Should patients receiving such treatment be eligible for hospice admission? When should the person with pneumonia be treated with medication, and when ought such an individual to be treated with nonchemical interventions? Who are eligible for admission to hospice programs and who are not? When eligibility is determined in part by the availability of a caregiver, what does that mean for citizens in a geographically mobile society where family members may live at great distances from one another?

As increasing numbers of people live to greater ages, there will be a larger number of potential hospice clients who live alone or with another individual who may be frail. Does a concern with the costs of hospice care dictate that we eliminate the very consumers who may be in greatest need? This is an area where innovative approaches are required, or surely hospice groups will be delivering care to those who already have many other social supports. If that is the case, history will judge the hospice movement a social movement that occurred in industrialized nations in the latter part of the 20th century and that was committed to improving the lives and deaths of a largely middle-class clientele.

## References

Ajemian, I., & Mount, B. M., *The R. V. H. Manual on Palliative/Hospice Care.* New York: Arno Press, 1980.

Brown University Division of Biology and Medicine, Section of Community Health (in association with the Hebrew Rehabilitation Center for Aged, Boston, MA, and Abb Associates, Inc., Cambridge, MA), *An Overview of the National Hospice Study.* Unpublished manuscript, 1980.

Chan, L-Y., "Hospice: A New Building Type to Comfort the Dying," *AIA Journal,* 1976, *65,* 42–45.

Corless, I. B., "The Hospice Movement—1979: Issues and Concerns." Forthcoming.

Corless, I. B., Incidental observation, St. Peter's Hospice, 1980–1981.

Davidson, G. (Ed.), *The Hospice: Development and Administration.* New York: Hemisphere, 1978.

Foster, Z., Wald, F. S., & Wald, H. J., "The Hospice Movement: A Backward Glance at Its First Two Decades," *The New Physician,* 1978, *27,* 21–24.

Hackley, J. A., "Full-Service Hospice Offers Home, Day, and Inpatient Care," *Hospitals, Journal of the American Hospital Association,* 1977, *51,* 84–97.

Hollander, N., & Ehrenfried, D., "Reimbursing Hospice Care: A Blue Cross and Blue Shield Perspective," *Hospital Progress,* 1979, *60,* 54–56, 76.

Knecht, B., *Social Services Within the Framework of Hospice Care—Utilization and Policy Paper.* Unpublished manuscript, 1980. (Available from Social Services Research Institute, 1015 18th Street N.W., Suite 810, Washington, DC 20036.)

Kron, J., "Designing a Better Place to Die," *New York Magazine,* 1976, *9,* 43–49.

Lack, S. A., & Buckingham, R. W., III, *First American Hospice.* New Haven: Hospice, Inc., 1978.

Mount, B. M., *Palliative Care Service: October 1976 Report.* Montreal: Royal Victoria Hospital/McGill University, 1976.

National Hospice Organization, *Preliminary Directory.* Unpublished manuscript, 1978.

Osterweis, M., & Champagne, D. S., "The U.S. Hospice Movement: Issues in Development," *American Journal of Public Health,* 1979, *69,* 492–496.

Paige, R. L., & Looney, J. F., "When the Patient is Dying: Hospice Care for the Adult," *American Journal of Nursing,* 1977, *77,* 1812–1815.

Parkes, C. M., "Determinants of Outcome Following Bereavement," *Omega,* 1975, *6,* 303–323.

Plant, J., "Finding a Home for Hospice Care in the United States," *Hospitals, Journal of the American Hospital Association,* 1977, *51,* 53–62.

*Report to the 1980 California Legislature on the Hospice Project.* Unpublished manuscript, 1980.

Rogers, J., Vachon, M. L. S., Lyal, W. A., Sheldon, A., & Freeman, S. J. J., "A Self-Help Program for Widows as an Independent Community Service," *Hospital and Community Psychiatry,* 1980, *31,* 844–847.

Ryder, C. F., & Ross, D. M., "Terminal Care—Issues and Alternatives," *Public Health Reports,* 1972, *92,* 20–29.

Stoddard, S., *The Hospice Movement.* New York: Stein & Day, 1978.

Vachon, M. L. S., Lyal, W. A., Rogers, J., Freedman-Letofsky, & Freeman, S. J. J., "A Controlled Study of Self-Help Intervention for Widows," *American Journal of Psychiatry,* 1980, *137,* 1380–1384.

Walter, N. T., *Hospice Pilot Project Report.* Hayward, CA: Kaiser-Permanente Medical Center, 1979.

# Epilogue

*Our Epilogue, fittingly enough, is by a former patient at St. Christopher's. Enid Henke reflects in an insightful and moving manner on the Biblical parable of the Good Samaritan. It is a story familiar to us all, and yet one about which we know surprisingly little. Who was the wounded man? Or his Samaritan helper? More importantly, what was the final outcome? We do not know, and in a larger sense—as Henke indicates—that is not the main point. What counts most of all is that someone cared and made a concrete effort to be available and to translate concern into practical action. What is important is that we are interdependent, in life and in death. Dying people and their grieving relatives will accept and forgive our limitations if they can see that we are honestly trying to do our best. They will welcome all of our professional skills—that is, all that are relevant and used wisely—and all of the humane contributions that we can bring to their aid. What they cannot and should not forgive is our lack of caring. There is a wounded Jew and a Good Samaritan in each of us. We must learn to accept and to fulfill both roles. It is our hope that this book will help us all to realize that potential through its exposition of principles and practice for hospice care.*

# The Purpose of Life

*Enid Henke*

*This chapter was dictated with some difficulty because of a speech defect by a young woman who was dying of a progressive paralysis. It was finished two weeks before she died and illustrates the peace she achieved during her four years of illness.* —Dame Cicely M. Saunders, D.B.E., M.A., M.D., FRCP, St. Christopher's Hospice, London

A friend and I were considering life and its purpose. I said, even with increasing paralysis and loss of speech, I believed there was a purpose for my life but I was not sure what it was at that particular time. We agreed to pray about it for a week. I was then sure that my present purpose is simply to receive other people's prayers and kindness and to link together all those who are lovingly concerned about me, many of whom are unknown to one another. After a while my friend said, "It must be hard to be the wounded Jew when by nature you would rather be the Good Samaritan."

It is hard: it would be unbearable were it not for my belief that the wounded man and the Samaritan are inseparable. It was the helplessness of the one that brought out the best in the other and linked them together.

In reflecting on the parable I am particularly interested in the fact that we are not told the wounded man recovered. I have always assumed that he did, but it now occurs to me that even if he did not recover the story would still stand as a perfect example of true neighborliness. You will remember that the story concludes with the Samaritan asking the innkeeper to take care of the man, but he assures him of his own continuing interest and support: so the innkeeper becomes linked.

If, as my friend suggested, I am cast in the role of the wounded man, I am not unmindful of the modern-day counterparts of the priest and Levite, but I am overwhelmed by the kindness of so many "Samaritans." There are those who, like you, have been praying for me for a long time and constantly reassure me of continued interest and support. There are others who have come into my life—people I would never have met had I not been in need who are now being asked to take care of me. I like to think that all of us have been linked together for a purpose which will prove a means of blessing to us all.

# Table of Selected Drug Name Equivalents*

| Generic (Approved) | United States | Great Britain |
|---|---|---|
| acetaminophen/paracetamol | Tylenol | Panadol |
| amitriptyline | Elavil | Tryptizol |
| aspirin + codeine | aspirin + codeine | Codis |
| bromhexine | not available | Bisolvon |
| chlormethiazole | not available | Heminevrin |
| chlorpheniramine | Chlor-Trimeton | Piriton |
| chlorpromazine | Thorazine | Largactil |
| cholestyramine | Questran | Cuemid/Questran |
| cyclizine | Marezine | Valoid |
| danthron + softener | Dorbane | Dorbanex |
| dextromoramide | not available | Palfium |
| dextropropoxyphene + paracetamol | Darvon = propoxyphene HCl | Distalgesic |
| diazepam | Valium | diazepam/Valium |
| dichloralphenazone | Midrin | Welldorm |
| dioctyl sodium sulphosuccinate | Colace | Dioctyl-forte |
| dipipanone + cyclizine | not available | Diconal |
| dothiepin | not available | Prothiaden |
| emepronium bromide | not available | Cetiprin |
| haloperidol | Haldol | Haldol/Serenace |
| hydromorphone | Dilaudid | hydromorphone |
| ibuprofen | Motrin | Brufen |
| levorphanol | Levo-dromoran | Dromoran |
| meperidine | Demerol | pethidine |
| methadone | Dolophine | Physeptone/Dolophine |
| methotrimeprazine | Levoprome | Veractil |
| metoclopramide | Reglan | Maxolon |
| morphine solution | various | Nepenthe |
| nitrazepam | not available | Mogadon |
| oxycodone pectinate | [oxycodone HCl is found in Percodan and Tylox] | Proladone |
| papaveretum | not available | Omnopon |
| pentazocine | Talwin | Fortral |
| phenazocine | Prinadol; not now available | Narphen |
| prochlorperazine | Compazine | Stemetil |
| scopolamine | scopolamine | Hyoscine |
| thioridazine | Mellaril | Mellaril |
| trimethoprim + sulfamethoxazole | Septra/Bactrim | Septrin/Bactrim |

*Editors' note: We are grateful to J. Joseph Gruber, R.Ph., for assistance in the preparation of this table.

# Index